Moving from COVID-19 Mathematical Models to Vaccine Design: Theory, Practice and Experiences

Edited by

Andrés Fraguela-Collar

Professor and Researcher in Applied Mathematics
Faculty of Physics and Mathematics
Autonomous University of Puebla
Puebla, Mexico

Moving from COVID-19 Mathematical Models to Vaccine Design: Theory, Practice and Experiences

Editor: Andrés Fraguela-Collar

ISBN (Online): 978-981-5051-90-2

ISBN (Print): 978-981-5051-91-9

ISBN (Paperback): 978-981-5051-92-6

First published in 2022.

Bentham Science Publishers Pte. Ltd.
80 Robinson Road #02-00
Singapore 068898
Singapore
Email: subscriptions@benthamscience.net

BENTHAM SCIENCE

Contents

FOREWORD I

Living and coping with COVID 19, the second pandemic of the millennia after the 2009 influenza pandemic, has posed unprecedented challenges. The world has dealt with pandemics before. Human history has been shaped by diseases that present themselves as epidemic, endemic or pandemic diseases. We have registered pandemics since well before the Christian era, and surely, although no registries are available, they have always accompanied humankind. Some remarkable pandemics, that changed the course of history were the Black Plague in the 14th century that killed a great proportion of the European population, and the Spanish Influenza, that occurred little more than a century ago in 1918-19, and killed well over 40 million people, although some scholars say the number of deaths might have reached more the 100 million.

Circumstances have changed and the world is quite different from what it used to be just a few decades ago. Knowledge, technology and communications have developed in an unprecedented speed in human history in the last century and especially in the last four decades. While these are great achievements, they also pose new challenges. Lifestyles have changed and the world faces global threats such as climate change, overpopulation, undernourishment, non-communicable diseases, the emergence of new potentially pandemic infectious diseases such as COVID-19, and many others that have pushed together the global community in efforts to deal with them in a coordinated fashion. Common targets such as the Sustainable Development Goals prove that leaders all over the world are concerned about the future of human kind, although not all to the same extent.

These efforts, however, have been insufficient, and COVID-19 has shown that much more than meetings, nice documents and good intentions are needed to face current challenges. ConfrontingCOVID-19 has risen several questions that need yet to be answered by scientists as well as politicians. For instance, what was the origin of SARS-CoV-2; how can we deal with health inequities such as differential access to vaccines, or why many governments and country leaders disregarded the World Health organization's recommendations.

In this very complicated scenario, any attempt to better understand and cope with COVID-19are welcome. This book will surely provide vast and comprehensive knowledge about the pandemic and its development, and the best ways to confront it.

Editor and author, Andrés Fraguela Collar, has brought together several contributors, from different Mexican institutions as well as from highly renowned institutions from other countries in a great effort to try to understand COVID-19.

In chapter 1, readers will find a very thorough and challenging description of the mathematical modelling of pandemics in general and of COVID-19, in particular.

Chapter 2 will guide them through key issues about the epidemiology of infectious diseases. They will get a comprehensiveview from chapter 3 about what was known at the time the book was written about how SARS-CoV-2 does its damage, how we, human beings, experience the disease and where were the possible treatment options at that moment.

Chapter 4 is devoted to mathematical modelling of epidemics. Chapter 5 will offer readers avery interesting discussion about the importance of data analysis, and the challenges faced when dealing with something new like COVID-19.

Chapter 6 deals with the epidemic progression of the diseases in a non-homogeneous population. Those who love Mathematics will enjoy this chapter. Chapter 7 leads the reader through the very important subject of social inequities and their role in the propagation of infectious diseases.

Chapter 8 will update the reader on the statistical approach to understand the severity and fatality of COVID-19.

Chapter 9 is devoted to the Cuban experience, on immunotherapy and the role played by mathematical models of disease progression at the individual level.

Chapter 10 and last explains in a very comprehensive manner many aspects of vaccine development and the challenges it poses.

Throughout the book, the reader will find many graphs, tables and formulas, and a very extensive bibliography in each chapter.This book is an example of a multidisciplinary endeavor. It is no easy reading for those who do not have statistical or mathematical background, but anyhow it will be highly enjoyable for any reader and particularly for those familiar with mathematical concepts and methods.

COVID-19 is evolving in many senses, and it is a challenge to health systems, and at the individual level, to both clinicians and researchers. Modelling it has proved to be a very difficult task and as we learn more about it, we discover that there are yet many things to unveil. With this disease, human kind is walking in unchartered territory.

I recommend the reader to follow on new every day developments, to stick to basic publichealth messages which have proven to be the best defense against the disease and to have in mind that this will not be the last pandemic we will face. There is a very high probability of a new pandemic in the future, although we do not know when or how it will occur. As someone said "the clock is ticking, but we do not know what time it shows..."

Enjoy this book, as it contributes to better understand COVID-19.

Pablo Kuri-Morales
Independent Health Consultant

FOREWORD II

Mathematical modeling of infectious diseases has a long history of being used as a tool to study the mechanisms by which a disease can spread within communities, to predict the direction of an outbreak in a population and to evaluate the effectiveness of therapeutic interventions (*e.g.*, vaccination programs) to control an epidemic. These mathematical models derive from basic theories, the collection of statistical data or both, and they help to define parameters for a variety of infectious diseases, and to estimate the effects of the different interventions.

The appearance of a new human viral infection which causes the disease known as COVID-19, constitutes both a challenge and a test to the usefulness and relevance of mathematical modeling. This coronavirus known as SARS-CoV-2 emerged suddenly in South Asia and rapidly disseminated around the globe. It represents a significant concern because, very few times before, the population of the whole world had to face a disease of such pandemic proportions, that has exposed the lack of preparedness of the health care systems to handle thousands of patients and the limited therapeutic interventions to counteract such disease. Fortunately, rapid action in the development of effective vaccines worldwide and the accelerated emergency approval of these therapeutics has let different countries to combat this disease, increasing survival and reducing the death toll.

Current and emerging problems during the pandemic, and the effectiveness of the vaccine platforms developed to cope with it, will define the future of outbreak control. For example, it is unknown whether this novel coronavirus will establish itself in an endemic form or will it eventually die out. Furthermore, the appearance of variants (also known as mutations in the viral genome of SARS-CoV-2) that increase the capacity of the virus to cause disease (*e.g.*, transmissibility), might increase the capacity of the virus to overcome vaccine protection. Therefore, continuous monitoring of the pandemic is required, not only to evaluate vaccine distribution and coverage, but also to follow up individuals who were infected by SARS-CoV-2, since they could be carriers viral variants that might disseminate through the population.

Mathematical modelling can help decide which interventions to avoid and which to test, or can predict epidemic or pandemic patterns, as well as help understanding the impact of vaccination programs. In this book entitled: "Moving from COVID-19 Mathematical Models to Vaccine Design: Theory, Practice and Experiences", the authors provide a perspective on how to attack a present problem in public health with mathematical tools, that can guide the decision making related to COVID-19 epidemiology and vaccine production and distribution. But why is this book different from others already published on mathematical modelling? First, the authors of this book are from different countries that are significantly affected by the disease. Second, the book presents a balance set of basic and applied chapters describing topics from disease progression and prevention to those models that could be used in different scenarios. The aim of the book is to present the COVID-19 pandemic as a complex public health problem, that requires the participation of multidisciplinary and interdisciplinary groups of experts to tackle the problems associated with the disease, and demonstrate the role mathematical and computational modeling had during the course and evolution of the pandemic.

The book is divided into 10 chapters. Chapters 1, 4 and 6 introduce mathematical and computational models that can be used to study the COVID-19 pandemic and understand the epidemiology of the disease. Chapters 2 and 3 describe the epidemiology and present the clinical manifestations associated with the disease. Chapter 5 discusses the importance of data science as a tool for COVID-19 informatics. Chapter 7 presents an important aspect of the pandemic that has to do with the impact in populations that lack proper health services or present pre-existing health conditions. Chapter 8 is an overview of the statistical methods that can be used to understand COVID-19 morbidity and mortality. Chapter 9 discusses the impact mathematical modeling and statistics can have in the treatment of COVID-19 patients. Finally, chapter 10 is an overview of all the experimental vaccines available to combat the COVID-19 pandemic. I hope this book becomes a referent for current and future generations of investigators interested in mathematical modeling and infectious diseases, and provides additional tools to understand the current pandemic.

Alfredo G. Torres
University of Texas Medical Branch
Galveston, Texas
USA

FOREWORD III

The pandemic of COVID-19, caused by the SARS-CoV-2 virus (Severe Acute Respiratory Syndrome Coronavirus 2), has shaken up our societies, with an intensity and effects not suffered by humanity for a long time. To date, there have been registered millions of deaths associated to COVID-19, and hundreds of millions of confirmed cases all around the world. Moreover, this pandemic has triggered not only a deep and global health crisis, but also an economic and social (without mentioning psychological, educational, *etc.*) crisis like never seen before.

In order to endure and overcome this major tribulation, the different human communities, guided by their respective administrations and governments, have been put to the test in multiple and severe ways, under the direct effects of the disease, and the performance of several therapeutical and non-pharmaceutical interventions and mitigation measures. Among others, we could mention: the severity of symptoms and disease evolution in serious and critical cases (including assisted ventilation), and the long-term effects; the lack of effective treatments, specially in the first stages; unstoppable death tolls and incidence rates, with increasing numbers of hospitalizations that press and even saturate the health care national systems; hygiene or sanitary measures (frequent hand washing, not touching the face, the generalized use of disinfection products, the use of masks, gloves, and glasses, *etc.*); the use of detection tests (as PCR); quarantines, home isolation and confinements; the implementation of severe social distancing and isolation measures (indeed curfews in some cases); mobility, travel, circulation and gathering restrictions, and closure of borders; reduction or suspension of nonessential activities, with loss of millions of jobs and increasing unemployment rates; total or partial closure of colleges and universities and the unequal and frequently improvised performance of on-line education; campaigns for tracing possible cases; vaccination programs; the psychological effects on mental health in the community; *etc.*

Hence, this picture entailed the scientific community to face to an unprecedented challenge, in order to appropriately assess and advise health authorities and decision-makers. Such a kind of complex phenomena appeals to multidisciplinary and interdisciplinary groups of experts to take their part in order to reach a comprehensive approach, able to deal with the many relevant and multifactorial aspects of COVID-19, as illness and as pandemic. Of course, topics as the epidemiological and clinical aspects of the disease are central, but not the unique ones. Other matters require to be understood, as the SARS-CoV-2 virology, or the COVID-19 pathophysiology and immunology; the study of temporal evolution of infected individuals and their contagiousness; the lack of preparedness of the health care systems and the rapid reaction in Medicine research, including the development and access to vaccines; the population heterogeneity and the effects of mobility and human behavior in the spread of the disease; the role of health and social inequities; *etc.*

In this context, the appearance of scientific works, which organize and summarize a great part of the scientific job carried out, is of great value. In particular, if the subject is approached from a comprehensive and multidisciplinary perspective, considering the individual and collective levels, and their temporal and spatial evolution, the biological, socioeconomic, technological aspects, *etc.*, and its consequences for the societies in which it occurs, as the current work does. In addition, the case of this scientific work is especially interesting, since it highlights the role that Mathematical and Computational Modeling can play together with other related areas such as Data Science and Statistics, when dealing with this type of multidisciplinary phenomenon, for which is an excellent reference for researchers and decision makers on how to deal with this type of problem.

Based on all that has been said above, I hope that this book will help researchers and decision makers to better understand and evaluate the situations that can arise in the context of a complex problem such as that caused by the COVID-19 pandemic and the way to face it.

Victoriano Gabriel Covarrubias Salvatori
Head of the Council of Science and Technology of the State of Puebla
Puebla, Mexico

PREFACE

This book is a multidisciplinary work, dedicated to the current problems around the COVID-19 pandemic and which has been carried out by a group of specialists from various scientific institutions in Mexico, United Kingdom, Spain, France, Russia, Cuba, Belgium and India.

Although the book does not exhaust the subject, it is however the result of the authors' effort to convey, to a certain extent, a comprehensive approach. Therefore, although not all possible points of view and relevant matters are addressed, which make up the multidisciplinary dimension of the research that has been carried out around the COVID-19 pandemic and its associated virus SARS-CoV-2 with its variants of concern, those that have proven to be essential and accessible to the authors' competence and resources have been included.

The first chapter aims to give a comprehensive view of results from different scientific perspectives that have been useful for building and studying epidemiological mathematical models for COVID-19. The conclusions and predictions provided by these results, have been the source of key recommendations to decision-making in several countries.

In later chapters, the problem is approached from the epidemiological and from the clinical point of view which together encompass its individual and societal dimensions. As in all health problems both points of view are essential although their methods and analytical tools are different. However, both approaches complement each other to provide the understanding of the measures that contribute to solving problems and their negative effects, which is indispensable for a global approach to the problem. Mathematical modeling, to different degrees and at different times, is present in both approaches.

The epidemiology of COVID-19 requires analyzing and dealing with large volumes of data, through mathematical and statistical models, which allow studying the problem of transmission as a complex problem, by means of theoretical and computational resources. All these conceptual and operational tools are present in the book under a general and global approach.

The exclusive epidemiological perspective, is however insufficient. Clinical aspects such as: pathophysiology, clinical manifestations, pharmacological treatment of COVID-19, among others, are also essential for understanding and coping with this disease. Chapters 2 and 3 attempt to provide a panoramic view of the epidemiological and clinical components of this multifaceted problem.

Chapters 4 and 5 attempt to advance in the direction of the modeling of epidemics and pandemics, by presenting and discussing techniques and procedures for analyzing and modeling data analysis, thus providing the conceptual and practical bases to solve or minimize the undesirable effects of the pandemic.

Chapters 4 and 6 introduce the reader to the modeling of epidemics through the use of mathematical models. Different perspectives and uses of the models are presented. Chapter 6 in particular is devoted to the study of the effect of population heterogeneity in the process of spread of COVID-19, which is essential for the study of the pandemic, and surprisingly relegated in the available literature, as compared with other topics. "Data Science" is addressed in chapter 5, and shows the process of transforming data into information, using standard procedures with a rich recent development. Data Science is an indispensable tool for a full understanding of the ways in which COVID-19 manifests itself, and the different interpretations.

Population heterogeneity is revealed not only by territorial distribution and demographic factors associated with different social groups, but also by existing social inequalities and biological factors that characterize the response of different individuals to COVID-19 such as age, sex, pre-existing comorbidities, *etc.* Chapters 7 and 8 are devoted to the study of these two interesting topics.

The scientific and methodological approach associated with the study of the presence of "social inequalities" in the evolution of the pandemic, provides essential methods to assess the influence of context in morbidity and mortality associated with COVID-19. Chapter 7 addresses this problem from a conceptual, methodological and practical point of view, showing examples of specific cases.

Chapters 8 and 9 combine quantitative measurement and a qualitative approach to assess and understand the severity, fatality, and impact (both short and long term) of a pandemic with explicit application to COVID-19.

In particular, for a better understanding of the impact of immunotherapy protocols with their modeling aspects, the Cuban protocol, implemented during the pandemic, is shown and developed as an example, of the role and application of mathematical and statistical models.

Chapter 10 addresses a fundamental strategy for the control and elimination of the pandemic, namely the production and application of vaccines. Two key problems are included:

- The conception, production and laboratory evaluation, through clinical trials in its various phases, including the extent and duration of immunity and protection, all encompassed by the clinical aspects of the problem.

- The massive application of strategies to control the disease, to anticipate new mutations and variants, and to build risk perception among the general population. This chapter shows the progress attained on an essential issue with a prospective view to curb and ultimately eradicate the pandemic.

At the end of the book we have included an appendix with a series of graphs, duly selected, that show relevant data on how the COVID-19 pandemic has evolved in different regions and countries of the world. Concretely, this group of charts show the time series of the rolling 7-day average of number of daily new confirmed COVID-19 cases and deaths in the countries with the largest number of accumulated confirmed cases of COVID-19 in the world, and some specific regions (the whole World, the European Union, and the continents of Asia, Europe, North America, South America, and Africa). These plots constitute a simplified snapshot of the pandemic, that would be useful to quickly summarize the whole picture.

The topics covered in the book will undoubtedly be useful for specialists from different areas who have been involved, either in scientific research or daily work, with the COVID-19 pandemic. Doctors from different specialties, epidemiologists, chemists, biologists, pharmacologists, immunologists, microbiologists, mathematicians, computer scientists, sociologists and specialists in data analysis, among others will be clear beneficiaries of the messages conveyed by the book.

It will also be useful to any reader who, without being a specialist in any of these areas, wants to have an overview of the extensive work that has been carried out, during the little more than a year and a half that has elapsed since the beginning of the pandemic today. The book provides a very complete picture of the meaning scope of multidisciplinary scientific work aimed at a common goal.

I must express deserved recognition and gratitude to all who, in one way or another, have made possible the final result of this multidisciplinary work, on a subject that is of fundamental importance for all humanity.

In the first place, our gratitude to all the authors, many of whom were immersed in their professional daily work of caring for COVID-19 patients in intensive care rooms in hospitals or in laboratories dedicated to the creation of vaccines and immunotherapeutic treatments, while they wrote their chapters.

We also want to thank the Council of Science and Technology of the State of Puebla (CONCYTEP) in Mexico and, in particular, the Head of the Council, Dr. Victoriano Gabriel Covarrubias Salvatori, who, on behalf of the State Government, provided his support for the fulfillment of this work.

Our thanks to the Scientific Directorate of the HM Hospitales of Spain, Research Foundation who provided us with an extensive database of their COVID-19 patients, which has been of great help in obtaining some of the results presented in this book.

A special recognition to Dr. Moisés Soto Bajo, for the valuable work done in the revision and composition of the book.

Andrés Fraguela-Collar
Professor and Researcher in Applied Mathematics
Faculty of Physics and Mathematics,
Autonomous University of Puebla
Puebla, Mexico

Dedication:

In memory of those who died as a result of the COVID-19 pandemic,

To all people, especially children, who have lost a loved one due to the pandemic,

To healthcare workers who have been on the front lines caring for COVID-19 patients,

To the scientists around the world, whose work has been the striking force that will ultimately control this pandemic.

List of contributors

Andrés Fraguela Collar, Ph.D., Dr.Sci.

Multidisciplinary Center for Mathematical and Computational Modeling

Faculty of Physical Mathematical Sciences

Autonomous University of Puebla

Puebla, Mexico

Raúl Felipe-Sosa, Ph.D.

Multidisciplinary Center for Mathematical and Computational Modeling

Faculty of Physical Mathematical Sciences

Autonomous University of Puebla

Puebla, Mexico

Moisés Soto-Bajo, Ph.D.

CONACYT Researcher Chairs Program

Multidisciplinary Center for Mathematical and Computational Modeling

Faculty of Physical Mathematical Sciences

Autonomous University of Puebla

Puebla, Mexico

María Eugenia Jiménez-Corona, M.D.,
Department of Epidemiology
National Institute of Cardiology
Mexico City, Mexico

Manlio F. Márquez-Murillo, M.D.
Deputy Director Clinical Investigation
National Institute of Cardiology
Mexico City, Mexico

Daniel Manzur Sandoval, M.D.
Cardiovascular Intensive Care Unit
National Institute of Cardiology
Mexico City, Mexico

Gustavo Rojas-Velasco, M.D.
Cardiovascular Intensive Care Unit
National Institute of Cardiology
Mexico City, Mexico

Efrén Melano Carranza, M.D.
Cardiovascular Intensive Care Unit
National Institute of Cardiology
Mexico City, Mexico

Camelia Cruz Rodr´ıguez, M.D.
Cardiovascular Intensive Care Unit
National Institute of Cardiology
Mexico City, Mexico

Arturo Arzate Ram´ırez, M.D.
Cardiovascular Intensive Care Unit
National Institute of Cardiology
Mexico City, Mexico

Francisco Javier González Ruiz, M.D.
Cardiovascular Intensive Care Unit
National Institute of Cardiology
Mexico City, Mexico

Gerardo Arteaga Cárdenas, M.D.
Cardiovascular Intensive Care Unit
National Institute of Cardiology
Mexico City, Mexico

María Alexandra López Polanco, M.D.
Cardiovascular Intensive Care Unit
National Institute of Cardiology
Mexico City, Mexico

Eduardo Alberto González Escudero, M.D.
Cardiovascular Intensive Care Unit
National Institute of Cardiology
Mexico City, Mexico

Edgar Garc´ıa Cruz, M.D.
Cardiovascular Intensive Care Unit
National Institute of Cardiology
Mexico City, Mexico

Luis Augusto Baeza Herrera, M.D.
Cardiovascular Intensive Care Unit
National Institute of Cardiology
Mexico City, Mexico

Luis Efrén Santos Martínez, M.D.
Cardiovascular Intensive Care Unit
National Institute of Cardiology
Mexico City, Mexico

Jorge X. Velasco-Hernández, Ph.D.
Institute of Mathematics
National Autonomous University of Mexico
Juriquilla, Querétaro, Mexico

Nicandro Cruz-Ram´ırez, Ph.D.
Artificial Intelligence Research Institute
Universidad Veracruzana
Xalapa, Veracruz, Mexico

Guillermo-de-Jesús Hoyos-Rivera, Ph.D.
Artificial Intelligence Research Institute
Universidad Veracruzana
Xalapa, Veracruz, Mexico

Sonia-Lilia Mestizo-Gutiérrez, Ph.D.
Faculty of Chemical Sciences
Universidad Veracruzana
Xalapa, Veracruz, Mexico

Horacio Tapia-McClung, Ph.D.
Artificial Intelligence Research Institute
Universidad Veracruzana
Xalapa, Veracruz, Mexico

Malay Banerjee, Ph.D.
Indian Institute of Technology Kanpur
Kanpur, India

Samiran Ghosh, Ph.D.
Indian Institute of Technology Kanpur
Kanpur, India

Vitaly Volpert, Ph.D., Dr. Habil.
Institut Camille Jordan
University Lyon 1
Villeurbanne, France

Jorge Bacallao Gallestey, Ph.D.

Atherosclerosis Research and Reference Center

University of Medical Sciences

Havana, Cuba

Alfonso Casado Collado, Ph.D.

Department of Preventive Medicine and Public Health

School of Medicine

Autonomous University of Madrid

Madrid, Spain

Armando Humberto Seuc-Jo, Ph.D.

National Institute of Hygiene, Epidemiology and Microbiology

Havana, Cuba

Elly Mertens, Ph.D. Institute

of Tropical Medicine

Antwerp, Belgium

José Luis Peñalvo, Ph.D.

Institute of Tropical Medicine

Antwerp, Belgium

Karina Garc´ıa-Mart´ınez, Ph.D.
Center of Molecular Immunology
Havana, Cuba

Patricia Luaces-Á lvarez, Ph.D.
Center of Molecular Immunology
Havana, Cuba

Lizet Sánchez-Valdés, Ph.D.
Center of Molecular Immunology
Havana, Cuba

Kalet León-Monzón, Ph.D.
Center of Molecular Immunology
Havana, Cuba

Tania Crombet-Ramos, Ph.D.
Center of Molecular Immunology
Havana, Cuba

Rolando Pérez-Rodríguez, Ph.D.
Center of Molecular Immunology
Havana, Cuba

Barbara Dema, Ph.D.
The Jenner Institute
University of Oxford
Old Road campus Research Building, Oxford, UK

Sthefany Pagliari, Ph.D.
The Jenner Institute
University of Oxford
Old Road campus Research Building, Oxford, UK

Arturo Reyes-Sandoval, Ph.D.
Instituto Politécnico Nacional, IPN
Mexico City, Mexico

CHAPTER 1

An Approach to COVID-19: Current Results, Perspectives and its Study with Mathematical and Computational Modeling Tools

Andrés Fraguela-Collar[*1], **Moisés Soto-Bajo**[12], **Raúl Felipe Sosa**[13]

[*] **Corresponding author:** fraguela@fcfm.buap.mx, Phone: +52 (222) 2295500 ext. 2129

[1] Autonomous University of Puebla, Puebla, 72570, Mexico

[2] CONACYT Researcher Chairs Program, Mexico City, 03940, Mexico

[3] CONACYT Postdoctoral Stays Program, Mexico City, 03940, Mexico

Abstract. This chapter presents the COVID-19 pandemic as a complex problem, which has resulted in multidisciplinary and interdisciplinary research of unprecedented magnitude at the international level. In particular, the important role that mathematical and computational modeling has played throughout the different phases of the evolution of the pandemic is analyzed. Some of the most notorious achievements and difficulties in obtaining results with the use of mathematical models and computational simulations are discussed, and some proposals are presented about relevant and still pending tasks.

Key words: COVID-19, epidemiological model, sensitivity analysis, bifurcations, parameter identification, controllability, stabilization.

1 INTRODUCTION

1.1 Importance

Today, mathematical and computational modeling is an indispensable tool for the study of complex systems and phenomena. Mathematical Epidemiology and its application to the study of the COVID-19 pandemic has been a relevant example of the usefulness of this tool.

In this chapter, we analyze and conceptualize some aspects of the pandemia from different perspectives, according to its relevance when studying and representing mathematically this phenomenon. We summarize relevant, and basically quantitative information about "model calibration and assessment".

We also review the mathematical and computational models which have been used to describe the pandemia and the main results they have yielded. This text has been written in such a way that the congruence between the first analysis phase and the second conceptual synthesis phase of modeling could be easily perceived, that, although arising in a disordered way, underlie all modeling processes.

Finally, without any pretensions to being exhaustive, we show some fundamental results achieved with these models until now, and we identify some relevant problems and suggest possible strategies for their solution from the perspective of mathematical and computational modeling.

This summary, dedicated to such a wide and complex topic, necessarily has to be brief, schematic, and incomplete. Consequently, the matter is developed without the deep insight devoted to different topics in the remaining chapters of the book, to which readers are redirected to deepen into each corresponding topic.

Therefore, the goal of this chapter is, on the one hand, to offer a review of the scientific work in relation to the COVID-19 pandemic, having as backbone the mathematical and computational modeling; and on the other hand, to show the close link between scientific results achieved along a widespread multidisciplinary research, the demands of the decision making in different stages of the pandemic, and the proposing and resolution of problems by using mathematical and computational models.

In this chapter, we will review from a methodological point of view, how mathematical models for the study of COVID-19 have evolved, based on basic principles. With the modeling of the phenomenon as a directing vector, relevant aspects will be discussed and how they have been taken into consideration. Among others, we can mention the inclusion of NPI (non-pharmaceutical interventions); population heterogeneity, including vulnerability and variability of human behavior; the effect of mobility; mitigation measures; the intra-domiciliary, extra-domiciliary and intra-hospital dynamics; limited immunity, after recovery from the disease, or as a result of the application of vaccines; vaccination strategies; the genetic variability of the virus and its characteristics regarding the transmission and severity of the disease, etc.

Despite the large number of important results that have been obtained so far, we will show that there are still many nonminor problems that require an answer. We will also discuss the need for new ideas to deal with them; on the one hand, to obtain models that better represent the dynamics of COVID-19, and on the other, a more in-depth qualitative analysis of the models is needed.

Frequently, using very particular models, general conclusions have been drawn only from numerical simulations, which reproduce certain incidence data in the study areas. In addition, on many occasions, to carry out numerical simulations, the information required by the models is used, which does not even correspond to the place where the results are applied. In this context, in addition to obtaining new results of a general nature, the qualitative study would allow to encompass and confirm a large number of results of this type.

With the support of more complete and reliable databases and numerical simulations of convenient scenarios, we will enhance our understanding of the behavior of the complex dynamics associated with this phenomenon. Applied to particular situations, this will make it possible to offer more accurate recommendations to health authorities and decision makers.

1.2 The COVID-19 Pandemic as a Complex Phenomenon

Epidemics have always accompanied mankind. The current COVID-19 pandemic (Coronavirus Disease 2019), produced by a mutant strain of a coronavirus, SARS-CoV-2 (Severe Acute Respiratory Syndrome Coronavirus 2), has generated a severe economic, social and health crisis, never before experienced on a global scale.

SARS-CoV-2 is a virus from the family known as coronaviruses, two of whose oldest strains are the cause of the common flu. In 2003, the first major mutation emerged, resulting in the SARS strain that appeared in China, with a total of 8,460 confirmed cases in 27 countries, and a fatality rate of 10% [1]. Subsequently, in 2012, another strain appeared as a result of a new coronavirus mutation in Saudi Arabia, giving rise to MERS-CoV, which produced 2,499 confirmed cases and a fatality rate of 37% [2].

The next major strain of coronavirus, SARS-CoV-2, originated in China at the end of December 2019, in the province of Hubei (Wuhan city), where 27 cases of pneumonia of unknown causes were reported, with seven seriously ill patients. After a year and a half of scourging humanity, the true origin of the virus is still not known for sure, although it is assumed that it was transmitted to man by pangolin, a mammal used as food in China, or some type of bat. The first case was reported on December 8, 2019 [3, 4]. On January 7, 2020, the Chinese Ministry of Health identified a novel coronavirus (nCoV) as a possible causal agent [3, 4]. By January 24, 2020, 835 cases were already reported in China, 534 of them in Hubei, and within a few weeks the epidemic spread to other parts of China.

The influence of the mobility of human beings in a highly connected world, with fast and massive means of transport, quickly turned this phenomenon into a global one.

The first case outside of China was reported in Thailand on January 13, 2020 [5]; on January 19, 2020, cases were reported in South Korea [6]; later, the virus spread to many countries around the world. The coronavirus reached the US on January 15, 2020, when a man who had visited Wuhan returned home to Washington State and tested positive on January 20, 2020 [7]. In Europe, the coronavirus apparently arrived through France, where the first three cases were confirmed on January 22, 2020 [8]. Italy reported its first case on January 31, 2020 [9], subsequently turning out to be the most affected country in terms of loss of life in the first phase of the epidemic. On February 27, 2020, the first positive case for COVID-19 was detected in Mexico [10].

This rapid spread of a new disease, totally unknown before, prompted WHO (World Health Organization) to announce it as a public health emergency of international concern on January 30, 2020. Shortly thereafter, on March 11, 2020, its Director General, Dr. Tedros Adhanom Ghebreyesus, declared it a new global pandemic, which was called COVID-19 [11].

The COVID-19 pandemic has had devastating global effects, due to which humanity is still suffering. According to the statistics from the Coronavirus Resource Center of the Center for Systems Science and Engineering (CSSE) at Johns Hopkins University (JHU) [12], as of July 8, 2021, the global death toll from COVID-19 has already exceeded 4 million. The dimension of the tragedy can be better grasped if we consider that the populations of Hong Kong or New York barely double these figures. Moreover, the crisis continues to be a real challenge, despite vaccines, due to the appearance of new variants of the virus, highly contagious and more resistant to treatments and vaccines.

This situation has generated an unprecedented joint response from the global scientific community, including the development of vaccines in record time for a disease that did not exist a short time before [13, 14].

The objective of this book is to offer a global vision of the multidisciplinary and interdisciplinary research endeavor, which has been deployed around this scourge of humanity, and which has represented a colossal effort, to reach the current level of knowledge and understanding. It is impossible to cover all edges of such a complex problem and many of its components will remain unaddressed. However, we want to illustrate the diversity of apparently unrelated issues involved such as the application of classical mathematical models of the Kermack and McKendrick type [15–20] to try to understand the spread of the epidemic, the development of vaccines (see Chapter 10), and how they relate to each other in the quest for answers that help decision-making. We hope that this first chapter shows the way to perceive the common thread of such an impressive journey.

The main objective of Epidemiology is to study epidemics as a process of propagation of a disease in a community, taking into consideration all factors, known or under investigation, possibly contributing to the phenomenon in question. That is why perhaps, of all branches of knowledge that have intervened in the research about COVID-19, Epidemiology is at the center (see Chapter 2 of this book). Among these contributing factors, in the case of COVID-19, we must highlight, among others, the genetic variability of the SARS-CoV-2 virus, which has led to variants that are increasingly infectious and more resistant to existing treatments and vaccines; the nonexistence of preventive and / or curative drugs for the disease; the variability of human behavior; the heterogeneity of the populations and their demographic distribution, in relation to vulnerability and capacity to recover from the disease; human mobility and the adverse effects of confinement on people's mental health, and the development of essential and daily socio-economic activities.

The results derived from the study of those factors should advice health authorities and decision makers on how to control epidemics and mitigate their negative effects. From a scientific perspective, it is necessary to detect the origins of the disease, understand the causes of its evolution at the individual level and its community spread, as well as explain the underlying mechanisms associated with its evolution and its consequences, to assess its impact on the affected populations. In this way it is possible to predict, and subsequently to foresee scenarios and to design strategies, based on qualitative and quantitative conclusions drawn from the process that gives rise to the phenomenon.

The situation becomes even more complex when the epidemic situation cannot be controlled at the community or country level, and becomes a problem at the international level; that is, in a pandemic, as is the case of COVID-19.

Epidemics are a complex phenomenon since, to understand how an infectious disease spreads, it is necessary to consider the combined effect of all its contributing factors. In general, the study of each component separately does not provide enough information to attack the problem in all its multidimensionality.

Currently, despite the great achievements in the development of vaccines, there is still a lot of uncertainty regarding the future of COVID-19. This is so since completing the vaccination scheme does not exempt people from becoming infected, becoming ill, or even dying, due to the appearance of new variants of the virus, which increasingly have greater transmission capacity and impact on human health, and less responsiveness to treatments. On the other hand, the limited immunity produced by the effect of vaccines and the restrictions on their acquisition in many countries, coupled with vaccination policies that are not always designed based solely on scientific criteria, cause long periods of vaccination campaigns. This results in the reemergence of populations of susceptible individuals who have already completed their period of immunity since they were first vaccinated. If an efficient and sustained control of these dynamics is not sought, it is possible to fall into endless cycles or states of endemic equilibrium, which will continue to endanger the world population (see Chapters 4 and 6).

It is not yet possible to predict a clear picture regarding the control of this disease, due, among other factors, to the frequent appearance of new variants of the virus and the unknown duration of immunity provided by recovery from infection and the effect of vaccines [21].

This limited knowledge and uncertainty, coupled with the constant variation of the conditions in which the disease manifests and spreads, renders endless the task of biologists, chemists, infectologists, virologists, pharmacologists, pathophysiologists, immunologists, pneumologists, cardiologists, hematologists, and other specialists. In this list of specialties in which some of the most important social consequences of the epidemic also fall, we must also include sociologists, economists, psychologists, and so on.

In response to these difficulties, comprehensive solutions are needed, the result of a systemic analysis, which includes as many contributing factors as possible and their most relevant interactions, and this is not possible from a unidisciplinary perspective. It is precisely in this integrating context, where mathematical and computational models, together with the corresponding mathematical and numerical tools required for their study, become a very useful instrument for epidemiology.

1.3 Mathematical and Computational Modeling in Epidemiology

Mathematical Epidemiology is a branch of Epidemiology that, based on the tools provided by Mathematical Sciences, seeks to build and study mathematical models of epidemiological processes, which allow useful conclusions to be drawn, for the better understanding and management of an epidemic. The working paradigm of mathematical epidemiology is framed within mathematical and computational modeling. Stated schematically, the researchers observe the epidemiological phenomenon, analyze the available data and the literature on the matter, try to understand the phenomenon and the main mechanisms that govern it, together with their interactions and, based on this, they build mathematical models that can be studied theoretically and used to draw informed conclusions.

The role of mathematical and computational modeling is of utmost importance in mathematical epidemiology, as it allows indirect analysis and experimentation on phenomena, which otherwise would not be possible, due to the great variety of contributing factors. In a particular epidemic, the only information available is a very limited amount of data which is expensive to collect, often contaminated in multiple ways, and impossible to reproduce. Consequently, the data must be used with great caution and the results they yield them must be subject to cross-validation.

In this framework, there are two complementary perspectives: the adjustment of data with parameterized models (curve fitting) and the study of mathematical models generated ad hoc, based on a deep and detailed analysis of the phenomenon. In the first case, the results will be conditioned by the quality and representativeness of the available data and the adequacy of the model used. In the second case, the information provided by the data can be modulated with a priori knowledge about the phenomenon. Only in the second case, is there sufficient generality to obtain qualitative conclusions of great importance for decision makers.

In modeling, the acquisition of a deep and adequate understanding of the underlying mechanisms that generate epidemiological dynamics is of utmost importance. Only by explicitly including in the models the fundamental principles that govern these mechanisms and their interactions, can the conclusions be useful for decision-making. Otherwise, if they are not taken into account by the models, they will ignore their effects and, when these effects are relevant, the conclusions of the model will not be consistent with reality. In this process of analysis of the different facets of the phenomenon, the role of multidisciplinary and interdisciplinary groups in which experts in different areas combine their knowledge, techniques, and methodologies, is essential.

We conclude from all this that a deep and comprehensive understanding of the problem, from the biological and epidemiological perspective, is essential, especially at the beginning and at the end of the mathematical modeling process. Such an understanding is required to:

- Correctly represent the characteristics of the phenomenon under study.
- Properly formulate the questions to be answered, so that the study of the models offers answers with practical sense.
- Correctly interpret the information available when calibrating the models and doing simulations.
- Correctly interpret the results obtained from the numerical simulations and the analysis of the models within the framework of the problem under study.

However, the models are not only used to draw conclusions from numerical simulations or the simple stability analysis of their equilibrium states. The qualitative analysis of the models, using appropriate mathematical tools, allows, in addition, to extract relevant information on the behavior of the associated dynamics, by varying the parameters with biological sense in admissible ranges and, formulating many particular results, obtained from the measurements, in a unified context.

This underscores the importance of theoretical studies. Among them, we can cite here the following ones: the identifiability analyses of the models and their uniqueness to reproduce a certain type of dynamic behavior; the study of sensitivity and bifurcation of the solutions when varying the parameters of the model; obtaining controllability and stabilization conditions for certain desirable dynamics, together with an estimate of their cost; and the establishment of problems of simultaneous optimization, which result in measures to reduce the transmission of the epidemic, affecting as little as possible other important sectors such as the economy. The theoretical analysis generates results of great practical importance, which are impossible to predict a priori.

To describe how the mathematical and computational modeling tool has worked in the study of COVID-19, we will begin by discussing in Section 2, the specific characteristics of the different biological, temporal, and spatial scales through which the disease and the pandemic pass, together with the measures and interventions that have been sought during this evolution. This description is essential for the construction and analysis of mathematical and computational models, according to the objectives to be pursued. This is particularly important in the current period, with the introduction of vaccines. In Section 3, the construction scheme of the mathematical models that have been used so far will be discussed and the fundamental contributions that have been obtained with them will be analyzed, as well as its relationship with each of the evolution phases of the pandemic. At the end of this section, some new perspectives of work with mathematical models will be raised, and the need to deepen their qualitative analysis. The chapter ends with a concluding section and the bibliography.

2 DIFFERENT PERSPECTIVES FOR THE STUDY OF THE DISEASE AND THE COVID-19 PANDEMIC

Whether considered as a disease at an individual level or as a pandemic, COVID-19 is a highly complex phenomenon, in which a multitude of factors of diverse nature converge and interact in a nontrivial way. Among them, it is necessary to highlight its manifestation at different biological, temporal, and spatial scales, which are closely related. Consequently, it is a difficult phenomenon to understand and model. This circumstance is aggravated by the limited knowledge about the virus and the disease since the beginning of the pandemic, around which many questions remain unanswered.

The COVID-19 pandemic can be analyzed from several different perspectives, taking into consideration:

- The different scales of biological organization, in which the interaction of the SARS-CoV-2 virus and its variants with the human organism is revealed.
- The temporal evolution of the disease at the individual level.
- The temporal evolution of the pandemic at the country level and at the global level; the role of human mobility.
- The collateral consequences for human health, society, and economy.

In what follows we will address these issues, trying to draw conclusions and identify data that may be useful for the planning and study of mathematical models of COVID-19, and as a source of practical problems that can be solved within the framework of these models. To underscore these findings and data, we have highlighted the corresponding paragraphs of the text in italics.

2.1 Action of the Virus at Different Scales of Biological Organization

Considering the action of SARS-CoV-2 at different scales of biological organization, the pandemic can be analyzed from several scientific disciplines:

- On a cellular scale, the nature of the SARS-CoV-2 virus itself is studied, its structure and interaction with different types of cells and tissues of the human body, and its consequent effect on the organs. The study is carried out from the point of view of Cell Biology, Physiology, Virology, and Immunology;
- On an individual scale, in which the COVID-19 disease itself and the complications that it usually entails for the health of the patient are studied, as well as the effect of the application of different medications and treatments. This is studied from the point of view of Medicine, Pathophysiology, and Immunology;
- On a global or collective scale, the contagion process (transmission of the virus from one person to another) is studied, as well as the study of its consequences in a human community. This is the field study of Epidemiology and its associated disciplines.

In each of the previous scales, a large number of factors, characteristics, and effects converge, which are analyzed in a different way.

2.1.1 On a Cellular Scale

SARS-CoV-2 is one of the three coronaviruses that affect humans and are highly pathogenic. It belongs to the family of β-coronaviruses, which are single-stranded ribonucleic acid (RNA) viruses, with positive polarity, enveloped, non-segmented, with a genome of 27 to $32kb$ and a size of $80 - 160nm$. They are the largest RNA viruses so far discovered and belong to group IV of the Baltimore classification [22].

Studies on this biological scale have been developed around the viral replication process and the causes that affect some organs such as the lungs and kidneys and the cardiovascular system, including the appearance of acute inflammatory processes, among others. For more information on this, see Chapter 3.

Regarding the nature of the virus, the fundamental difficulty has been its great capacity for variation. Although the terms strain, mutant, and variant have been used interchangeably when expressing the genetic variability of the virus, they do not represent the same thing [23].

So far, SARS-CoV-2 is the only strain associated with COVID-19. From this strain, new variants associated with one or more mutations have emerged and managed to expand, and have been detected in certain groups of people in different countries. This has occurred on multiple occasions in many parts of the world, but so far the variants that have most concerned researchers, due to their greater infectivity, transmissibility, severity of the disease, and/or resistance to the effect of treatment or vaccines, are the British, South African and Brazilian variants, also known as Alpha, Beta and Gamma variants, and more recently, the Indian variant, also known as Delta, with its new Delta plus variant, detected until July 2021 in a large number of countries [24], as well as the Epsilon variant, found for the first time in California, United States, in early 2021, and which has already been detected in 34 countries, according to information from WHO [21, 25]. The highest infectivity is evidenced by the fact that a person needs to inhale less amount of the virus to become infected; greater transmissibility translates into an increase in the amount of virus shed by a person; the highest fatality, as a consequence of more serious manifestations of the disease; and resistance to the effect of treatment or vaccines is due to the fact that they evade more easily the immune system, according to information from WHO [21, 25].

Some researchers have predicted that, by September 2021, around 90% of COVID-19 infections in Europe could be caused by the Delta variant, which is characterized by being 40% more infectious than the original version of the virus [26].

For a new strain to originate, the virus would have to undergo a drastic mutation in its gene chain, which has not happened so far. However, it is clear that as more viruses that are circulating, the greater the likelihood that mutations will occur and that new variants will emerge. Therefore, low vaccination rates, in addition to representing a higher risk of acquiring the disease, also increase the risk of emergence of new potentially more dangerous variants emerging.

Some new variants of the virus are more transmissible than the original variant detected in China. The number of secondary infections produced by an infected person is called the reproduction rate of the disease.

It is estimated that a person infected with the original SARS-CoV-2 virus infects an average of 2 or 3 more people, while with the Alpha variant an infected person can transmit the infection to 4 or 5 people, and with the Delta variant to 8 or 9 people. That is, the reproduction rate of COVID-19 has increased from values 2-3 to 8-9, and if we compare it with the reproduction rate of influenza, which is 1.4, we conclude that SARS-CoV-2 is one of the most contagious respiratory viruses. People infected with the Delta variant of the virus have a viral load 10 times higher, an infectivity of the order of 2.6 times higher than those infected by the original variant, and a transmission capacity of the order of 40%-60% more than the Alpha variant [27, 28]. See Fig. 1 for a comparison of the effects of different reproduction rates.

Immunity to disease is a measure of the body's readiness to respond to the next exposure to the disease-causing microorganism.

The term "group immunity" defined almost 100 years ago by WC Topley and GS Wilson [29, 30], was used to explain that in some infections the spread slowed as more individuals in the affected population were immunized either naturally or through the application of a vaccine. Currently, the expression "herd or group immunity" refers to the proportion of immunized people among all individuals in a population.

Usually, a threshold of 70% of individuals immunized against COVID-19 is considered necessary to "stop or at least slow the progress in the spread of this disease".

However, there is still a lot of uncertainty surrounding this hypothesis. Indeed, the difficulty in reaching a group immunity threshold is due to different factors:

- Existing vaccines do not interrupt transmission, although they appear to reduce it.
- The limited duration of natural immunity and that produced by vaccines.

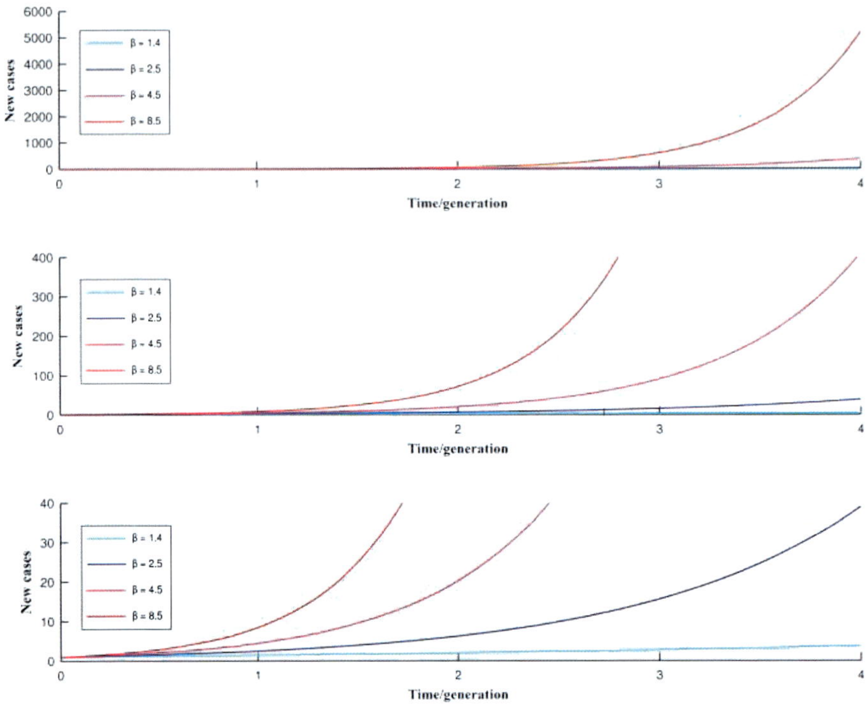

Figure 1: Comparison of different reproduction rates. The curve $C(t) = e^{t \log \beta}$ satisfy the relation $C(t+1) = \beta C(t)$ for any t. In the figure above, several choices of $\beta = 1.4, 2.5, 4.5, 8.5$ are plotted, showing the very different evolution for different values of β. The second and third graphics are zooms of the first one

- The long time that poorly designed vaccination campaigns are occupying and the unequal distribution of vaccines among countries.
- The possibility of reinfection even after having been vaccinated.
- Improper human behavior such as rejection of vaccines and reluctance for self-protection.
- Existence of more transmissible, infectious and lethal variants of the virus that modify the required immunity threshold.

According to the criteria of some specialists, such as Dr. Jaime Sepúlveda, Distinguished Professor in Global Health at the University of California - San Francisco, and Dr. Carlos del Río, Distinguished Professor of Medicine and Epidemiology at Emory University, due to the increasingly predominant circulation of the Delta variant, it is possible that the so-called "group immunity" can only be achieved when 90% of the total population is immunized. In conclusion, it seems to be a difficult goal to try to achieve group immunity only by vaccination; global control of the pandemic is required and has not yet been implemented [31].

2.1.2 At the Individual Level

At this scale, studies are aimed at the combined process of infestation of susceptible cells and viral replication in the presence of the action of interleukin 6 (IL-6), which intervenes in the triggering of inflammatory processes, and of type 1 interferon (IFN 1) which participates in the inhibition of viral replication. The models that represent this process play a fundamental role in proposing treatments to attack the two fundamental phases of the disease; the first, in which it is necessary to stop viral replication, and the second, in which the inflammatory process is exacerbated [32] (see chapters 3 and 9).

However, with respect to the COVID-19 disease, its complications and treatment continue to be a challenge for the medical community, without a specific treatment, yet, beyond therapeutic measures to alleviate symptoms and maintain vital functions. There are physiological factors that can be decisive in the outcome of COVID-19. These include natural immunity, age (older people are more susceptible to severe or severe episodes of COVID-19, with a greater propensity to a fatal outcome), gender (men), certain preexisting conditions (diabetes, cardiovascular disease, hypertension, chronic lung disease, kidney disease, cancer, immunosuppression, obesity, or pregnancy).

2.1.3 Collectively

The main properties that characterize the collective effects of the virus on the host are the following (see [33]):

- The transmissibility or ability of the agent to spread from one host to another.
- The infectivity or ability of the microorganism to invade and multiply in a susceptible host.
- The pathogenicity or ability to induce disease in the infected.
- The virulence or relative ability of a microorganism to cause severe damage in the infected.
- The immunogenicity or ability to induce a specific and lasting immune response in the host.

From the point of view of Epidemiology, focused on the study at a collective scale, it is essential to consider the transmission mechanisms of the virus, considering two fundamental factors: the way in which the virus is transmitted from one human to another, and the ability of the virus to infect the recipient human.

In this chapter, we are more interested in analyzing the COVID-19 pandemic from an epidemiological point of view. Therefore, we will refer to these issues to illustrate the level of difficulty in modeling the contagion process between people.

Since the beginning of the pandemic, many scientists have argued that the SARS-CoV-2 virus is spread rapidly through the cough or respiratory secretions of infected people, and through close contact with sensitive people.

Today it is known that respiratory droplets of more than five microns are capable of being transmitted at a distance of up to two meters, and hands, fomites, and air contaminated with these secretions, introduce the virus to the recipient, through contact with the mucosa of the mouth, nose, or eyes. In general, the virus is transmitted through droplets of saliva and aerosols produced during breathing, conversation, sneezing, and coughing, hence the importance of the use of masks [34–37].

There is a competition between certain physical properties of these droplets and aerosols, which depend on their size, inertia, gravity, and evaporation, which determine how far they can travel and stay in the air.

The droplets, due to their size, fall rapidly on surfaces that are immediately contaminated and are the basis of transmission by direct contact. The virus can remain on average between one or two days on cardboard surfaces, or three to four days if it is plastic or metal and, even more than four days, if there are low temperatures with humidity. Contagion occurs when someone touches an infected surface and put their hands on their face [3].

There is also transmission by direct contact between people, for example, through greeting if one of them has the virus on their hands [3].

On the other hand, aerosols can reach the air up to 6 feet beyond the person who emits them, while droplets of saliva settle 1.5 to 2 feet around. However, sometimes small aerosols do not have time to fall due to gravity, as they evaporate very quickly, causing the virus to float in the air and move with air currents, leading to transmission by inhalation of the air [38].

Note that these are three different contagion schemes, which in principle require different types of modeling, and which have been studied in great detail under laboratory conditions.

On the other hand, the size of the respiratory droplets influences the severity of the disease. For example, when aerosols with sizes of less than one micron are breathed, they end up deeper in the alveolar region of the lungs, where there is very little immune response, and therefore their effect is more severe, although they do not produce symptoms immediately. In general, the virus spreads rapidly to the pharynx and from there to other parts of the body, before the immune response is activated and produces symptoms [39].

When the virus has replicated sufficiently in the body, and a higher viral load is produced, people begin to transmit the virus, without yet having a noticeable manifestation of symptoms. This makes the potential transmissibility of this disease even higher, because infected people can be highly contagious for several days before symptoms appear (if they do). Suffice it to say that, in the Wuhan outbreak, an estimated 79% of infections were due to undetected cases of infected individuals.

Person-to-person transmission is related to the number of times an infected person exhales, speaks, or sneezes during contact with another. For example, during one minute of loud conversation by an infected person, aerosols containing more than 1000 virions can be generated. Furthermore, some individuals called superspreaders can generate up to a few hundred times more contaminating material than average spreaders.

In a macrostudy carried out by the Charité Hospital in Berlin (Germany), with more than 25,000 participants, under the direction of Dr. Christian Drosten [40], the existence of invisible superspreaders was confirmed. Research shows that people infected by the coronavirus reach their peak viral load in the throat between one and three days before the onset of symptoms, but among them there are some that stand out for their contagion capacity, closely related to their high viral load. A normal sample, taken from the throat of a sick person, contains 2.5 million copies of the virus genome, but nearly 9% of those infected have 1 billion copies or more, the study shows.

The conclusions are consistent with other recent studies. A study published on May 10, 2021 [41], with 1,400 positive cases without symptoms, identified at the University of Colorado in Boulder (USA), suggests that 2% of those infected carry 90% of circulating viruses. The authors, led by virologist Sara Sawyer, speak of "viral supercarriers and possibly also superspreaders". Another study published in November 2020 in India [42] found that 71% of 85,000 infected people did not transmit the virus to anyone else, while an analysis of 1,200 cases in China in January 2021 [43] found that 15% of those infected caused 80% of the infections.

Given that the new variants of the virus produce a viral load in infected people, up to 10 times higher than that produced by the original virus, it is logical to think that they also generate a greater number of superspreaders.

When speaking in the open air, the emitted aerosols can travel farther due to air currents, and the propagation can reach greater distances. This type of spread of the virus through air currents can affect people who are at a distance greater than that stipulated by the measures of social distancing programs. This can undermine the effectiveness of testing, tracking, and social distancing programs, although the probability of this type of long-range contagion is much lower. It is also known that the virus can be spread by cigarette smoke, as far as the smell of smoke reaches, due to a diffusion process that is independent of transport by air currents.

It is not yet well known whether the SARS-CoV-2 virus can be inactivated by ultraviolet radiation, or whether it is sensitive to variations in ambient temperature or relative humidity, or to the presence of other atmospheric aerosols in contaminated places, nor if it can adhere to other dust and pollution particles, which could change its aerodynamic characteristics and increase its dispersion. An important problem to study, since the virus can remain in the air for prolonged periods, before being inhaled by people, are the factors that lead to the loss of infectivity of the virus over time in different atmospheres in the free air.

In a closed room with patients, aerosol concentrations may increase over time and the probability of infection is greater (especially in asymptomatic patients and if precautions are relaxed). That is why, in closed spaces, ventilation, the number of people gathered, and the length of stay are essential drivers of transmission.

A crucial aspect, which still requires the attention of the scientific community, is the minimum viral load necessary for a person's infection. It is reasonable to assume that this minimum viral load could vary considerably from one person to another. This is related to the infectivity of the virus, but also to the pathogenicity, virulence, and immunogenicity, which are also relevant aspects in modeling, especially if it is required to qualitatively analyze the health damage in the population (beyond the number of infected).

2.2 Temporal Evolution of COVID-19 Disease at the Individual Level

Those infected by COVID-19 go through five important periods or phases that do not occur in strict in chronological order, but correspond to different states of the subject with respect to the disease process and its infective capacity, which may overlap each other. See Fig. 2 for an orientative time schedule showing the different states of a mild symptomatic case of COVID-19.

2.2.1 Incubation

This period, which is defined for the case of symptomatic patients, corresponds to the time that elapses from the moment of exposure to the virus until the appearance of the signs and symptoms of the disease for the first time; that is, the time required for the viral load to reach the threshold necessary to generate symptoms.

The incubation period can last between 1 and 14 days, although it has been found that in 95% of cases it occurs between 4.5 and 5.8 days, with an average of 5.1 days, and 97.5% of those infected develop symptoms within a period of 11.5 days after the date of exposure to the virus [44–47]. These data are important for mathematical models, since the statistical distribution of the transition from one stage of the disease to another can significantly affect the dynamics of its temporal evolution (see chapter 4).

This is also important to determine the duration of quarantine to avoid transmitting the infection to other people. From these calculations, experts have recommended a quarantine period of 14 days. Although countries like Spain and Germany have proposed to reduce it to 10 and 5 days, respectively [48].

It is understandable, then, that the probability function of the incubation period is a sigmoid function, which starts from the value 0 at time zero, and grows asymptotically to the value of probability 1, with curvature increments between days 2-3 and 11-12, and with an inflection point between days 5-6 [49].

2.2.2 Latency

It is the period from the moment the pathogen is acquired, until the person becomes contagious. In several epidemiological observations, it has been shown that the mean serial interval for COVID-19 is less than the incubation period (see Chapter 4).

On the basis of these observations, and the analysis of cases detected in contact studies, it could be concluded that the transmission of the infection began 1 to 2 days (possibly up to 3) before the onset of symptoms [50, 51]; that is, for COVID-19, the latency period is strictly contained in the incubation period. This fact is relevant for the dynamics of the epidemic, and therefore for modeling.

People who are infectious before symptoms develop are called presymptomatic. The existence of presymptomatic patients in COVID-19, coupled with the fact that the peak of the viral load of this disease occurs a few days after the onset of symptoms, marks a fundamental difference between COVID-19 and SARS or MERS, for which the peak of infectivity occurred many days after the first symptoms (between 10 and 14 days for SARS and 7 to 10 days for MERS, from the onset of symptoms) [52]. This explains why the transmission of these two diseases could be contained effectively, through the immediate location and isolation of the people who showed symptoms. And it also explains why it is so difficult to contain COVID-19, as it expands very quickly in the early stages of infection. Indeed, when it is possible to detect cases that had contact with individuals infected with COVID-19, they have generally already become silent propagators. In this way, the chain of transmission can become so great that it is impossible to stop the contagion only with quarantine measures.

It has been proven that, when there are more than 100 infected in a community, it is practically impossible to trace the chain of infection, and even if those detected are isolated, the transmission cannot be stopped.

2.2.3 Disease Development

If the virus carrier is symptomatic, this period corresponds to the time elapsed from the moment the symptoms begin, until they disappear and the person recovers.

A patient with COVID-19 is considered recovered, when at least 10 days have elapsed from the onset of symptoms and, after 24 hours without fever and without using medications, a noticeable improvement is observed [44].

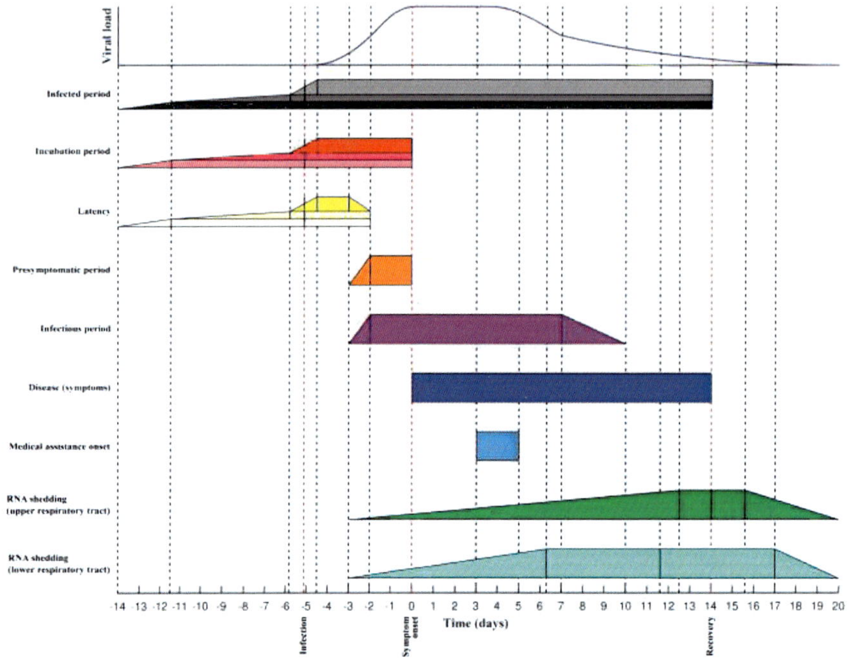

Figure 2: Time schedule showing the different states of a mild symptomatic case of COVID-19, according to data in the literature (see the text and references therein). Note that time zero refers to the symptom onset, which is the main time guide. Skew lines represent the underlying probability distributions and mark some guiding values (for more details, see the text). The viral load curve is merely orientative. RNA shedding could persist until 83 and 59 days, and it is related to PCR testing, according to Cevik et al. [52]

However, there are infected people who never have symptoms, or suffer from very mild symptoms during the entire period of their disease. These people are called asymptomatic. The rest of those infected, at the end of their incubation period, are called symptomatic and are classified as mild, moderate, severe, and critical, according to the intensity and nature of their symptoms.

The set of presymptomatic, asymptomatic, and mildly symptomatic, known by the acronym PAMS, are often called silent propagators. They play a decisive role in the COVID-19 spread process, since they usually are a not detected source of virus transmission, as they do not show symptoms that warn of their infectious condition [53–56]. The role of the infected among PAMS class becomes even more evident since, as confirmed in [41], more than a third of patients with very high viral loads, that is, superspreaders, belong to this class. In Wuhan, China, 86% of infected individuals were found to be mildly symptomatic or asymptomatic prior to travel restrictions, and 79% of infections of severe symptomatic cases were due to them [57].

The rest of those infected with high viral load and, therefore, superspreaders, are patients in serious and critical condition who, in general, are hospitalized until their recovery or death, and therefore do not pose a great infectious threat (except for the health personnel who treat them).

According to the WHO, the following characterization of the four symptomatic categories of COVID-19 disease is given (see [58]):

- The disease is "mild" when the patient meets the COVID-19 case definition, but does not present with pneumonia or hypoxia. These patients do not require hospitalization and must be treated in isolation.

- The disease is "moderate" when the patient has clinical signs of mild pneumonia. The cases of adolescents or adults and children are distinguished, taking into consideration other additional clinical signs. Moderate patients may not require hospitalization, but should be treated in isolation.

- The disease is "serious" when pneumonia shows signs of severity, differentiating adolescents or adults from children by the appearance of other additional symptoms. These patients require the inclusion of oxygen therapy in their treatment.

- The disease is considered "critical" when acute respiratory distress syndrome appears, which occurs in the week following the detection of pneumonia, resulting in poor oxygenation of the patients. Acute and life-threatening complications can appear, giving rise to different variants of critical illness, among which are acute organ dysfunction (septicemia), septic shock, and acute thrombosis. Critical patients require assisted ventilation, which may be noninvasive, but in extreme cases endotracheal intubation with implementation of mechanical ventilation may be required.

According to [3] (and the references therein), the average time from the onset of symptoms to recovery from COVID-19 disease is a maximum of 2 weeks, when the disease has been mild or moderate and, 3 to 6 weeks, when it has been serious or critical. People who develop severe symptoms of the disease require hospitalization within an average of 1 week from the onset of symptoms. Those who reach the critical phase are generally seriously ill patients who present with acute respiratory distress syndrome on the eighth day after the onset of symptoms. Respiratory distress can be overcome or persist and worsen, in which case the seriously ill patient must be referred to assisted ventilation, which corresponds to the critical state of the disease. This generally occurs, in the case of hospitalized patients, during the second week after the onset of symptoms; that is, the week after being hospitalized for having contracted the severe form of the disease. Finally, critically ill patients who cannot recover, die as a result of the disease in a period of 2 to 8 weeks from the onset of symptoms.

It is very difficult to compute the percentage of seriously ill patients who become critical, nor the percentage of critically ill patients who die, nor the total time spent by COVID-19 patients in hospitals, figures that are essential to understand the dynamics of the population of hospitalized patients (intra-hospital dynamics). This is so since generally patients who pass the critical phase of the disease, require a recovery time in the hospital, which is unpredictable, before being discharged. These percentages depend on the preexisting comorbidities in patients admitted to the hospital, the availability of resources in the hospitals, and the effectiveness of the treatments applied. They also depend on the properties of new variants of the virus, which in some cases are more contagious, more resistant to treatment, and/or more lethal. The improvement in the treatments and the increasing understanding of the complications, which can occur throughout the evolution of the disease, have a significant impact on the reduction of the transition percentages from severe to critical, and from critical to deceased.

It is estimated that asymptomatic patients represent between 30% and 70% of all infected (although in the case of infected children they can reach up to 95% of the total). It is also estimated that, of 100% of symptomatic people with COVID-19 at any time, around 70-80% of them suffer from the disease in a mild or moderate way (including patients with mild pneumonia), from 14% to 25% suffer from the severe form of the disease, and from 4% to 5% the critical form [59, 60]. See Fig. 3.

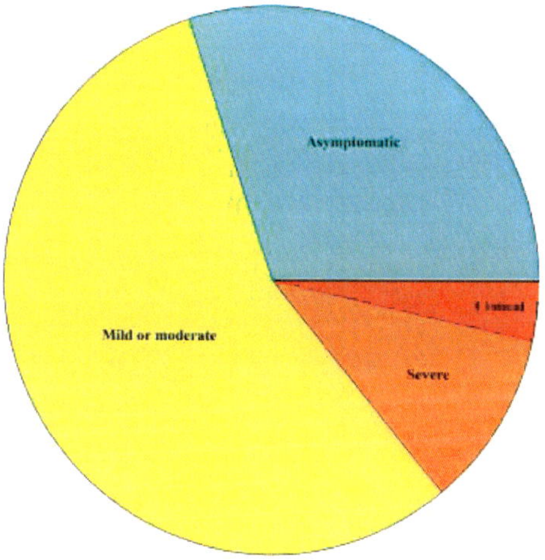

Figure 3: Estimated rounded percentages of asymptomatics (30% in the graphic), mild or moderate cases (56%, 80% of symptomatic cases in the graphic), severe cases (10.5%, 15% of symptomatic cases in the graphic), and critical cases (3.5%, 5% of symptomatic cases in the graphic)

Although at the beginning of the pandemic up to 80% of critically ill patients died, this percentage, as well as the average length of stay of patients in hospitals, was gradually reduced in many countries, until new virus variants began to appear; in particular, the Delta variant, which again increased the incidence, mortality, and hospital demand rates.

There are people who report renewed or recurring symptoms for weeks or months, even after being discharged from the hospital, and show symptoms and signs related to COVID-19 sequelae.

This has been called persistent COVID-19 or Long COVID [3], and may be a cause of death even after negative results for virus tests.

Summing up, patients may die due to the direct consequences of the critical period of the disease, or as a result of persistent COVID-19.

Unfortunately, not all those who suffer a critical form of the disease have access to hospitals, either because there is no hospital infrastructure in their places of residence, or because it is saturated. These cases of serious or critical infections, not detected by the health system, contribute a large number of deaths that are generally not registered in the statistics. This affects the forecasts that can be made from the analysis of data and mathematical models, and their usefulness for decision-making. It is also clear that the percentage of cases in this situation is difficult to estimate and may vary temporarily, especially in the case of saturation of health systems.

2.2.4 Infectiveness

It corresponds to the period during which the infected person can transmit the virus and infect others. The risk of transmission by an infected person is positively correlated with the viral load.

The time window for virus transmission is the result of adding the period of silent contagion to the time patients already experience the symptoms of the disease. During the presymptomatic period, people continue to carry out their usual social activities, without seeking medical attention. In addition, the longer it takes an infected person to receive medical care, the more likely it is that they will develop a severe or critical form of the disease and require hospital care.

For people with mild or moderate disease, the contagious period begins 1 to 3 days before the onset of symptoms and can last 7 to 10 days more, which is precisely the period in which symptoms develop, which depends on the intensity of their viral load [44]. Since the recovery period of these patients is almost 2 weeks after the onset of symptoms, it turns out that in the last days of recovery the sick person is no longer contagious, whether or not they have symptoms. This makes a fundamental difference with other viruses that continue to spread long after the symptoms of the infected person disappear, but, in that case, the recovered person knows that they must stay away from other healthy people for a certain time to avoid contagion. What's more, in general, persons with COVID-19 look for medical assistance and start their treatment between days 3-5 after symptom onset, when 5-7 days have passed in which they have potentially been transmitting the disease without knowing it.

The SARS-CoV-2 virus behaves like the influenza virus, which is characterized by increasing its infectivity around, or even before, the onset of symptoms.

Some persons have suggested three fundamental differences between symptomatic and asymptomatic with respect to their viral load:

- *In PCR tests, asymptomatic patients and, in general, PAMS, are detected, on average, 5.1 days after the maximum viral load, while to detect symptomatic patients, an average of 2.4 more days are required [40].*
- *Asymptomatic patients have a significantly longer duration of viral shedding than symptomatic patients [61].*
- *Asymptomatic individuals have a weaker immune response to SARS-CoV-2 infection than symptomatic individuals [61].*

Next, we deal with the detection of the virus in the body. "Serology" is the study of antibodies in the blood serum. "Antibodies" are part of the body's immune response to infection. Antibodies that act against SARS-CoV-2 can generally be detected in the first weeks of infection. The presence of antibodies indicates that the person was infected with SARS-CoV-2, regardless of whether they had severe or mild illness, or did not have any symptoms.

"Seroprevalence studies" are performed to estimate the magnitude of an outbreak or the extent of infection in a given population group. Using "serological tests", it is possible to detect the presence of antibodies against a given virus and calculate the amount of antibodies produced after infection, which makes it possible to determine whether a person was previously infected with

SARS-CoV-2. Furthermore, they make it possible to differentiate between new infections that occur through community transmission and those that may be occurring within households [62].

The initial seroprevalence of any new virus in a population is assumed to be low or nonexistent, since the virus has not previously circulated. In the case of SARS-CoV-2, there is almost no information on seroprevalence in the population, and therefore it is not easy to make more realistic estimates of the proportion of asymptomatic patients.

The test consists of a rapid determination of antibodies in the blood by immunochromatography, which is obtained from a finger prick, and which provides information to know if the person has been infected. This can be done at home or in a health center, depending on the evolution of the epidemic and the circumstances of each family. To ensure the reliability of the results and apply the maximum methodological rigor, it is highly recommended to obtain a serum sample from all patients who give their consent with the same technique that is routinely used to perform blood tests (venipuncture, that is, a puncture arm), and are analyzed using a more sophisticated and accurate serological technique than rapid tests. There are many tests that can be done, for example, IgM which shows whether there is blood infection, or IgG which shows if there was an infection, but does not identify the presence of the virus. When IgM concentration is low, it is mandatory to do a PCR [63].

When a new disease such as COVID-19 appears, initial surveillance and detection strategies focus primarily on molecular testing to measure acute infections, and the care of patients with severe disease, who are the ones seeking and in need of health care. This can often miss mild or asymptomatic infections, which do not require medical attention, and therefore the full extent of the infection is unknown in the early phase of an outbreak. In this context, seroprevalence studies offer a more complete picture of how this population has been infected with SARS-CoV-2 and allow the detection of unknown cases that were not identified by systematic or active surveillance.

On the other hand, "molecular tests", including polymerase chain reaction (PCR) tests, allow for the detection of the genetic material to determine if the person is currently infected with that virus. Serologic tests should not be used to diagnose acute SARS-CoV-2 infection, since antibodies appear a few weeks after infection [64, 65].

PCR tests are capable of detecting the virus in the body since the first day that the infected person is contagious, which occurs approximately the third day after infection, while rapid antigen tests are reliable since the beginning of the symptoms. If a person takes either of the two tests before the indicated period, the result is likely to be a false negative. On the contrary, after 14 days of infection, the test may be positive, because it detects fragments of the virus in the body, but the person is no longer infectious and we would be in the presence of a false positive.

Through contact tracing studies and simulations, it has been possible to determine that the peak of the viral load in infected people and, therefore, the maximum level of contagiousness, occurs in the first 5 days after the onset of symptoms [43, 66].

Hence, the importance of identifying people who may have been in a contagious area, and being able to carry out the PCR test 48 hours after the event has occurred.

In this way, the infected persons who must be kept isolated are identified, thus being able to determine who are asymptomatic. Asymptomatic patients are kept in isolation for 10 days, from the moment of detection of infection, and symptomatic patients up to 14 days.

In turn, when a person begins to manifest symptoms, it is not necessary to carry out a screening test, but it is enough to remain isolated for 10 days under observation until it is no longer contagious, or has a complication that requires hospital care. In general, asymptomatic patients do not present complications.

These recommendations, however, do not apply to people with more severe symptoms of COVID-19, or to those who are immunosuppressed, even if they have recovered from the disease. Indeed, it is estimated that this type of person can be contagious up to more than 20 days after the symptoms of the disease appear [3].

A remarkable result in [54] is the estimate that at least 50% of new SARS-CoV-2 infections are caused by asymptomatic and presymptomatic patients.

To obtain this result, an analytical model was used, in which it was assumed that the maximum infectivity occurred in the median of the onset of symptoms, and that 30% of infected people were asymptomatic, and 75% as infectious as symptomatic ones. Under these assumptions, the model resulted in the asymptomatic representing approximately 24% of all transmission and the presymptomatic 35%. By varying these assumptions over a wide range of values, it could be estimated that more than 50% of infections are produced by silent contagiers [54].

In general, although vaccination does not completely prevent infection and/or transmission, it does significantly reduce the amount of virus that an infected person can shed through the nose or mouth, and it shortens the time it takes to eliminate the virus. Consequently, vaccination reduces the risk of infecting others and of suffering from a severe form of the disease.

However, if a vaccinated person is infected with a new, more infectious and lethal variant of the virus, such as the Delta variant, although reinfection is unlikely, they could manifest the disease more severely, and have a greater probability to infect other people with these new variants. This means that vaccines will probably take longer to reduce transmission and promote herd immunity than if these new variants had never emerged [67].

2.2.5 Natural Immunity, Immunity Caused by Vaccines, and Reinfection

Immunity to any viral disease is a process that occurs as a result of recovery from infection, or as a consequence of the application of a vaccine against the disease.

During this process, the immune system produces different types of molecules and cells, including antibodies, B cells, and T cells of the CD4+ and CD8+ types, which are the main components of the body's innate and adaptive immune responses, and which contribute to the protection of people against disease and reinfection. For more information see Chapter 9.

Knowledge about the magnitude, quality, and durability of immune responses, natural or mediated by vaccines, against SARS-CoV-2, determines the epidemiological dynamics of COVID-19, and allows defining more efficient strategies for the protection of the population, including vaccination campaigns.

The study by Dan et al [68] concluded that approximately 95% of the people who have been infected, retain their immunological memory to SARS-CoV-2 for a minimum of 6 months, and in some cases, up to 8-12 months, after recovery from infection. The time of immunity increases if the person who gets sick is vaccinated after they have recovered. It is estimated that the period of immunity for a person who has been vaccinated without having previously contracted the disease is at least of the same order of 6 months as in the case of people recovered from the infection. It still takes time to know for sure if some vaccines can offer longer protection. During the period of immunity, reinfection is unlikely, at least with the same variant of the virus.

On the other hand, the higher the viral load in infected people, the greater the stimulus to the immune system to produce an immune response, and the greater the amount of antibodies that is produced. That is why the asymptomatic or those who have had a mild form of the disease, produce fewer antibodies and are more likely to be reinfected than those who have suffered from a severe variant of the disease.

Although some cases of reinfection have been described, studies to date show that the immune responses, natural or elicited by the vaccine, that have been generated after the first infection, can be long-lasting, and successfully protect the majority of patients from subsequent infections, generating T and B cells that reach a stable plateau after six months [69, 70].

It has been observed that, in the few cases of reinfections studied, both in people recovered from the first infection and in vaccinated people, the disease has been milder, because they already have an immune response memory.

However, one of the concerns raised by specialists is the duration of the immune responses (natural or caused by the vaccine) to the new variants of SARS-CoV-2 identified. The answer to this question will be key to the management of the pandemic, since it will determine the true level of herd immunity required and the need or not for revaccination [69].

2.3 Temporal Evolution of the COVID-19 Pandemic at the Country Level and at the Global Level; the Role of Human Mobility

With regard to epidemics, there is no single classification of the chronological phases of their evolution. The classifications made for COVID-19 include between 4 and 6 phases and the difference lies in whether or not some periods are integrated under the same concept. To conceptualize this evolution, we have preferred to consider 6 chronological phases for COVID-19, which are described below. There is no a priori linear sequence that indicates the duration of each phase or clear-cut limits of its beginning and end. Other classifications have been proposed in different countries. For example, in Spain, at the beginning of May 2020, after 50 days of strict confinement, four phases (0, 1, 2, and 3) were proposed, which would follow one another gradually and asymmetrically in each territory, presumably reaching "the new normality" - at the end of June 2020 [71]. The reality turned out to be quite different.

As an example and without much detail, we will report some measures that have been taken in some countries, in the periods corresponding to the respective phases, mainly in Mexico and Spain.

2.3.1 Phase 1: Import

It is characterized in each country by the arrival of positive cases imported from other countries, producing second-generation transmission and family outbreaks of dozens of cases. In Mexico, the first phase began on February 28, 2020, a day after the first case of a man who arrived infected from Italy was detected, and was not immediately detected by health authorities. The first patient registered in Spain with COVID-19 was German, detected on January 31, 2020. Nine days later, another case of COVID-19 was detected in Palma and it was not until February 24 when the virus jumped to the peninsula, where the first cases were reported in the Community of Madrid, Catalonia, and the Valencian Community. This date can be considered as the beginning of Phase 1 in Spain [72].

2.3.2 *Phase 2: Community Dispersion*

In this phase, third-generation and higher transmission already appears. It is characterized by community outbreaks, with hundreds of reported or estimated cases. For this reason, regulations are being established through measures to control or mitigate the epidemic, fundamentally aimed at reducing the number of infections. On the one hand, there are hygiene or sanitary measures, whose objective is to reduce the presence of viruses in the environment that can cause contagion, hindering their arrival at the recipient. Among them, the recommendation of frequent hand washing or not touching the face, the disinfection of objects before handling them and places of public access, or the use of masks, gloves, and glasses or other protective devices.

An effective measure at this stage is the detection of cases and the tracing and confinement of contacts. In the case of COVID-19, when there are more than 100 detected cases, it becomes impossible to trace the chain of infection, and only people can be isolated and massive activities avoided, but the transmission cannot be contained. In Mexico, this phase was declared on March 24, 2020. In Spain, there was an uncontrolled growth of cases as of March 8, 2020, progressing very quickly in community dispersal. This motivated that, by March 9, 2020, the Ministry of Health had to decree a level of reinforced containment to try to contain the epidemic, which marked the beginning of a 50-day of strict confinement.

2.3.3 *Phase 3: Epidemic Spread*

It is characterized by regional outbreaks and nationwide spread of the disease, with tens of thousands of cases recorded. According to the World Health Organization (WHO), phase 3 occurs when the disease is present in most of the national territories, and a large part of the infections are community-based. For this reason, at this stage, confinement is vital, and it is necessary to increase the distancing measures. The aim is to reduce as much as possible the contact between people that can lead to new infections [71].

In this group of measures, we can cite quarantine, home isolation, restriction of mobility (between countries or regions), maintaining interpersonal distance, limiting meetings, activities, and social events in public and private spaces (demonstrations, activities of leisure, festivities, family gatherings, etc.) and the temporary interruption of nonessential activities, including some work activities, among others.

However, in many countries much stricter isolation measures have been required, such as curfews, suspension of economic and cultural work and school activities, closing of establishments and shops, suspension of public events, mainly in closed places, and restriction of all activities that are not essential, prohibiting people from leaving their homes (home confinement).

In Spain [71, 72], this stage of more strict confinement began in March, while in Mexico, it began on April 21, 2020 [73], and was extended until May 30, 2020, although it was impossible to predict its duration. An important regulation was established as of March 23, 2020, in which the National Healthy Distance Day was declared, which lasted 70 days, culminating on May 30, 2020. On May 20, 2020, the Gradual Plan towards the New Normality in Mexico City was established, which included epidemiological traffic lights and its operating rules [74].

Immediately after concluding the National Day of Healthy Distance in Mexico, on June 2, 2020, CONAGO (National Confederation of Governors) and SEGOB (Ministry of the Interior), agreed the rules of operation of the Epidemiological Risk Traffic Light extended to all country, which were published on June 7, 2020 [75]. The Epidemiological Risk Traffic Light to move towards a new normality was created as a monitoring system to regulate the use of public space, according to the risk of contagion by COVID-19.

In phase 3, the proper organization and availability of hospital care is essential, since, in this phase, the main risk is the saturation of the hospitals. For this reason, studies on how to plan their occupation and mitigation measures to avoid the massive entry of people, were so important. In Mexico, there were at that time an average of 687 COVID hospitals, with around 14,368 beds available for serious cases.

During phase 3 in Spain, the massive confinement and the state of alarm played a determining role. The measures that were taken were summarized in two large groups: those of the dance phase, which consists of the application and relaxation of the measures to maintain the reproductive number R_t oscillating around 1 (note that it would be impossible to keep it always less than 1, since that would imply having the entire population locked up almost permanently, with severe consequences of a different nature), and those of the hammer phase, where the objective is to flatten the contagion curve when it grows too large.

2.3.4 Phase 4: Exit of the First Outbreak (Wave) and Start of the Second and Subsequent Waves

It generally began to appear 3 to 9 months after the third phase ended, mainly due to the fact that imported cases appeared again, reinforcing the epidemic that had not yet concluded. In this phase, international agreements are required to stop the spread.

During this stage, vaccination campaigns are already in place, but the efficacy shown by the vaccines and the appearance of new variants of SARS-CoV-2, has made many specialists think about the possibility of reaching a chronic endemic state, and it is not possible to definitively predict the disappearance of the disease. At present, Asia is caught between a third and fourth wave of COVID-19, the fourth and fifth waves are spreading across Europe, the United States is on the verge of a fourth wave, and a third wave is expanding across Latin America, which has already arrived in Mexico.

2.3.5 Phase 5: Recovery

To reach this hypothetical phase, which we have not yet reached, it is necessary to give a global response to the possible appearance of a state of emergency, with the objective, according to the WHO, of coordinating multisectoral resources, to mitigate social and economic repercussions, as well as to assess the need for external assistance to meet the humanitarian needs of some countries [76–78].

In this case, the fundamental study of the models should be aimed at proposing measures that allow, at least, to guarantee the stabilization of the endemic state, and that a critical situation is not generated again, simultaneously proposing measures aimed at economic recovery.

2.3.6 Phase 6: End of the Epidemic

Currently, it is impossible to predict the arrival of this phase, which must be decreed by the supranational organizations such as the World Health Organization (WHO) or the Pan American Health Organization (PAHO), when in the vast majority of countries the contagion situation has been controlled.

A great difficulty that must be overcome in this phase is the fact that, apart from these organizations, fundamental decisions of a health or political nature are usually made at the national level, and to a lesser extent regional, by the governments of different countries and regions, and by the agencies to which they delegate. This is basically due to the fact that the population of each country and region has its own peculiarities and, for that reason, the development of the COVID-19 epidemic is generally quite different in each of these spatial units, fundamentally delimited by political and administrative divisions. However, the abyss marked by political and cultural divisions, and social and economic inequalities between countries, must also be considered. Chapter 7 deals with this topic.

2.4 Collateral Consequences for Human Health, Society and the Economy; Final Comments

In addition to all above, it is relevant to analyze the consequences of the pandemic, beyond the direct effects of the disease (see Chapter 7). These consequences are very varied and include very diverse aspects, starting with the fact that the sequelae derived from COVID-19 for human health, known as persistent COVID-19 or Long COVID, are not yet fully known.

It is important to highlight the economic impact of the pandemic. At the macroeconomic level, the national economies of practically all countries of the world have suffered severely, due to the reduction of activities. There are also effects at the microeconomic level, due to the closure of thousands of companies and the loss of millions of jobs, which has substantially impacted the family economy worldwide, especially in the most vulnerable and low-income segments of the population. This has undoubtedly accentuated social inequality, which, in turn, has hardened the effects of the pandemic in the most economically affected sectors of the population.

The academic lag that has occurred due to the total or partial closure of colleges and universities is evident, and will possibly have negative effects on the training of students, with differences among socio-economic strata to the detriment of the poorest.

From the point of view of the social impact of the pandemic, it is also necessary to consider the impact (pending analysis) that social distancing and isolation measures have caused in other important aspects, such as mental health and psychological effects in the community. These decisions can be traumatic for the population, both in infected and uninfected individuals, leading to consequences that are impossible to predict. Furthermore, this leads to an inevitable alteration of human behavior, which, in turn, affects the possibility of controlling the epidemic.

On a social scale, the variability of human behavior and population heterogeneity significantly influence the socio-economic activity carried out by different population groups, and the vulnerability to disease, according to age groups, sex, pregnancy in women, and preexisting comorbidities in the population (see Chapter 6).

Facing these difficulties, still immersed in a pandemic that does not end, represents a challenge for all humanity, since eradicating an infectious disease is not an easy task, and it can be an unattainable goal, at least in the medium term. In particular, it represents a great challenge for decision makers, a task in which science plays a decisive role.

To date, the WHO has declared only two viral diseases officially eradicated, smallpox and rinderpest. In particular, smallpox has been one of the deadliest diseases known to humans, and it is also the only disease that has been eradicated with vaccination, although some outbreaks have occurred in recent years. Suffice to mention that smallpox caused more than 300 million deaths in the 20th century, until its eradication in the 1980s. In terms of geographic distribution and scope, it is comparable to the current COVID-19.

In the case of smallpox, the vaccine cut the transmission of the virus, which was the key factor in its eradication. However, the COVID-19 vaccines developed so far are not capable of preventing the infection, but only of attenuating it and making the disease less serious, but vaccinated people can still transmit the virus. This is why many experts believe that COVID-19 will become an endemic disease, which has been supported by some mathematical models. This means that it will continue to circulate for the next few years, within certain ranges of infected people in groups of the world population.

This is not surprising since, as is known, influenza viruses and the four coronaviruses that cause common colds are endemic. The WHO estimates that each year between 290,000 and 650,000 people die worldwide from the flu and its consequences. However, influenza and common colds are manageable, and their symptoms can be treated with quite effective drugs, the vaccine does not require refrigeration, and the effects are observed immediately.

Many scientists and some governments hoped at some point that the same could be achieved with COVID-19, and for this reason they came to propose that the objective should be to learn to live with the disease, and not fight against it, since they ensured that the virus would remain, although people would develop some immunity through vaccination and natural infections. Consequently, there would be fewer severe cases and far fewer hospitalizations and deaths due to the disease.

However, it must be taken into account that viruses constantly mutate as part of their evolutionary process, becoming resistant to treatments and vaccines, and thus being able to continue spreading. Such is the case with the influenza virus, which makes it necessary to review the composition of influenza vaccines annually, while other diseases such as tetanus require periodic booster shots.

In the case of SARS-CoV-2, statistics have shown that vaccination has been effective against the Delta variant. For example, in Spain, despite the presence of the Delta variant and the growing increase in infections, only 5% of those infected had both doses of the vaccine, and another 83%

of those infected were unvaccinated, or had only received one dose.

The insufficient application of complete vaccination systems and the presence of new variants of the virus, have forced several countries to reintroduce travel and circulation restrictions, due to the increase in the rates of infections and hospitalizations, with consequent social and economic repercussions, including rising unemployment. This means that governments are faced with the dilemma of carrying out confinements and closing their borders, with their usual economic consequences, given the need to protect their population from the virus.

There has been a poorly coordinated global effort, given the international situation of unequal distribution of vaccines. The European Union (EU) has advanced in this regard, having implemented the COVID Digital Certificate, currently recognized by the 27 members of the EU, as well as by Iceland, Norway, and Switzerland. This distinction allows citizens and residents to move within the continental bloc, without being subject to restrictions, if they have been vaccinated, have a valid negative test, or have recently recovered from the disease.

The need to achieve an equitable distribution of the vaccine, which favors developing countries, is not the only a humanitarian issue, because millions of people vulnerable to the virus are being abandoned to their fate. It is also a way to reduce the likelihood that new variants of the virus will emerge. On June 30, 2021, in an open letter, the heads of the WHO, the International Monetary Fund (IMF), the World Bank, and the World Trade Organization (WTO), have warned of this danger [79].

Until July 5, 2021, only a little more than 1 billion people have been vaccinated with the complete schedule worldwide, which represents less than 15% of the world population, a figure still very far from what is desirable to reach worldwide group immunity. Within this framework, there is an open debate on the suspension of patents on vaccines, or some other alternative options, as effective measures to accelerate the vaccination process worldwide [80–85].

During the most recent G7 summit, held in England on June 11-13, 2021, the leaders of the world's seven largest advanced economies (Canada, France, Germany, Italy, Japan, the United Kingdom, and the United States) discussed two big topics: global warming and the COVID-19 pandemic. One of the summit agreements was the commitment to send 1 billion doses of vaccines to developing countries. However, below the estimated 11 billion doses that WHO considers necessary to meet the needs of the world's poorest population [86, 87] and to have an equitable distribution of vaccines in the world. If the virus continues to circulate in the near future, which seems to be the most likely scenario, access to vaccines will be a sine que non condition to expand the required immunity globally.

3 MATHEMATICAL AND COMPUTATIONAL MODELING OF COVID-19: RESULTS AND PERSPECTIVES

The mathematical modeling of the dynamics of infectious diseases has a rich history, dating back to over 100 years and encompassing a wide variety of methods, which are not necessarily comparable nor were they designed for the same purpose. Their assumptions and limitations are also different, and must be taken into account, in order to avoid erroneous conclusions that detract from the reliability and correctness of mathematical models.

In what follows, we will analyze the field of applicability of mathematical models in epidemiology and will present some of the most important results they have yielded for the study of the propagation dynamics of COVID-19. We will include several subsections, presenting the methodology for the construction and analysis of mathematical models of infectious diseases and the process of drawing conclusions. We will end with a brief discussion of some problems, mainly of a conceptual nature, related to the study of models.

3.1 Main Characteristics of Forecasting and Compartmental Models and the Basic Assumptions that Support Them

Modeling studies of COVID-19, like other infectious diseases, generally follows one of the two approaches which we will refer to as forecasting models and compartmental models. Although there are hybrid approaches (see [88] where compartmental models are combined with machine learning) and other computational approaches such as cellular automata [89] and agents [90], and complex network models [91, 92], which we do not discuss in this chapter, the two basic models mentioned address different issues, relative to an epidemic, on different scales of time, deal differently with uncertainty, and are vastly comprehensive.

Forecasting models are often statistical in nature. They fit a certain curve to a time series of data and then use its analytical expression to extrapolate the behavior pattern of the data to the near future, ignoring the dynamics of the process that produces the pattern.

Normally they use cumulative data, start from an initial value, and evolve as time passes, towards an asymptotic value, limited by the size of the population. This sigmoidal behavior, which is logistic, is simulated by a Gompertz-type curve, the simplest expression of which depends on two or more real parameters given by the number of inflection points to be identified. The parameters are based on the fit to the data. In this way, accumulated epidemiological data on active infected persons, hospital admissions, deaths, etc. are used, either from the near past or from different settings, but with similar characteristics to that of the study area. Using analytical tools such as machine learning and regression, reasonable short-term forecasts are made.

Most prognostic models can barely make projections not much more than a week in advance. In [93], a video is available on the application of statistical and simulation models to predict healthcare resources in Spanish hospitals during the pandemic.

A controversial example of the application of forecasting models was the original version of a model from the Institute for Health Metrics and Evaluation (IHME), which extrapolated the shape of the epidemic curve of outbreaks in China and Italy, to fit data from other places where the epidemic was just beginning, with the purpose of making projections of its evolution.

On the other hand, compartmental epidemic models can be used to describe the spread of infectious diseases and to forecast or simulate future scenarios under various assumptions about the parameters that govern the transmission and evolution of the disease, as well as about the immunity that is generated in recovered people.

The most commonly used compartmental models are the SIR (Susceptible-Infected-Removed) models, which are a simplified version of the general Kermack-McKendrick model, proposed in his famous works [13, 14] since 1927 and the extension to SEIR models (Susceptible-Exposed-Infected-Removed) of Heathcote [94] in 2000, which considers the incubation period of some infectious diseases, during which, as in the case of COVID-19, infected people may be transmitting the disease before showing symptoms of it.

These models can be considered in a deterministic or stochastic way. Deterministic models, which are no more than limit mean-field models corresponding to stochastic models, assume that the factors involved in the epidemic process can be controlled and that their results can be accurately predicted in an explicit and generally numerical way.

Stochastic models consider the impossibility of controlling the factors that intervene in the epidemic process, which can be as unpredictable as human behavior, and the results are expressed only in terms of a probability distribution.

The classical SIR or SEIR-type models do not consider the possibility of reinfection or many other factors that determine the behavior of each particular epidemic.

A description of some fundamental results that follow from these models and some of their simpler variants can be found, in addition to the original sources, in Chapter 4, and a global discussion on infectious disease modeling can be found in several comprehensive texts on the subject [95–104].

The elegance and simplicity of the classic models suggest that they can be easily adapted to real situations, simply by adding new compartments obtained by disaggregating the states of the basic SIR or SEIR schemes, to reflect certain specific characteristics of an epidemiological problem. This apparent simplicity generally masks subtle, but very important and complex situations, related to the structure, parameterization, and practical applicability of "realistic models" that can hardly be discussed within the framework of the aforementioned texts.

In realistic compartmental models, the infection process of susceptible individuals is usually modeled using the concept of **Infection Force**, which is expressed as a function of the different categories of infected individuals that can be found in a population and that represent the sources of infection of its susceptible people. It is assumed that, at each instant of time, the number of new infected individuals is directly proportional to the number of contacts between susceptible individuals and individuals of the different categories already infected (also considered infectious) and inversely proportional to the total number of individuals that interact with each other.

In addition, it is considered that the total population is homogeneously mixed, so that the hypotheses of the **Law of Mass Action** are satisfied, to represent the contacts between susceptible and infected as a product of the total number of susceptible individuals and the force of infection.

The constants of proportionality that appear in the expression of the infection force are usually interpreted as instantaneous per capita infection rates, which in some way measure the capacity of an infected individual of a certain class to infect other susceptible individuals, per unit of time.

On the other hand, SIR models also assume the existence of transition rates between different compartments of the model. These rates are defined as the quotient between the fraction of individuals from one compartment that move to another (for example, from infected to recovered, or from infected to deceased), divided by the mean transition time. This assumption is possible only when the probability distribution of the random variable corresponding to the transition time is an exponential function $F(t)$ of the form:

$$F(t) = Prob(\text{transition time} \leq t) = \begin{cases} 1 - e^{-\mu t} & \text{for } t \geq 0\,, \\ 0 & \text{otherwise}\,. \end{cases}$$

There are other magnitudes related to infection rates such as the **Reproductive Number (Basic and Effective)** [105] and **Intervals (Generational and Serial)** [106–108] of the disease, for which there are methodologies for calculation established from epidemiological evolution data. Furthermore, it is also possible to obtain transition rates directly from the “processing” of certain epidemiological data without using the models. When this is done, there is a risk that, when the model is subsequently completed with the epidemiological parameters obtained, it will not reproduce the data that were used to get the parameters.

A summary of the importance of obtaining the distribution of the generational and serial intervals, as well as other distributions related to residence times, which are necessary for the study of transition rates, is presented in Section 3 of chapter 4.

That is why an important step to make predictions from the data is the process of building an "adequate" compartmental model to study the epidemiological situation of interest. On many occasions, this modeling process is "predetermined" to a certain extent due to the number of parameters that can be obtained from the available data. It is common to state that "a more complex model would be more appropriate, but there are not enough data to obtain the required parameters". However, it is assumed that the model that is finally proposed, which we will call the "generic model" (because the parameters required to carry out the simulations have yet to be determined), already includes all compartments that are considered necessary for the study, together with their interactions. It also incorporates a generic proposal of the components of the force of infection that can include the effects of human behavior, as well as terms that stand for nonpharmaceutical interventions such as the use of masks, physical distancing and selective quarantine of some social groups, or for pharmaceutical interventions such as vaccines, and some processes inherent to the epidemiological dynamics in question, such as the effect of immunity, reinfection, the appearance of new variants of the virus, etc.

3.2 Renewal Equations: Another Scheme for the Construction of Compartmental Models

Although the modeling scheme of the spread of an infection through generalization of the SIR model has historically proven its usefulness, it is important to bear in mind, as mentioned in Chapter 4, that the two hypotheses, of a homogeneous mixture of the population and of the exponential probability distribution for the transition times between compartments, in general, are not fulfilled.

Another way of introducing compartmental models in epidemiology is through the **renewal equations** that appear in continuous models of population dynamics with age structure (see Chapter 7 of [99]). When applying this compartmental modeling scheme to the study of the dynamics of infectious diseases, a partition of the total population is established in n demographic groups indexed by $k = 1, \ldots, n$, for example, n groups with disjoint age ranges, and the evolution of the **daily incidence** $i_k(t)$ (that is, the number of new infected individuals) is studied, where the population of susceptible individuals is represented by $S_k(t)$, in the k-th demographic group. The functions $S_k(t)$ and $i_k(t)$ are related by the dynamic equation (1.1):

$$S'_k(t) = -i_k(t)\,. \tag{1.1}$$

Note that, in the SIR-type models, the population of **active infected** individuals is considered instead of the daily incidence of infected individuals.

The incidence satisfies the renewal equation

$$i_k(t) = R_t \frac{S_k(t)}{S(t)} \sum_{j=1}^{n} \alpha_{k,j} \int_0^\infty K_{serial}(\tau) i_j(t-\tau)\, d\tau\,, \tag{1.2}$$

where it can be assumed that the function $K_{serial}(t)$ has compact support contained in an interval $[0, T]$, where T is the maximum time that a person can be infectious since the moment they are infected.

In (1.2), R_t is the time-dependent effective reproduction number, $S(t) = \sum_{k=1}^{n} S_k(t)$ is the total susceptible population, $K_{serial}(t)$ is the probability density function of serial intervals, and $(\alpha_{k,j})$ is the matrix of contact rates between the susceptibles in group k and the infected in group j, which is assumed to be constant as is the total N_k of individuals in group k, throughout the entire epidemic.

In general, the system of equations (1.2) is studied with $k = 1, \ldots, n$, expressing the effective reproduction number R_t in terms of the basic reproductive number, a forcing factor $F(t)$ (which may have a seasonal or human behavior origin), a mitigating factor $M(t)$ (which may be due to applied nonpharmaceutical interventions and/or risk perception), and the fraction of the total susceptible population $S(t)/N$ with $N = \sum_{k=1}^{n} N_k$. That is,

$$R_t = R_0\, F(t)\, M(t)\, R\left(\frac{S(t)}{N}\right),$$

where $R(1) = 1$.

In particular, in [109] it is considered that $R(S/N) = S/N$ and, in [110], the forcing and mitigation factors are not taken into account, that is, $F(t) = M(t) \equiv 1$, and the case $S/N \approx 1$ is considered, which is valid when the total population is large and there are not many infected persons and then, by linearizing the effective reproductive number around $1 - S/N$, we obtain

$$R_t \approx R_0 \left(1 - \lambda \left(1 - \frac{S}{N}\right)\right),$$

where the coefficient λ is called the **immunity factor**.

In [56], this modeling scheme is applied in the case in which the total population is divided into two large demographic groups, symptomatic and asymptomatic, with the aim of studying the influence of asymptomatic patients on the spread of COVID-19.

3.3 Methodology for the Application of Compartmental Models of the SIR-Type

Aside from the relevant assumptions associated with SIR-type compartmental epidemiological models, let us analyze the methodology frequently applied in specific epidemiological contexts.

First, it is necessary to determine the properties of the set of parameters (rates), that fit satisfactorily to the data and that will be used to complete the model.

In practice, a great difficulty related to the estimation of the rates are the coefficients unknown a priori in the models that, in fact, keep varying continuously over time due to a series of factors, among which the most salient are the perception of risk by the population [111, 112] and human behavior.

To simplify this complex behavior, it is decided to use estimations, generally constant, of the rates that are obtained directly using data from epidemiological evolution. When models are used to identify the parameters that reproduce the data, the problem of lack of uniqueness arises, that is, there are many sets of parameters that can fit "equally well" to a given set of data, which is nothing more than a consequence of the fact that there are much more data than parameters to calculate. However, it is known that different sets of parameters can alter the predictions of the model as time passes. This makes it necessary to have ways of **quantifying the uncertainty** produced by the data in the predictions of the model, which increases as a function of the intended time of the prediction.

This happens because we want to obtain models with constant transition rates and, at most, usually take into account only infection rates which depend on the temporal variability of the measures of mitigation and human behavior, including the perception of risk.

If the problem of "identification of coefficients" were correctly posed in the appropriate classes of functions whose images are contained in the admissible ranges of rates, this problem would not exist. It is precisely this observation that makes the information provided in Section 2 of this chapter relevant, where we highlight the information on ranges of certain magnitudes associated with the pandemic, which are required to obtain the admissible ranges of rates.

As an example, the following Fig. 4, which refers to the case of Mexico during the period from Mar 2020 to Sep 2021, during which three large waves of the COVID-19 epidemic have occurred, the last one in full development, which are located at intervals of time that coincide with the reckless behavior of the population, during the festive or vacation seasons. In this case, the temporal variability of human behavior is reflected in the temporal variability of the rate of contagion, what produces the oscillating behavior of the curve.

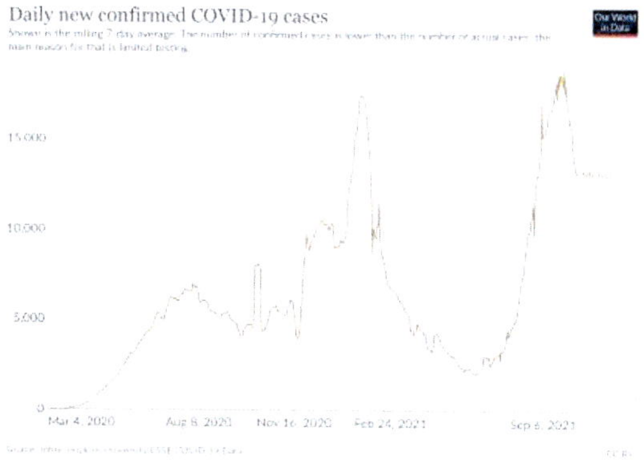

Figure 4: Epidemic curve of new daily confirmed cases in Mexico [113]

It should be noted that there is a variety of theoretical work on SIR models with variable rates, mainly due to the dependence of some epidemics on seasonal variability [114–119].

One way of reducing uncertainty is through the use of Bayesian statistics, since they yield the posterior distribution of the model parameters as a function of their prior distributions and the posterior predictive distributions. All possible epidemic curves compatible with the data can be obtained, thus providing more robust forecasts in probabilistic terms. In some cases in which there are not enough data to obtain the rates, we resort to the use of rates that have been obtained in similar contexts, or consider values that make a reasonably logical sense.

Finally, simulations are carried out with the models to quantify the uncertainty in the predictions and draw conclusions in a practical sense. An example of the application of this methodology can be seen in Mena et al [120].

3.4 What Are Compartmental Epidemiological Models Useful for and What Are Their Limitations?

SIR-type epidemiological models and their generalizations are sufficiently useful to describe the dynamics of transmission in some concrete situations and lead to a qualitatively significant understanding of the disease spreading process.

Despite this, the classic SIR or SEIR models cannot describe the dynamics of an epidemic in the face of a sudden drop in the number of contacts, as occurs during confinement, or in the presence of focal super-dispersion events such as those that occur in bars, parties and family events, where the transmission is much higher than the model can account for.

Something to be expected from the more realistic models is the possibility of making predictions of the size of the disease and its duration, as well as the magnitude and the moment in which the maximum peaks of infected or dead people could be reached. From a decision-making perspective, the prediction of the maximum peaks could warn the health system to prepare for the arrival of the critical stage of the epidemic.

However, all attempts to chronologically visualize the future of the COVID-19 epidemic by means of calculations made with mathematical models, have been very inaccurate. Suffice it to mention the case of the model of Youyang Gu, a data scientist graduated from Massachusetts Institute of Technology (MIT), which has been used by the United States Center for Disease Control and Prevention, which made estimates of the reproductive number for Mexico [121] and predicted a range of 81,256 to 124,386 deaths (in the worst case scenario), culminating in November 2020, reaching the peak of the epidemic on July 25, 2020, with a cumulative total of 1,898,795 confirmed cases and a range between 530,000 and 3 million 165 thousand cases, while the peak of deaths would occur on August 6, 2020, with 1,009 deaths on that day and a range between 285 and 1,685 deaths.

As can be seen, the proposed ranges are too wide, and they include any probable number of confirmed or deceased cases. In fact, if the predicted ranges are compared with the official figures, it turns out that the actual amounts are in the aforementioned ranges, considerably above the predicted values, the peaks are reached on very different dates, and the worst of the predicted scenarios for the deceased has already been doubled by August 2021, even without including the excess of deaths during the pandemic.

Actually, the only thing that can be expected, in terms of long-term forecasts through the use of models, is to show what the course of the epidemic would be like if some assumptions and interventions, which can be reflected in the structure of the model, are strictly fulfilled or vary in a certain range.

For example, when there are no vaccines or effective treatments, only four basic public health policy options remain to control an infectious disease such as COVID-19, which are hygiene and personal protection measures (such as frequent hand washing, use of antibacterial gels and masks and maintaining a healthy distance), effective isolation of symptomatic individuals, the tracing and quarantine of their contacts, and the performance of serological tests for the detection of asymptomatic patients. In this case, the models should reflect the application of these interventions.

In this sense, a good attempt to apply a modeling scheme to monitor the COVID-19 epidemic in

Mexico was carried out by PADeCI (Project for the Analysis of Decisions in Uncertain Contexts), a multidisciplinary group that emerged in the Center for Research and Economic Teaching (CIDE) of Mexico, who created, in collaboration with experts from Stanford University in California-United States, the SC-COSMO model (Stanford-CIDE COronavirus Simulation Model) [122].

This mathematical epidemiological model was set out to measure the effectiveness of different interventions, and was used to project the behavior of the pandemic under the National Day of Healthy Distance Journey (Sana Distancia Day), that was decreed in Mexico in February 2020, and contemplated the different ways in which different demographic groups interact in the population on which projections are to be obtained, considering the socio-cultural patterns of coexistence that directly influence the way in which the number of contagions can be extended.

With the SC-COSMO model, four different scenarios were projected:

1. Without intervention (if there had been no distancing measures).
2. With Sana Distancia Day until May 31.
3. With Sana Distancia Day until June 30.
4. With Sana Distancia Day until August 31.

Finally, in Mexico, only the second option was considered, for which it was predicted that the peak of the epidemiological curve would occur on June 21, with 28,757 new cases confirmed on that day and the total number of confirmed cases accumulated at the end of the projection would be of 680,008. However, official figures show that by June 21, 2020, there were a total of 23,567 active cases and at the end of the projection the total accumulated confirmed cases was only 90,664.

We can conclude that, in addition to randomness, the ignorance of many influencing factors has been so great that it has been impossible to make reliable quantitative predictions, although the qualitative conclusions drawn from these results are essential to design control measures that decision makers can implement. In the case of COVID-19, a fundamental difficulty has been the ignorance of the level of protection of the population and its level of immunity.

From all this, the importance of careful use of the results derived from mathematical models can be deduced, since any alternative action taken on the basis of them could lead to an incorrect interpretation and mismanagement of the disease with disastrous consequences.

For this reason, five questions must be answered before considering the results of the models in decision-making: [123]

1. What is the purpose of the model and what is the time interval of validity of its conclusions? It is important to distinguish between a purely statistical model destined to provide short-term forecasts or a compartmental model of SIR type that allows to investigate future scenarios, since both types of models have different limitations.

2. What are the basic assumptions of the model? For example, what is assumed about immunity and asymptomatic transmission or under what considerations contact rates are included.

3. How is the uncertainty shown and quantified in model projections? In the case of statistical models, it is necessary to verify how confidence intervals are calculated and displayed, and for compartmental models of the SIR-type, which parameters are changing, and whether their range of variation makes sense for the study problem.

4. In case the model parameters are obtained by fitting the model to certain data, it is important to ensure the quality of the data. In general, the models adapted to data on confirmed cases of COVID-19 are not reliable, due to the existence of a large number of undocumented cases. It is more advisable to adjust the model to hospitalization or death data, as long as the reliability of the source of origin is confirmed.

5. Are the results of the model of a general nature or do they reflect a particular context? In the second case, it is important to know the spatial scale (national, regional, or local) for which the results are valid.

Some of the important problems that are investigated with the models are: the effect of vulnerability, the role of different components of the population in the force of infection, due to population heterogeneity, important factors such as age, sex, comorbidities, work activity, socio-economic level, etc., the disease transmission process under confinement conditions (intra-domiciliary, intra-hospital, etc.), and how mitigation and reinforcement measures, along with other pharmaceuticals measures (such as therapeutic treatments and vaccination) influence this process.

Models are used to draw inferences on how to control spread. In the case of COVID-19, most results have been obtained from simulations and from the analysis of an analytical expression of the basic or effective reproductive number in simple models.

We will exemplify this situation in Section 3.6, while, in Section 3.7, we will show that much more can be done through qualitative analysis of the models, and by varying the approach of the methodology for its practical application, based on inverse problems instead of forward problems as has been done so far.

3.5 How Are the Components of an Epidemiological Compartmental Model Constructed in Correspondence with the Application It Is Intended for?

The simplest compartmental epidemiological models assume that individuals are in one of at most three possible states: susceptible (S), infected (I), and removed (R). The most important models of this type are the so-called SI, SIS, and SIR, which, as we have already seen, can be considered in a deterministic or stochastic way, and a common assumption is that the interaction between individuals is random. The validity of these models depends on certain assumptions that we already discussed in subsection 3.1. Many childhood infectious diseases are modeled using a SIR model since recovery from infection leads to lifelong immunity. For most sexually transmitted diseases, the SIS model is most appropriate, since only a small number of these diseases produce immunity after infection. HIV is a clear exception and it can still be adequately described, at least in the Western world, by an SI-type model. [124].

All these three models assume that the total population remains constant and the SI and SIS models only consist of two equations. See Fig. 5, 6, and 7 for the corresponding flow diagrams. For SI they are considered:

$$\begin{aligned} S'(t) &= -\beta\frac{S(t)I(t)}{N}\,, \\ I'(t) &= \beta\frac{S(t)I(t)}{N}\,. \end{aligned} \tag{1.3}$$

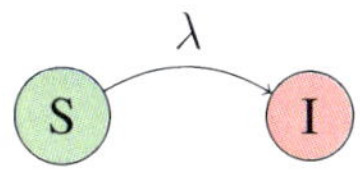

Figure 5: Flow diagram for a SI model

For SIS, the term $\gamma I(t)$ is appropriately added and subtracted, where the constant γ represents the rate at which individuals continue to be susceptible, after recovering from the disease, assuming that there is no mortality as a consequence of the disease. That is,

$$\begin{aligned} S'(t) &= -\beta\frac{S(t)I(t)}{N} + \gamma I(t)\,, \\ I'(t) &= \beta\frac{S(t)I(t)}{N} - \gamma I(t)\,. \end{aligned} \tag{1.4}$$

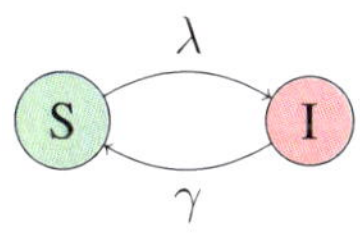

Figure 6: Flow diagram for a SIS model

The SIR model is composed with the same equation of the SI model for the variable S, the equation of the SIS model for the variable I, and the difference is that the term $\gamma I(t)$ becomes part of the equation for the class of individuals removed, and the constant γ now represents the removal rate which is equal, in this case, to the sum of the recovery and mortality rates associated with the disease, which are generally different. Hence,

$$\begin{aligned} S'(t) &= -\beta\frac{S(t)I(t)}{N}\,, \\ I'(t) &= \beta\frac{S(t)I(t)}{N} - \gamma I(t)\,, \\ R'(t) &= \gamma I(t)\,. \end{aligned} \tag{1.5}$$

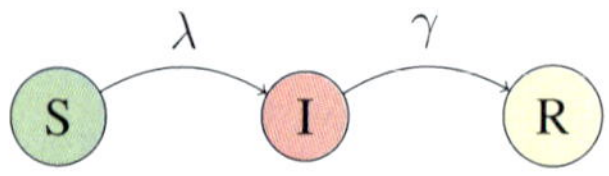

Figure 7: Flow diagram for a SIR model

When analyzing the long-term behavior of a SIR model, it is necessary to include the natural birth and death rates of the population, which must be equal to a certain value μ under the assumption that the total population remains constant. See Fig. 8 for the corresponding flow diagram. In this case, the term $\mu(N-S)$ is added to the equation for the variable S in the SIR model, and the terms $-\mu I$ and $-\mu R$ are added to the equations for the variables I and R respectively. Hence,

$$\begin{aligned} S'(t) &= -\beta \frac{S(t)I(t)}{N} + \mu(N - S(t)), \\ I'(t) &= \beta \frac{S(t)I(t)}{N} - \gamma I(t) - \mu I(t), \\ R'(t) &= \gamma I(t) - \mu R(t). \end{aligned} \tag{1.6}$$

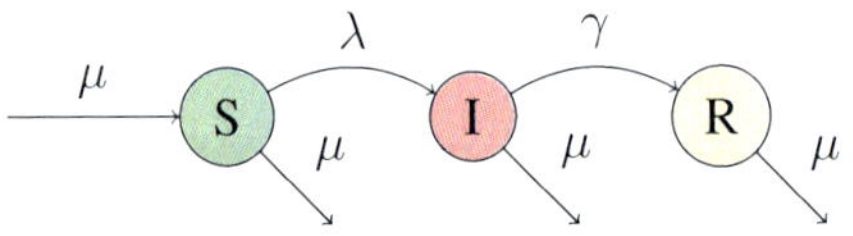

Figure 8: Flow diagram for a SIR model with demographics

The influence of these new terms in the SIR model is something much studied and appears in many texts, but we recommend consulting references [95, 124, 125], which focus on the discussion of these simple models, and Section 2 in chapter 4 of this book. In particular, in the case of the SIR model with birth and mortality rates, the existence of an equilibrium point corresponding to the **endemic state** is demonstrated. The course of the disease is studied and rests on the analysis of the stability of the equilibrium point. This analysis is based on the interpretation of the reproductive number, which, in these cases, is explicitly calculated in a very simple way.

The following generalization of the SIR model corresponds to the SEIR model, where the class E of **exposed** individuals is added, which are those that correspond to the latency period of the disease and that, as we have already commented on several occasions, are of particular importance in the case of COVID-19 since, during a certain interval of time, individuals exposed to COVID-19 are transmitting agents of the disease without even having presented symptoms. See Fig. 9 for the corresponding flow diagram.

To build a SEIR model, a new equation for the variable E is added to the SIR model. As a result, a new term is incorporated to the model, associated with a parameter σ, which represents the incubation rate of the virus. If the population birth and death rates μ continue to be considered in the SIR model, we obtain the following system of differential equations for a basic SEIR-type model which includes demographic analysis:

$$\begin{aligned} S'(t) &= -\lambda(I(t))S(t) + \mu(N - S(t)), \\ E'(t) &= \lambda(I(t))S(t) - (\sigma + \mu)E(t), \\ I'(t) &= \sigma E(t) - (\gamma + \mu)I(t), \\ R'(t) &= \gamma I(t) - \mu R(t), \end{aligned} \tag{1.7}$$

where $S(t) + E(t) + I(t) + R(t) = N$. Here, $\lambda(I)$ denotes the force of infection, which in the case of classic models of SIR-type (1.3), (1.4), (1.5), (1.6) depends linearly on I; concretely, $\lambda(I) = \beta I/N$.

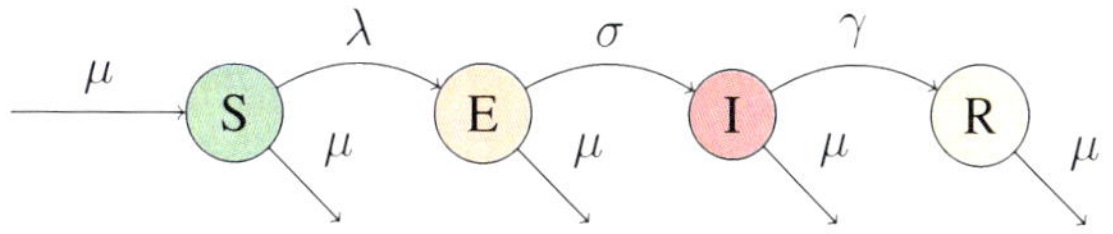

Figure 9: Flow diagram for a SEIR model with demographics

The basic (R_0) and specific (R_t) reproductive numbers, *defined as the average number of secondary cases that are generated by an infected individual, in a totally susceptible population (in the case of* R_0*) or, in a population in which not all persons are susceptible (in the case* *of* R_t*)*, are possibly the most important quantities to extract useful information from the study of compartmental epidemiological models, in particular, regarding the stability analysis of their equilibrium states [125]. See also [126] where the importance of R_0 for public health applications is analyzed.

There are statistical methods that, based on the analysis of data corresponding to the evolution of an epidemic, allow the calculation of approximate values of R_0 and R_t. However, in the case of simple models like SIR or SEIR, as shown in (1.5), (1.6), and (1.7), there are analytical methods to calculate R_0. For instance, the **next generation matrix method** [125, 127, 128]) or the **graph theoretic method**. [129].

On the other hand, although the reproductive number estimated from the epidemic model can also be used to measure the effectiveness of intervention strategies such as social distancing and quarantine, it sometimes happens that obtaining other magnitudes related to R_0, directly from epidemiological data, reveals that R_0 derived from the model has been underestimated or overestimated.

Using the next generation matrix method, we get the value of

$$R_0 = \frac{\beta\sigma}{(\gamma + \mu)(\sigma + \mu)}$$

for the SEIR model, and for the SIR model with demographic analysis we obtain

$$R_0 = \frac{\beta}{\sigma + \mu}.$$

The fact that R_0 is lower for the SEIR model than for its corresponding SIR model is due to the fact that some individuals die before getting infected and belong no more to class E.

Note that, although in model (1.7), the term $\lambda(I)$ that corresponds to the **force of infection**, is generally taken to be equal to the term that appears in the SIR model, that is, $\lambda(I) = \beta I/N$, we write it in a more general way to facilitate the understanding of the generalizations of this model to the study of some epidemics and, in particular, the one caused by SARS-CoV-2. Indeed, model (1.7) represents the basic modeling scheme for COVID-19, to which many new components have been added as a result of the disaggregation of classes S, E, and I, thus obtaining generalizations and refinements of the model, applicable to specific situations, as we will see below.

In particular, the expression of the force of infection can vary remarkably depending on the properties of the infectious disease in question, the mitigation and reinforcement measures that are taken, and the way in which different components of the class of infected individuals I interact with certain subsets of the class of susceptible individuals S, which can lead to very serious complications for the study of the models.

One of the simplest cases arises in the presence of an **external force of infection** to the study area. If we represent it by J, the **rate of influx** of infected individuals to the study area (which can be constant or variable), then

$$\lambda(I(t)) = \beta\frac{I(t)}{N} + J(t)$$

and, in this case, R_0 cannot be calculated explicitly. When J is very small with respect to the term $\beta I/N$, we can first obtain the expression of R_0 for $J = 0$ and later an approximate expression of $R_0(J)$ using the classical asymptotic procedure of the theory of regular disturbances.

Taking into account the characteristics of the disease transmission process, there are two main ways of considering the infected population in the expression of the infection force $\lambda(I)$, which are essentially different when the population size is variable. This happens when natural birth and death rates are different, or when the disease can cause death.

These two forms are called ***"frequency dependent"*** *and* ***"density dependent"****, and are differentiated by the impact that infected individuals can cause on the susceptible persons, according to the characteristics of the disease. It is frequency dependent if $\lambda(I)$ is independent of population size and depends solely on the number of infected persons, and it is density dependent if it depends on the fraction of persons that are infected in the total population.*

In the first case we would have, for example, $\lambda(I) = \beta I$ and, in the second case, $\lambda(I) = \beta I/N$.

Density dependent transmission is used primarily to model the force of infection in diseases in which the virus is transmitted directly through the air, such as measles and influenza and currently

COVID-19.

Although, in most cases an expression of the force of infection directly proportional to I or I/N is used, there is a large amount of literature in which nonlinear formulations of the force of infection are studied, which appear in other contexts such as infection by parasites and transmission of rabies, which we will not consider in this text.

The **level of risk** or **vulnerability** of different population groups is a fundamental factor to take into account when defining the force of infection and its consequences on the fatality rate due to infection. The risk depends, to a large extent, on the social activity in which individuals are involved, which in turn is related to their work or school activities and their mobility, but also depends on other factors such as age, sex, preexisting comorbidities, and socio-economic level. Almost all of these factors are, in some way, correlated with some measure of **activity level** and **age**.

Section 3 of Chapter 4 discusses a criterion for measuring the level of activity and analyzes its influence, together with age, on the force of infection.

In chapters 5 and 8, the influence of comorbidities on the level of vulnerability and on the determination of predictors of COVID-19 fatality is particularly discussed, using Artificial Intelligence techniques and statistical analysis, respectively.

Chapter 7 establishes the conceptual and methodological bases to measure socio-economic, socio-demographic, and socio-cultural inequalities in health, along with some applications to the current COVID-19 pandemic. These metrics are an indispensable tool for the inclusion of social inequalities in the description of the force of infection.

On the other hand, the influence of human mobility has been taken into account in the study of COVID-19, in computational models of agents [90], and in compartmental models from a Lagrangian perspective, through the concept of **residence time** [130].

In particular, human mobility has been studied using GPS data from mobile phones. Such is the case of the BBC Pandemic Project, and of censuses of ***workflows****, using the so-called* ***gravity models****, that require the construction of* ***source-destination flow matrices*** *[131].*

The application of mitigation measures (see subsection 3.4 of this chapter), together with the **perception of risk** by the population are reflected in a decrease in the **effective rates of contact** and, consequently, in the force of infection. In [111, 112], a proposal is made for modeling the perception of risk, based on the assumption that the increase in deaths from the disease will cause people to protect themselves more from situations of risk. However, in the case COVID-19, human behavior has not been consistent with the severity of the pandemic situation.

This need to reflect the different components of the level of risk in the force of infection, leads in turn to the need of introducing **population heterogeneity** in the compartmental epidemiological models, as well as their **contact patterns**, which are also discussed in Section 3 of chapter 4.

In Chapter 6, a heterogeneous population is considered, distributed in different spatial patches, each composed of different subpopulations, which communicate with each other through the mobility of individuals. It is also assumed that there may be **reinfections**, that is, after some time, those recovered from each patch may become susceptible again. The reinfection term is expressed in terms of a reinfection rate that is the inverse of the **mean time of immunity**. As regards models, this implies the subtraction of the term ηR in the equation for the recovered ones and its addition to that of the susceptible ones. It is shown in Chapter 6 that reinfection in a heterogeneous population distributed in spatial patches, can give rise to the existence of an endemic equilibrium point that may be stable.

This is precisely one of the risks associated with COVID-19, while there are no vaccines that provide permanent immunity, either by themselves or by a booster dose.

In practical terms, considering population heterogeneity in a spatial region implies partitioning the total population of size N into n subpopulations, with N_k people each, with $N = \sum_{k=1}^{n} N_k$. Each subpopulation has its own susceptible, exposed or latent, infected, recovered, and deceased individuals. According to the population heterogeneity criterion to be included in the study, each of these subpopulations are divided into subgroups.

In the case of COVID-19, it is natural to subdivide the class of susceptible persons according to criteria related to the level of risk, such as age, sex, comorbidities, work activity, socio-economic level, etc. In infectious patients, the presymptomatic, symptomatic, and asymptomatic and, on occasion, superspreaders are separated. When confinement measures are applied, susceptible persons are usually divided between those who are confined and those who are not.

In the case of certain subclasses such as the population of people admitted into the categories of serious, critical, those requiring mechanical ventilation, recovered, and deceased, each group of susceptible persons within a subclass is associated with an infection force, which is generally defined as a convex linear combination of the infection forces, exerted on that susceptible group by all infected groups corresponding to each of the subpopulations into which the total population was divided. The coefficients of this convex linear combination must reflect the level of risk of the group susceptible to contagion by each of the groups of infected with whom it interacts.

3.6 Some Important Results Obtained on COVID-19 with the Use of Compartmental Mathematical Models

In this Section, we will describe some important results obtained through mathematical models, many of which have been used for decision-making for the control of the pandemic.

In each of the works that we will mention, some variant of the compartmental epidemiological model is introduced, which is studied with the aim of obtaining conclusions about the epidemiological dynamics or to deal with specific problems related to the pandemic, such as transmission control. Subsequently, the methodology and results are exemplified in the specific situation of a specific country.

It is not our interest to show the results in detail, nor to talk about the specific applications, but only to emphasize its meaning and relevance.

The importance of this section is that:

- All results can be extended to more general models and can be applied to local situations of interest in any country.
- The applications that are derived from some of these works confirm several of the main

results that were highlighted in Section 2 of this chapter and that, in some way, can be used as a priori information for the solution of inverse problems associated with the models.

- For obvious reasons, the objective of these works have been to provide answers to specific pressing situations derived from the pandemic. However, at the same time, many of them constitute the basis for new mathematical approaches and qualitative analyzes that, without doubt, will result in new knowledge to cope with future pending challenges.

Next, we will divide the text into three subsections, trying to show the chronological evolution of mathematical models through some notorious examples.

3.6.1 The First Mathematical Models for COVID-19

Three of the first important models for the spread of COVID-19 were developed by Joel Hellewell [48], Alberto Aleta [90], and Neil Ferguson [132], and collaborators. These models followed the classic scheme of SIR models, incorporating certain additional elements that represented, in a very simple way, the object of study. However, despite their relative simplicity, these types of models have been used since the first months of the pandemic, to make projections in the short and medium term of the evolution of COVID-19. These projections have been very useful for designing strategies and making decisions aimed at slowing the spread of the epidemic, especially while vaccines were not available. An example of this has been the website designed at Los Alamos National Laboratory [133]. For an analysis of the results of these three models, we refer to Holmdahl et al [123].

These models were introduced to measure the efficacy of certain types of nonpharmaceutical interventions. Their applicability was very limited by the lack of knowledge of the characteristics of the virus and its transmission.

In [48], a parameterized stochastic transmission model was developed with respect to data from confirmed COVID-19 cases. The model was used to quantify the potential effectiveness of contact tracing and case isolation to control transmission. One of the problems of this study was the use of data from confirmed cases to parameterize the model, rather than data from hospitalized or deceased, which, as demonstrated in [134], are more reliable. Assumptions were also made that isolating people interrupted transmission and that immunity fully protected against infection for at least one to two years, a period that coincided with the duration of the simulation. This last assumption is also made in [90, 132].

Under these conditions, in [48] random simulations were carried out, keeping some parameters of the model fixed and varying others such as the initial cases and the basic reproductive number R_0. From these simulations, conclusions of the following types were drawn: "simulated outbreaks that start with five initial cases, $R_0 = 1.5$ and a transmission of 0% before the onset of symptoms, can be controlled even with a low probability of contact tracing, while, the probability of controlling an outbreak decreases with the number of initial cases, when R_0 is in the range 2.5-3.5, and there is also a higher transmission before the onset of symptoms".

In [90], it is assumed that, although severe social distancing measures have been shown to be effective in curbing the pandemic, second wave scenarios are likely to emerge as restrictions are lifted. To study the effect of lifting restrictions, a detailed compartmental stochastic epidemiological model was used, and simulations were carried out with transmission data obtained from agent-based models using anonymized and geolocated mobility data, together with data from the census and demographics of the metropolitan area of Boston in the United States.

The important conclusion of the study was that a period of strict social distancing, followed by a solid level of testing, contact tracing, and home quarantine, could keep the disease within the capacity of the health system and allow the reopening of economic activities. Hence, the importance of having a response system based on improved tests and tracking of contacts to be able to relax the social distancing interventions in the absence of herd immunity against COVID-19.

In [132], a modification of an epidemiological model developed for influenza was used to evaluate, through simulations, the potential of some public health measures, recognized as nonpharmaceutical interventions, which are applied with the objective of reducing the contact rates in the population and, consequently, reducing the transmission of the SARS-CoV-2 virus.

Two fundamental strategies of **mitigation** and **suppression** were simulated.

Mitigation consists of slowing, without necessarily stopping, the spread of the epidemic. It combines isolation of suspected cases, home quarantine for those who live in the same home as suspected cases, and social distancing from older adults and others who are at risk of serious illness. This is intended to reduce the demand for medical care while those most at risk of serious infection are protected.

Suppression, through widespread social distancing, combined with home isolation of the entire population, is a drastic measure that aims to reverse the growth of the epidemic, reducing and keeping the number of cases at low levels. Generally, suppression is complemented by the closure of schools and universities and the interruption of nonessential work activities, all of which have a negative impact on society.

In terms of the reproductive number R_t, suppression is equivalent to reducing the reproductive number to values lower than 1, while mitigation only seeks to reduce the reproductive number to manageable levels around but not lower than 1.

One conclusion of the study is that, to achieve a significant impact in reducing transmission, a combined strategy of both interventions is required, since the effectiveness of either of the two isolated interventions can be very limited.

An important result was that mitigation policies can reduce the maximum demand for medical care by $2/3$ and deaths by half, although the mitigated epidemic can still produce thousands of deaths and collapse health systems, especially intensive healthcare systems. It was also concluded that intensive suppression measures would be unavoidable as long as a vaccine that offers prolonged immunity is not available, which, until now, has not been possible.

3.6.2 Some Later Models

Almost at the same time as this first group of studies, a second group emerged, where essential results were also obtained, based on compartmental models and models of age of infection [56, 88,

109, 120, 135–140].

The study in [56] uses the framework of the renewal equations to model the daily incidence of infected individuals, that is, the rate at which new infections occur in the population, based on the previous incidence, and how the infectivity of individuals varies during their infection. In the model, birth and loss of immunity are neglected on the time scale of an outbreak.

The incidence is divided into two components, corresponding to symptomatic and asymptomatic cases. Using the model, the expected effects of asymptomatic transmission on the basic reproduction number R_0 are evaluated, as well as the fraction of new secondary cases attributable to asymptomatic individuals.

If the distribution of the generational interval of asymptomatic transmission differs from that of symptomatic transmission, the estimates of the basic reproduction number that do not explicitly take into account asymptomatic cases may be systematically biased. Specifically, if asymptomatic cases have a shorter generation interval than symptomatic cases, R_0 will be overestimated, and if it is longer, then it will be underestimated.

In [88], an epidemic model is proposed, which the authors call SuEIR, which is a variant of a SEIR model with a reinterpretation of the variables I and R. The variables S and E have the same meaning as in a classical model SEIR, but in the SuEIR model, variables I and R represent only infectious and recovered individuals who are detected by the health system. That is why it is assumed that the transition from class E to class I corresponds to only a fraction $0 < \mu < 1$ of all those exposed who become infectious.

To determine the value of μ, machine learning techniques supported by the model were used to make short-term predictions of confirmed cases and deaths from COVID-19 and to predict the peak date of active cases, as well as to estimate the basic reproduction number R_0. In particular, the forecasts based on the model suggested that the peak dates in the United States, New York State, and California would be 06/01/2020, 05/10/2020, and 07/01/2020, respectively, which clearly did not coincide with the number of cases that were reported.

The most interesting part of the study was the methodology developed, but it was too simple to reflect the complex problem associated with the evolution of the epidemic. Furthermore, it seems to be risky making such accurate forecasts.

In [135], a compartmental model called SEAIR is used, in which the asymptomatic class A is already explicitly incorporated into the SEIR model as a new variable. The model is inspired by two characteristics of COVID-19 infectivity: the late onset of symptoms compared to the onset of infectiousness, or even their total absence.

The chosen SEAIR model has a built-in delay, which means that the infected person does not start spreading the disease right away. This makes it possible to address the contagions of the disease in different phases and captures the presence of undetected propagators.

An interesting point is that it is a simple model that can be approached in a completely analytical way. For example, the roles of the main eigenvalue and eigenvector of the matrices obtained by linearization of the model around the equilibrium states in the spread of the epidemic are studied. It is already known that the main eigenvalue determines the epidemic threshold and, therefore, determines stability [141, 142], but in [135] it is shown that this eigenvalue with its associated eigenvector play an important role in estimating the risk of infection.

Although the SuEIR and SEAIR models seem very similar, there are some subtleties that distinguish them, mainly the fact that among the undetected infectious cases there are not only asymptomatic, but also presymptomatic persons.

In [136], a much more complete model than the previous ones is studied, especially due to the number of compartments it includes, distinguishing between the total number of infectious and the undetected infectious ones, and considering the different sanitary and infectious conditions of hospitalized people, as well as sick people who are quarantined at home. The model is called θ-SEIHRD, and as in the SuEIR model, a parameter θ is introduced ($0 < \theta < 1$) which has the same meaning as the parameter μ of that model.

In this study, the parameter θ is estimated in a different way than μ in [88], and the impact of asymptomatic transmission on the total number of infected cases is studied. It also provides estimates need for hospital beds.

The results were applied to the case of China, and it revealed that, during the study period, around 51% of all infected cases were undetected (asymptomatic) and they caused around 37% of infections.

In references [109, 120], predictive posterior distributions are used to account for all possible epidemic curves compatible with the data, thus allowing for a better forecast in probabilistic terms.

In [109] a model of the age of infection, modulated in time, was introduced, which leads to the system of renewal equations (1.1) and (1.2) (see Section 3.2). This is based on the evolution of the daily incidence of COVID-19 in certain groups of susceptible individuals, and includes the effect of certain mitigation strategies, fundamentally capturing the implementation of a strict isolation measure (Stay-at-Home) and scenarios for its eventual release.

The model is applied to the State of Illinois in the United States, assuming that the total population in each of the population groups of susceptible individuals considered, at different regional levels within the state, remains constant, and that the duration of immunity to COVID-19 is greater than the time scale in which the epidemic is simulated and, therefore, there can be no reinfection.

Since the daily number of susceptible individuals and the daily incidence of infected cannot be directly observed, the authors emphasize the importance of calibrating the model, using daily data from other indicators, like total and hospital deaths and the occupation of beds in hospitals and ICUs, for patients admitted with COVID-19. To avoid biases resulting from COVID-19 test data, which are not uniform or constant and are difficult to parameterize, data from positive cases are not considered for model calibration.

Bayesian estimation of the model parameters is carried out using Monte Carlo Markov Chains (MCMC) methods. Subsequently, a detailed analysis of the calibration and robustness procedure is carried out, as well as of the scope and predictive capacity of the model, based on a set of forward simulations that sample the posterior distribution over the model parameters.

The final objective of the study is to make predictions of the daily evolution of new infections, occupied hospital beds, occupied ICU beds, and in-hospital and out-of-hospital deaths. Future model predictions provide robust estimates of the maximum position and gravity and they also allow to forecast regional results dependent on the release of Stay-at-Home orders by the government. The results provide reliable estimates of the progression of the epidemic in the short term and allow to suggest scenarios for sustainable monitoring and control of the epidemic.

A work with similar objectives and methodology to [109] but with applications to Mexico City, is [120]. The main differences between the two studies lie in the fact that, in [120], a classic SIR-type compartmental modeling scheme is used, instead of an age of infection model, and a somewhat different methodology is applied to carry out the Bayesian estimation, of the posterior distribution over the model parameters.

Finally, let us consider in this subsection the works [137–139], where different practical approaches regarding the influence of the control of human mobility on the transmission of COVID-19 are studied.

In [137], a compartmental model of the SIR-type is introduced, to which the classes of individuals in confinement and those who died as a result of the disease are added. Using a really very simple model, the work draws interesting conclusions about the impossibility of predicting the turning point and the end of a spreading epidemic. The conclusions are obtained from the analysis of the explicit expression of the basic reproductive number R_0, which is explicitly calculated from the model, and from its Bayesian fit to the COVID-19 pandemic in Spain, at the time it was conducted the investigation.

An important conclusion of the work, at that time when many countries dared to predict the peak and end of the epidemic, was the proposition that **better data were necessary, but were not enough** to make accurate forecasts with the models. Short-term forecasts can be made, but they must be accompanied by a measure of their uncertainty.

In many countries, the measure of compulsory confinement of the inhabitants in their homes was applied, and it helped to suppress the transmission of COVID-19, but with devastating social and economic consequences, which can lead to disruptions in financial markets, including the banking systems and securities markets. The study in [138] proposes exit strategies from the confinement, which allow for sustainable, albeit small economic activity.

To this objective, a SEIR-Erlang model is proposed to which epidemiological measures are added and, based on the model, a stepwise cyclical strategy is proposed to define the confinement periods. Authors argue that this type of strategy produces better results than confining the population each time a critical epidemiological situation is reached.

The basic idea is to keep the effective reproduction number R_t of the disease below 1, since, in that case, the number of infected people decreases exponentially. To reduce R_t below 1, a cyclical program with k continuous days of work followed by n continuous days of confinement is proposed. The cycle pushes R_t below one by reducing the exposure time, drawing from the latency period of the virus, so that those infected during the work days, reach the peak of infectivity during the days of lockdown. As shown in [138], 4 days of work followed by 10 days of confinement is a reasonable cycle that allows a repetitive schedule every 2 weeks, without neglecting basic epidemiological measures.

This type of strategy can be combined with other interventions and can become an auspicious option for decision makers. It could be applied to organize the orderly return to schools and, in general, to organize the activities of the entire population, except those infected in quarantine and people in risk groups.

The study in [139] starts from the same incentive as [138] on the need to relax blocking restrictions and social distancing while protecting public health, given the negative impact they have on the economy.

For this, a modified SEIR model is also built, from which modified blocking and social distancing restrictions are designed that allow to reduce overall death rates and at the same time increase economic activity. This new proposal of stepwise liberation policy is compared with the reference policy of simultaneously releasing all social groups over a predetermined time.

The results suggest that properly designed stepwise release policies may work better than simultaneous release policies, in terms of protecting the most vulnerable members of the population, reducing risks to general health, and increasing economic activity.

During the early phases of COVID-19, many outbreaks were associated with a history of travel, from a region where the epidemic had already evolved. This situation was considered in [140].

However, most of the population models that consider this situation assume a homogeneous infected population, without considering that imported and secondary cases, produced by imported cases, may present different risks for community dissemination.

Taking this observation into account, in [140] a SIR-type metapopulation model is proposed that includes a matrix of mobility rates of infected individuals between different nodes (cities) of a network, and that distinguishes between the dynamics of imported infected and the corresponding secondary and locally infected. The model is used together with the cumulative number of secondary cases, to determine the probability of community spread.

To calculate the number of imported cases, it is assumed that infected cases could pass border control or relocate to other settings only during their incubation period, since otherwise they would be detected and quarantined.

The study made it possible to evaluate the effects of border control and quarantine measures on the appearance and global spread of COVID-19 in a fully connected world, using the dynamics of secondary cases.

As an example, the 10 most visited cities of Wuhan in China were considered. It was shown that the arrival time and the dynamics of the outbreaks in these cities could be predicted successfully with a reproduction number $R_0 = 2.92$, and an incubation period $\tau = 5.2$ days, which, by other means has already been confirmed to coincide with the mean incubation period of the disease.

As we can see, the study of the dynamic processes on networks, and particularly in metapopulation networks, is of major importance to understand the behaviour of many complex phenomena, such as the global propagation of epidemics, rumours and opinions. However, the multiscalar nature and the intrinsic heterogeneity of the underlying networks, hinders the prediction of the evolution of the dynamic processes taking place in them and the localization of the causes that originate them. In addition, in many times the behavior at certain network nodes is not necessarily originated in spatially closer nodes. This happens, in particular, when studying the spatio-temporal dynamics of the contagion, produced by an infectious disease, among different localities composing a network. In this last case, it is not the geographic distance that determines propagation but flow of people among nodes.

In this framework, a proposal is elaborated in [143] about how contagion can be spread among different countries by estimating connectivity between each two countries by means of weights. The latter is performed by using the volume of air traffic between them. The distance d_{mn} from node m to node n is defined as the daily average number of total passengers traveling from node m to node n (note that, in general, d_{mn} is different to d_{nm}). Hence, the distance between nodes m and n through a path $n_1 = m, n_2, n_3, \ldots, n_k = n$ that connects them, is defined as the sum of the successive distances between two consecutive nodes in the path, $\sum_{j=1}^{k-1} d_{n_j n_{j+1}}$. Finally, the effective distance between nodes m and n is given by the shortest path length connecting nodes m and n, in the previous sense.

The above notion of distance is not a metric in a strict mathematical sense, but allows to compute the speed of the disease spread and its arrival times to each node, as well as determine functional relations among epidemiological and mobility parameters in the network. Furthermore, this concept of distance possess the following fundamental property: propagation is concentric with respect to the nodes where outbreaks occur. This allows to locate satisfactorily, with enough degree of approximation, the nodes responsible for propagating the epidemy. This is illustrated for the cases of the SARS epidemic in 2003 and the H1N1 influenza pandemic in 2009.

Moreover, a general theoretical framework is considered in [144] for studying the influence of the complex network topology in the propagation dynamics of spatio-temporal signals through the network, when signals are the result of reactions originated at each node and spread through their connections. In the particular case of epidemics in metapopulation networks, contagion plays the role of the propagated signal, and the network models the transmission of contagion from one node to another as a result of mobility between them.

Concerning the previously mentioned topic, we refer to [145] for an exhaustive review of the extensive research activity about the study of epidemic processes occurring in complex networks of diverse nature. This compilation addresses also a detailed examination of the most successful theoretical approaches along with their constraints and assumptions.

3.6.3 More Recent Models

Much more recently, new realistic elements have been incorporated into the models, which have made it possible, in the first place, to weaken the basic assumptions of homogeneity required in the original SIR-type models and to add other interventions such as the use of masks and the application of vaccines.

In [146], the presence of asymptomatic infections and the main policies that had been adopted so far to contain the epidemic were taken into account simultaneously; that is, social distancing, isolation of a part of the population, quarantine as strict isolation applied to infected confirmed cases, and testing for infected individuals.

The model included the proportion of people in isolation, the level of reduction in contact rates, and the rate of testing, as control parameters that can be variable over time, representing policies that can change at different stages of the epidemic. Using the model, the basic reproductive number R_0 is expressed as a function of epidemiological parameters and control policies, and in this way the effect of isolation measures and tests for the detection of confirmed cases on the evolution of the epidemic can be quantified, as well as simulations of different realistic scenarios.

From this analysis, it was deduced that the detection of asymptomatic patients through tests and their consequent isolation are fundamental actions for the control of the epidemic, and should be carried out as soon as possible to increase their effectiveness, which is supported by the flattening of the infection curve.

The studies in [110, 147] consider, from a conceptual point of view, the incorporation of population heterogeneity in epidemiological models, with the purpose of weakening the hypothesis of homogeneity, which is fundamental for the formulation of the classic compartmental models of the SIR- and SEIR-types.

These studies consider an important problem related to population heterogeneity, which has characterized the COVID-19 epidemic, namely, a **disproportionate dispersion** in which a great proportion of the transmission is driven by a minority of infected individuals. Indeed, **short-term overpropagation** events, as well as the **extreme rate of virus dissemination** by each individual in peak infectivity, while attending a large number of meetings without adequate protection, have caused a marked departure from the assumptions of homogeneity, typical of traditional well-mixed compartment models.

Finally, this heterogeneity can be of biological or social origin, and assuming that these two factors are independent, it is demonstrated how they can be incorporated into a wide class of epidemiological models. For this, two fundamental components of heterogeneity are considered, which correspond, on the one hand, to short-term superpropagation events, and on the other, to **persistent** or **long-term heterogeneity** of individual susceptibility or infectivity.

The previous work shows the role played by superspreaders and events of superpropagation, during the beginning of an outbreak and, from the proposed model, a nonlinear dependence of the effective reproduction number R_t is obtained with respect to the fraction of susceptible population S.

This dependence allows us to infer three important consequences of persistent heterogeneity in contrast to short-term overscattering effects:

- It gives rise to a significant change in the dynamics of the epidemic in the early stages;
- It significantly suppresses the threshold of herd immunity;
- It significantly reduces the final size of the epidemic.

In the works [148, 149], compartmental models are used to study the impact of the use of masks and vaccination in the transmission of COVID-19, considering the presence of new variants of the SARS-CoV-2 virus.

In [148], the model is used to compare the spread of infection within a homogeneous mixed population that uses different types of masks, it discusses when the policy about their use should be mandatorily applied, and analizes the consequences of noncompliance.

The results suggest substantial reductions in the size of the epidemic and the mortality rate in at least 75% of the mask wearers, and it shows how strict adherence to the use of moderate quality masks at the beginning of an epidemic, can achieve mortality reductions similar to those of minor compliance, with the use of high-quality masks, after the epidemic takes off. It is concluded that a critical mass of 84% of the population using masks, can completely stop the spread of the disease.

As it was exposed in [150], from the decade of 70s of the past century, some important results concerning the epidemics control through the use of vaccines have been established by using SEIR type simple models with constant rates. These results were successfully applied to the design of vaccination strategies for many diseases, for which immunity, natural or vaccine-induced, persists for a long time. This is the case of mumps, measles, rubella and chickenpox, but not of COVID-19.

In [150] is shown that if the basic reproductive number R_0 is greater than 1, and a fraction p of population is vaccinated (preferably soon after birth), and hence immunized, where $1 - 1/R_0 < p < 1$, then the basic reproductive number reduces to $R_0(1-p)$. Consequently, if p is chosen such that $R_0(1 - p) < 1$, it turns out that the disease tends to disappear.

In the long term, statistics of many common childhood illnesses show fluctuations, as a consequence of depletion and renewal of individuals in the susceptible class, giving place to inter-epidemic periods. This is reflected in the damped behavior of the solutions of the associated SEIR models, which asymptotically approximate to certain equilibrium states.

All this kind of diseases possess a duration time much lower than host life expectancy, so the estimated value for the oscillation period is $T = 2\pi(AD)^{1/2}$, where D stands for the sum of latency and infection periods and A is the reciprocal of the force of infection, which equals the average age at which individuals acquire the infection.

The following estimation for the necessary fraction p is also provided in [150],

$$p > \frac{1 + V/L}{1 + A/L},$$

where A is as before, V stands for the average age at which individuals are vaccinated, and L is life expectancy (which turns to be the reciprocal of death rate).

From all above results it is concluded that for attaining complete eradication for a disease with a high basic reproduction number, it is necessary to increase p, in order to reach a colective high immunity level, and reduce V by vaccinating as soon as possible. Note that $V < A$ is required, since $p < 1$. This analysis applies obviously just in case such effective vaccines providing long time immunity are available, as is the case with measles. In this context, it is important to estimate the inter-epidemic periods in order to design appropriately vaccination schedules, taking into account the population birth rate. Current vaccination strategies for common childhood illnesses are based on these principles.

However, the case of COVID-19 is much more complex, mainly due to its novelty. Regarding vaccines availability, the work developed in laboratories around the world has already produced several ones, validated by WHO, some of them by means of emergency use authorization and/or to be applied in a restricted way, and much many candidates. Notwithstanding this extraordinarily fast development of vaccines for COVID-19, many questions still remain unanswered, and there are no effective vaccines against a broad spectrum of SARS-CoV-2 variants or able to provide long-term enough immunity. Not to mention problems concerning unequal distribution or patent waiver on COVID-19 vaccines.

In recent years, some works consider mathematical models including a greater number of compartments, in order to distinguish among different population classes, such as presymptomatic and asymptomatic individuals, hospitalized, deceased as a result of the disease, etc. In the review [151] some of them are collected, from classical mean-field epidemiological models, in which an homogeneously-mixed population is considered but ignoring human behavior, to more recent and sophisticated models, which take into account human behavior and population heterogeneity according to spatial distribution and social factors, as well as their corresponding non linear interactions with the disease dynamics.

For the study of these latest models, methods of Statistical Physics are used, as well as their associated analytical supports. Modeling is strengthened with data coming from different digital resources about the epidemics evolution. Vaccination is also considered. All this mathematical and computational machinery allows to simulate real scenarios and provide useful information for decision-making.

In [149], a mathematical model is proposed, which is called θ-ij-SVEIHQRD, which is capable of simulating the possible impact of the contagiousness of new variants of the virus SARS-CoV-2, and the efficacy of vaccines, during the application of different types of vaccines to the population.

The model is applied to the particular case of Italy, as a case study. It is concluded that vaccines can reduce infections, but may not be enough to prevent a new wave with the current vaccination rates expected in that country, if control measures are relaxed. In addition, it is shown that a more contagious variant could significantly increase the number of cases, becoming the most common form of contagion. Even with the slowdown in pandemic cases (with a lower than 1 effective reproduction number), where the disease seems to be under control, the number of effective reproduction corresponding only to the new variant can be greater than 1 and, eventually, the number of infections would increase towards a new wave of infections. Therefore, a rigorous monitoring of the evolution of the number of infections with respect to any new variant, potentially more dangerous, is of utmost importance at any stage of the pandemic.

Shortly after the previous text, another interesting work was published [152]. Therein, optimal vaccination strategies were proposed, arisen from epidemiological models. It is considered the case in which there is a limited availability of vaccines, each one providing different degrees of effectiveness.

The last two models may be of interest to policy makers, as a tool to evaluate different possible future scenarios and for decision-making in regards to vaccination policies.

3.7 Some Pending Issues in the Collection and Analysis of Data and in the Study of the Mathematical Models, Associated with COVID-19

We will divide the exposition into three subsections.

3.7.1 Data Collection and Analysis

We have already seen that having complete and reliable data related to the evolution of the pandemic is not enough to answer the questions that arise about the prediction of the peak of infection or the final size of the pandemic, and not even to predict, with an acceptable level of certainty, the impact of the application of a measure in the long term. However, it is a necessary condition if good predictions are to be made in the short and medium term.

Many efforts have been made in this direction, but they should be systematized.

In the first place, an analysis is required on whether the attributes provided by the databases, which are put into the public domain in many countries, are sufficient to monitor the behavior of the epidemic dynamics in different strata of the population, and to create clusters with individuals who, although they belong to different strata, have a homogeneous behavior with respect to their response to the disease.

For example, what characteristics, with respect to age, comorbidities, and sex, do all individuals who have been hospitalized with COVID-19, have shown recovery times or mortality that fit the same probability distribution? Furthermore, will it be possible to partition the set of variables "age, sex, comorbidities, and others", in such a way that each class is characterized by respective probability distributions for recovery times and mortality?

On the other hand, the existence of asymptomatic cases will continue to be an impediment to making more reliable predictions on the models. It is known that tests are required to detect these cases, but how many, at what times, and with what samples from the population? The rest would depend on the possibilities and determination of governments and their health systems.

3.7.2 A New Way of Posing Mathematical Problems with Models, to Obtain Results that Can Be Applied to Decision Making

Until now, mathematical models have been used with a FORWARD approach to respond to the problems that are intended to be solved with them and, without doubt, very interesting and useful results have been obtained, but it would be convenient to pose the same problems with an INVERSE approach.

In all studies that we analyzed in the previous section, once the model is built, trying to incorporate the factors whose effect is to be studied, the model is calibrated using data from the previous evolution of the epidemic and, at most, some parameters are left "free" to analyze the consequences of different simulated scenarios. When it is possible to express the reproductive number by means of the parameters involved in the model, something more can be said from the qualitative point of view, but this is not always possible.

Subsequently, in some cases, Bayesian statistics are used to quantify the uncertainty of the predictions. In other works, it is a matter of going further, posing some type of **optimization problem**, to devise the **best possible strategy** within a set of possible options that, in general, is very limited.

The INVERSE approach entails asking the questions as follows: Given a certain model, a desirable dynamic for the evolution of the epidemic, a time interval, and a reasonable set of possible coefficients for the model defined from certain a priori information, how should the unknown coefficients (within the given set) be identified so that the corresponding model reproduces the preestablished ***desirable dynamics****, during the pre-set time interval?*

This approach may seem trivial at first glance, but it really is not.

First, it implies that, in a way, we **rely on the model** to describe the epidemic situation. For this reason, it is essential that the models are capable of adequately reflecting the epidemiological situation of interest, taking into account all relevant factors and that, in addition, they are theoretically grounded, so that they can incorporate the lack of homogeneity, which is present due to population heterogeneity and multiple social and biological factors that determine it.

It is also important that the models adequately incorporate the terms that represent the interventions which will be implemented during the period of time.

On the other hand, the following considerations must be taken into account, to adequately define the set of coefficients, where those that reproduce the desirable dynamics are sought:

- This set must be carefully defined, taking into account some characteristics that emerge from the epidemiological basis of the model. For example, if the sought coefficients correspond to rates in the model, their values, not necessarily constant, must fall within ranges determined by extreme values of the rates already established for the disease.
- The selected set must be such that it satisfies the condition of uniqueness, regarding the desirable dynamics that they are going to reproduce; that is, there must be a single set of coefficients in that set that reproduces the desirable dynamics.
- That set must satisfy certain additional conditions that allow the construction of an algorithm for the stable solution of the identification problem; that is, they should allow to obtain the solution with a preestablished range of uncertainty, during the entire time interval in which the desirable dynamics is reproduced.

Once this identification problem has been solved, the practical application of the results consists in determining how to apply a concrete strategy to reproduce the temporal variability of the identified coefficients. For example, if the model reflects the application of a vaccination campaign, how should the vaccination strategy be applied to reproduce the temporal evolution of these coefficients?

It must be taken into consideration that any strategy or intervention manifests itself directly in the behavior of certain specific coefficients of the model.

In this way, many longer-term recommendations can be made to be applied by decision makers. With this procedure, the economic, social and other costs associated with the implementation of the strategy can be added, which is an important element to be taken into account by those who make the decisions.

There should be no fear that there will be some disturbance in the application of the strategy that reproduces the identified coefficients and, therefore, a deviation from the desirable dynamics. In fact, these small variations are already contemplated by the stable solution algorithm of the identification problem, described in the third consideration above.

Finally, it should be noted that the usual methodology already solves inverse problems to identify the parameters (generally constant) of the model, based on certain data from the **past epidemiological dynamics**. This leads to a problem of loss of uniqueness in identification and the need to quantify the uncertainty of the forecast. In our proposal, the past epidemiological dynamics is replaced by a desirable dynamics that is about to unfold.

In addition, the uniqueness problem is solved, replacing the parameter spaces (constants) with sets of functions, and the need to quantify the uncertainty is replaced by the introduction of a **regularization strategy**, and the possible time interval in which the desired result is obtained, which is preset in advance.

3.7.3 Some Pending Theoretical Work on Mathematical Models

Much interesting theoretical work has been done with compartmental epidemiological models. We have cited some of them (see, for example, [115–119]). We also argued that many of the works, such as those mentioned in Section 3.6, constitute the basis for new mathematical approaches and qualitative analysis of the models involved.

In a study [95], it is shown how the theoretical study of a simple compartmental model, in this case the stability analysis of its endemic equilibrium state, directly impacts the understanding of the propagation phenomenon of some childhood infectious diseases. Here, we obtain relationships between the parameters of the model that determine the temporal evolution of the propagation of the disease, and that constitute indicators of the appearance or not of an epidemic outbreak, which are used in the evaluation of the impact of the control measures that have been taken, and in the proposal of optimal control strategies.

Logically, the success of this approach will depend on whether we are using the appropriate model, in the sense that its formulation reflects in the most realistic possible way the fundamental factors that determine the evolution of the disease. In addition, it is important that mathematical problems, no matter how abstract, are based on criteria and objectives that have as a reference the epidemiological problem in question and, finally, that the conclusions drawn from the mathematical results contribute to the solution of concrete problems.

In what follows, we present a list of some mathematical problems in epidemiological models, which reflect this approach:

1. Systematize inclusion in models of population heterogeneity, in terms of levels of susceptibility to the disease and its transmissibility, as well as the problem of propagation in complex networks. The objective at this point is to continue deepening the conceptual bases, to transcend the principle of homogeneity that limits the range of application of classical compartment models.

2. Study of the dynamics of models with the purpose of identifying parametric regions for which such dynamics reflect states consistent with the behavior of an epidemic in certain phases, such as, for example, endemicity or recurring or periodic behaviors. One of the objectives, in this case, is to obtain such parametric regions in terms of systems of mathematical inequalities which represent relationships between the parameters and that can be interpreted as, for example, conditions for the occurrence of an epidemic outbreak. In this case, the tools of bifurcation theory should be exploited in finite-dimensional dynamical systems and, in particular, the existence of Hopf and backward bifurcations.

3. Study of the dynamics of the disease, considering models with coefficients dependent on the time variable, whose evolution presents a periodic behavior. The question in this case is when

these conditions translate into a recurrent behavior of the contagion dynamics, analogous to that of the coefficients.

4. Study the problem of the existence, uniqueness, and regularization of the identification of coefficients in the models from previously processed data, to eliminate the inherent instability of the identification process. In this case, it is important to consider that the coefficients are functions of time, which represent the human behavior, and the frequency with which certain periodic social activities are carried out that lead to human mobility.
5. Study of control problems to determine the optimal strategy for vaccination, in the presence of simultaneous variants of the virus and the division of the susceptible population into vulnerable and less vulnerable to the disease.
6. Complement the study of the multiobjective control problem, already partially studied, which corresponds to reducing the number of infected individuals, in the presence of a vaccination campaign, and fully developing the activities which have maximum priority for the development of a country.
7. Another interesting problem that is indirectly related to the propagation behavior of the disease, is the proposal and study of a model that describes the response of the immune system to disease or vaccines. At this point, two objectives are proposed: first, to determine the optimal treatment application strategy in the two important periods of the disease (viral replication and inflammatory period), seeking to reduce the mean period of infectivity and the mortality rate. Second, to study at the individual level the effect of vaccines, according to the components of the immune system that they reinforce, to be able to include estimates of the time that the immunity provided by them could last.

4 CONCLUDING REMARKS

We have divided the discussion in this chapter into three sections.

The first of them has been of an introductory nature and was dedicated to showing the principles that justify the need for mathematical modeling in Epidemiology.

Section 2 discusses the importance of conceptualizing the COVID-19 disease and the associated pandemic, from different perspectives ranging from the different stages of biological organization in which the interaction of the SARS-CoV-2 virus with the organism is manifested, the temporal evolution of the disease at the individual level and the evolution of the pandemic at the country level and worldwide, up to the collateral consequences of the pandemic for human health, society, and the economy.

The analysis of these perspectives allows to extract important information to compose the mathematical models that have been used during the pandemic and define the approach to many practical problems associated with them.

Finally, we dedicate Section 3 to describe the importance of the results that have been obtained through mathematical models and discuss some possible prospects for working with them.

We have emphasized the role of mathematical modeling, since nowadays Epidemiology requires a contribution, which is irreplaceable, from Mathematics, Statistics, and Data analysis, to establish strategies that allow facing the spread of a disease such as COVID-19, at different levels of the societal structure.

A mere analysis of data with calculations of trends, averages, and other indicators, albeit essential, is not enough to make predictions that support correct decisions, except in the very short term.

Only mathematical models can comprehensively include all important information that can influence the dynamics of the disease propagation process, allowing conclusions to be drawn about the role of prophylactic measures, vaccination campaigns, diagnostic tests, and the different therapeutic protocols treatments they play, at the population level.

The results obtained from these studies can potentially help to predict the incidence of infections, the need for hospitalization and ICU occupancy, and possible death.

Only on the basis of this type of information, it is possible to establish the best strategy to stop the spread of the virus.

Medications, treatments, and vaccines are essential to limit contagion, help patients recover, and reduce the likelihood of death. However, when all this arsenal of resources are used to contain the pandemic, global strategies are required that can only be designed and implemented with solid scientific foundations. In this framework, the study of mathematical models plays a fundamental role.

5 CONSENT FOR PUBLICATION

Not applicable.

6 CONFLICT OF INTEREST

The authors declare no conflict of interest, financial or otherwise.

7 ACKNOWLEDGEMENTS

Authors acknowledge CONACYT financial support of MSB through "Cátedras CONACYT para Jóvenes Investigadores 2016" program, and SEP financial support of RFS through Postdoctoral scholarship program.

References

[1] Thompson L. Inicio de una nueva epidemia, SARS. Revista Médica Herediana [Internet]. 2013 Jan 22 [cited 2021 Jul 1];14(2):49. Available from: https://doi.org/10.20453/rmh.v14i2.753

[2] Clinical decision support for health professionals [Internet]. Overview of coronaviruses - patient leaflets — BMJ best practice; [cited 2021 Jun 22]. Available from: https://bestpractice.bmj.com/topics/en-gb/3000165/patient-leaflets

[3] Ministerio de Sanidad. Información científico técnica. Enfermedad por coronavirus, covid-19. [Internet]. Madrid: [publisher unknown]; 2021 Jan [cited 2021 Jun 22]. 111 p. Available from: https://www.mscbs.gob.es/profesionales/saludPublica/ccayes/alertasActual/nCov/documentos/ITCoronavirus.pdf

[4] Maguiña Vargas C, Gastelo Acosta R, Tequen Bernilla A. El nuevo Coronavirus y la pandemia del Covid-19. Revista Médica Herediana [Internet]. 2020 Jul 31 [cited 2021 Jun 23];31(2):125–31. Available from: https://doi.org/10.20453/rmh.v31i2.3776

[5] WHO | World Health Organization [Internet]. WHO statement on novel coronavirus in Thailand; [cited 2021 Jun 22]. Available from: https://www.who.int/news/item/13-01-2020-who-statement-on-novel-coronavirus-in-thailand

[6] Yonhap News Agency [Internet]. S. Korea reports 1st confirmed case of China coronavirus | Yonhap News Agency; [cited 2021 Jun 22]. Available from: https://en.yna.co.kr/view/AEN20200120004500320

[7] AHO/WHO | Pan American Health Organization [Internet]. CD58/6 - la pandemia de COVID-19 en la región de las américas - OPS/OMS | organización panamericana de la salud; 2020 Sep 5 [cited 2021 Jun 22]. Available from: https://www.paho.org/es/documentos/cd586-pandemia-covid-19-region-americas

[8] Barberena FC. France 24 [Internet]. Francia confirmó tres casos de coronavirus, los primeros en Europa; 2020 Jan 24 [cited 2021 Jun 22]. Available from: https://www.france24.com/es/20200124-francia-confirm%C3%B3-dos-casos-de-coronavirus-los-primeros-en-europa

[9] BBC News Mundo [Internet]. Cómo Italia se convirtió en el foco de coronavirus más grande de Europa y en el origen de los casos de México y Brasil-BBC News Mundo; [cited 2021 Jun 22]. Available from: https://www.bbc.com/mundo/noticias-51647372

[10] El Médico Interactivo [Internet]. Primer caso confirmado de Covid-19 en México; [cited 2021 Jun 22]. Available from: https://elmedicointeractivo.com/primer-caso-confirmado-de-covid-19-en%20mexico/

[11] WHO|World Health Organization [Internet]. WHO Director-General's opening remarks at the media briefing on COVID-19 - 11 March 2020; [cited 2021 Jun 22]. Available from: https://www.who.int/director-general/speeches/detail/who-director-general-s-opening-remarks-at-the-media-briefing-on-covid-19---11-march-2020

[12] Johns Hopkins Coronavirus Resource Center [Internet]. COVID-19 map - Johns

Hopkins coronavirus resource center; [cited 2021 Jun 22]. Available from: https://coronavirus.jhu.edu/map.html

[13] Moon JY, Yoon DY, Hong JH, Lim KJ, Baek S, Seo YL, Yun EJ. The most widely disseminated covid-19-related scientific publications in online media: a bibliometric analysis of the top 100 articles with the highest altmetric attention scores. Healthcare [Internet]. 2021 Feb 23 [cited 2021 Jun 22];9(2):239. Available from: https://doi.org/10.3390/healthcare9020239

[14] Else H. How a torrent of COVID science changed research publishing—in seven charts. Nature [Internet]. 2020 Dec 16 [cited 2021 Jun 22];588(7839):553. Available from: https://doi.org/10.1038/d41586-020-03564-y

[15] A contribution to the mathematical theory of epidemics. Proceedings of the Royal Society of London. Series A, Containing Papers of a Mathematical and Physical Character [Internet]. 1927 Aug [cited 2021 Jun 22];115(772):700–21. Available from: https://doi.org/10.1098/rspa.1927.0118

[16] Kermack W, Mckendrick A. Contributions to the mathematical theory of epidemics–II. the problem of endemicity. Bulletin of Mathematical Biology [Internet]. 1991 [cited 2021 Jun 22];53(1-2):57–87. Available from: https://doi.org/10.1016/s0092-8240(05)80041-2

[17] Kermack W, Mckendrick A. Contributions to the mathematical theory of epidemics–III. Further studies of the problem of endemicity. Bulletin of Mathematical Biology [Internet]. 1991 [cited 2021 Jun 22];53(1-2):89–118. Available from: https://doi.org/10.1016/s0092-8240(05)80042-4

[18] Kermack WO, McKendrick AG. Contributions to the mathematical theory of epidemics IV. Analysis of experimental epidemics of the virus disease mouse ectromelia. Journal of

Hygiene [Internet]. 1937 Apr [cited 2021 Jun 22];37(2):172–87. Available from: https://doi.org/10.1017/s0022172400034902

[19] Kermack WO, McKendrick AG. Contributions to the mathematical theory of epidemics: V. Analysis of experimental epidemics of mouse-typhoid; a bacterial disease conferring incomplete immunity. Journal of Hygiene [Internet]. 1939 May [cited 2021 Jun 22];39(3):271–88. Available from: https://doi.org/10.1017/s0022172400011918

[20] Kermack WO, McKendrick AG. Contributions to the mathematical theory of epidemics–I. Bulletin of Mathematical Biology [Internet]. 1991 Mar [cited 2021 Jun 22];53(1-2):33–55. Available from: https://doi.org/10.1007/bf02464423

[21] WHO|World Health Organization [Internet]. Tracking SARS-CoV-2 variants; [cited 2021 Aug 28]. Available from: https://www.who.int/en/activities/tracking-SARS-CoV-2-variants/.

[22] Bennett JE, Dolin R, Blaser MJ. Mandell, Douglas, and Bennett's Principles and Practice of Infectious Diseases. 9th ed. Churchill Livingstone: Elsevier; 2020

[23] Villarreal LP. Viruses and the evolution of life. Washington DC: ASM Press; 2005. 395 p.

[24] BBC News Mundo [Internet]. Delta plus: lo que se sabe de la nueva variante de Covid-19 detectada ya en 10 países - BBC News Mundo; 2021 Jun 23 [cited 2021 Jun 24]. Available from: https://www.bbc.com/mundo/noticias-57581280

[25] Redacción. El Financiero [Internet]. Epsilon: esto es lo que sabemos sobre la variante del coronavirus y cómo evade las vacunas; 2021 Jul 6 [cited 2021 Aug 28]. Available from: https://www.elfinanciero.com.mx/salud/2021/07/06/epsilon-esto-es-lo-que-sabemos-sobre-la-variante-del-coronavirus-y-como-evade-las-vacunas/

[26] CNN [Internet]. Variante delta en Europa: peligran las reaperturas ante la versión; [cited 2021 Aug 3]. Available from: https://cnnespanol.cnn.com/2021/07/12/variante-delta-covid-reapertura-europa-trax/.

[27] BBC News Mundo [Internet]. Las autoridades en EE.UU. advierten que la variante delta es tan contagiosa como el sarampión y puede ser transmitida por los vacunados - BBC News Mundo; 2021 Jul 30 [cited 2021 Aug 3]. Available from: https://www.bbc.com/mundo/noticias-internacional-58034383

[28] Nius Diario [Internet]. Los epidemiólogos advierten: "Otras variantes contagiaban a dos personas de media, delta a cinco"; 2021 Jul 6 [cited 2021 Jul 6]. Available from: https://www.niusdiario.es/sociedad/sanidad/epidemiologos-advierten-otras-variantes-contagian-dos-personas-delta-puede-infectar-cinco_18_3165495970.html

[29] Topley WW, Wilson GS. The Spread of Bacterial Infection. The Problem of Herd-Immunity. Journal of Hygiene [Internet]. 1923 May [cited 2021 Aug 11];21(3):243–9. Available from: https://doi.org/10.1017/s0022172400031478

[30] Jones D, Helmreich S. A history of herd immunity. The Lancet [Internet]. 2020 Sep [cited 2021 Aug 3];396(10254):810–1. Available from: https://doi.org/10.1016/s0140-6736(20)31924-3

[31] The Conversation [Internet]. La inmunidad de grupo: ¿es la solución a todos los problemas pandémicos?; 2021 May 24 [cited 2021 Jun 22]. Available from: https://theconversation.com/la-inmunidad-de-grupo-es-la-solucion-a-todos-los-problemas-pandemicos-161193

[32] Stebbing J, Phelan A, Griffin I, Tucker C, Oechsle O, Smith D, Richardson P. COVID-19: combining antiviral and anti-inflammatory treatments. The Lancet Infectious Diseases

[Internet]. 2020 Apr [cited 2021 Sep 22];20(4):400–2. Available from: https://doi.org/10.1016/s1473-3099(20)30132-8

[33] Gil Cuesta J, Vaqué Rafart J. Aspectos básicos de la transmisibilidad. Vacunas [Internet]. 2008 Jan [cited 2021 Sep 22];9(1):25–33. Available from: https://doi.org/10.1016/s1576-9887(08)71918-6

[34] Madas BG, Füri P, Farkas Á, Nagy A, Czitrovszky A, Balásházy I, Schay GG, Horváth A. Deposition distribution of the new coronavirus (SARS-CoV-2) in the human airways upon exposure to cough-generated droplets and aerosol particles. Scientific Reports [Internet]. 2020 Dec [cited 2021 Jun 22];10(1). Available from: https://doi.org/10.1038/s41598-020-79985-6

[35] Rosti ME, Olivieri S, Cavaiola M, Seminara A, Mazzino A. Fluid dynamics of COVID-19 airborne infection suggests urgent data for a scientific design of social distancing. Scientific Reports [Internet]. 2020 Dec [cited 2021 Aug 2];10(1). Available from: https://doi.org/10.1038/s41598-020-80078-7

[36] Issakhov A, Zhandaulet Y, Omarova P, Alimbek A, Borsikbayeva A, Mustafayeva A. A numerical assessment of social distancing of preventing airborne transmission of COVID-19 during different breathing and coughing processes. Scientific Reports [Internet]. 2021 May 3 [cited 2021 Jun 22];11(1). Available from: https://doi.org/10.1038/s41598-021-88645-2

[37] Crawford C, Vanoli E, Decorde B, Lancelot M, Duprat C, Josserand C, Jilesen J, Bouadma L, Timsit JF. Modeling of aerosol transmission of airborne pathogens in ICU rooms of COVID-19 patients with acute respiratory failure. Scientific Reports [Internet]. 2021 Jun 3 [cited 2021 Jun 22];11(1). Available from: https://doi.org/10.1038/s41598-021-91265-5

[38] SESA – Sociedad Española de Sanidad Ambiental [Internet]. 2021 Jul 23 [cited 2021 Aug 28]. Available from: https://www.sanidadambiental.com/wp-content/uploads/2020/09/Transmisi%C3%B3n-del-SARS-CoV-2-por-gotas-respiratorias-objetos-contaminados-y-aerosoles.pdf

[39] Transmission of SARS-CoV-2: implications for infection prevention precautions: scientific brief, 09 July 2020 [Internet]; 2020 Jul 1 [cited 2021 Jun 22]. Available from: https://apps.who.int/iris/handle/10665/333114

[40] Jones TC, Biele G, Mühlemann B, Veith T, Schneider J, Beheim-Schwarzbach J, Bleicker T, Tesch J, Schmidt ML, Sander LE, Kurth F, Menzel P, Schwarzer R, Zuchowski M, Hofmann J, Krumbholz A, Stein A, Edelmann A, Corman VM, Drosten C. Estimating infectiousness throughout SARS-CoV-2 infection course. Science [Internet]. 2021 May 25 [cited 2021 Jun 22];373(6551):1–14. Available from: https://doi.org/10.1126/science.abi5273

[41] Yang Q, Saldi TK, Gonzales PK, Lasda E, Decker CJ, Tat KL, et al. Just 2% of SAR-CoV-2-positive individuals carry 90% of the virus circulating in communities. Proceedings of the National Academy of Sciences [Internet]. 2021 May 10 [cited 2021 Jun 22];118(21):21. Available from: https://doi.org/10.1073/pnas.2104547118

[42] Laxminarayan R, Wahl B, Dudala SR, Gopal K, Mohan B C, Neelima S, Jawahar Reddy KS, Radhakrishnan J, Lewnard JA. Epidemiology and transmission dynamics of COVID-19 in two Indian states. Science [Internet]. 2020 Sep 30 [cited 2021 Jun 22];370(6517):691–7. Available from: https://doi.org/10.1126/science.abd7672

[43] Sun K, Wang W, Gao L, Wang Y, Luo K, Ren L, Zhan Z, Chen X, Zhao S, Huang Y, Sun Q, Liu Z, Litvinova M, Vespignani A, Ajelli M, Viboud C, Yu H. Transmission heterogeneities, kinetics, and controllability of SARS-CoV-2. Science [Internet]. 2020 Nov 24 [cited 2021 Jun 22]:2424. Available from: https://doi.org/10.1126/science.abe2424

[44] BBC News Mundo [Internet]. ¿Cuándo una persona enferma de covid-19 deja de ser contagiosa (tenga o no síntomas)? - BBC News Mundo; 2020 Nov 17 [cited 2021 Jun 24]. Available from: https://www.bbc.com/mundo/noticias-54828774

[45] Quesada JA, López-Pineda A, Gil-Guillén VF, Arriero-Marín JM, Gutiérrez F, Carratala-Munuera C. Incubation period of COVID-19: a systematic review and meta-analysis. Revista Clínica Española (English Edition) [Internet]. 2020 Nov [cited 2021 Jun 22]. Available from: https://doi.org/10.1016/j.rceng.2020.08.002

[46] Zaki N, Mohamed EA. The estimations of the COVID-19 incubation period: a scoping reviews of the literature. Journal of Infection and Public Health [Internet]. 2021 May [cited 2021 Jun 22];14(5):638–46. Available from: https://doi.org/10.1016/j.jiph.2021.01.019

[47] Ejima K, Kim KS, Ludema C, Bento AI, Iwanami S, Fujita Y, Ohashi H, Koizumi Y, Watashi K, Aihara K, Nishiura H, Iwami S. Estimation of the incubation period of COVID-19 using viral load data. Epidemics [Internet]. 2021 Jun [cited 2021 Jun 22];35:100454. Available from: https://doi.org/10.1016/j.epidem.2021.100454

[48] Ministerio de Sanidad, Consumo y Bienestar Social [Internet]. 2021 Jul 23 [cited 2021 Jul 23]. Available from: https://www.mscbs.gob.es/profesionales/saludPublica/ccayes/alertasActual/nCov/documentos/COVID19_Estrategia_vigilancia_y_control_e_indicadores.pdf

[49] McAloon C, Collins Á, Hunt K, Barber A, Byrne AW, Butler F, Casey M, Griffin J, Lane E, McEvoy D, Wall P, Green M, O'Grady L, More SJ. Incubation period of COVID-19: a rapid systematic review and meta-analysis of observational research. BMJ Open [Internet]. 2020 Aug [cited 2021 Jun 22];10(8):039652. Available from: https://doi.org/10.1136/bmjopen-2020-039652

[50] Anderson RM, Heesterbeek H, Klinkenberg D, Hollingsworth TD. How will country-based mitigation measures influence the course of the COVID-19 epidemic? The Lancet [Internet]. 2020 Mar [cited 2021 Jun 22];395(10228):931–4. Available from: https://doi.org/10.1016/s0140-6736(20)30567-5

[51] Hellewell J, Abbott S, Gimma A, Bosse NI, Jarvis CI, Russell TW, et al. Feasibility of controlling COVID-19 outbreaks by isolation of cases and contacts. The Lancet Global Health [Internet]. 2020 Apr [cited 2021 Sep 22];8(4):e488-e496. Available from: https://doi.org/10.1016/s2214-109x(20)30074-7

[52] Cevik M, Tate M, Lloyd O, Maraolo AE, Schafers J, Ho A. SARS-CoV-2, SARS-CoV, and MERS-CoV viral load dynamics, duration of viral shedding, and infectiousness: a systematic review and meta-analysis. The Lancet Microbe [Internet]. 2020 Nov [cited 2021 Jun 22]. Available from: https://doi.org/10.1016/s2666-5247(20)30172-5

[53] Role of asymptomatic infected people in the transmission of the SARS-CoV-2 coronavirus [Internet]. Galicia; 2020 Apr. Informe de Unidad de Asesoramiento Científico-técnico, Avalia-t, de la Agencia del Conocimiento en Salud (ACIS). Available from: https://coronavirus.sergas.gal/Contidos/Documents/290/CompilacResumos_Asintomaticos.pdf

[54] Johansson MA, Quandelacy TM, Kada S, Prasad PV, Steele M, Brooks JT, Slayton RB, Biggerstaff M, Butler JC. SARS-CoV-2 transmission from people without COVID-19 symptoms. JAMA Network Open [Internet]. 2021 Jan 7 [cited 2021 Jun 22];4(1):2035057. Available from: https://doi.org/10.1001/jamanetworkopen.2020.35057

[55] Wei WE, Li Z, Chiew CJ, Yong SE, Toh MP, Lee VJ. Presymptomatic Transmission Of Sars-Cov-2 – Singapore, January 23–march 16, 2020. MMWR. Morbidity and Mortality Weekly Report [Internet]. 2020 Apr 10 [cited 2021 Jun 27];69(14):411–5. Available from: https://doi.org/10.15585/mmwr.mm6914e1

[56] Park SW, Cornforth DM, Dushoff J, Weitz JS. The time scale of asymptomatic transmission affects estimates of epidemic potential in the COVID-19 outbreak. Epidemics [Internet]. 2020 Jun [cited 2021 Jun 27];31:100392. Available from: https://doi.org/10.1016/j.epidem.2020.100392

[57] Li R, Pei S, Chen B, Song Y, Zhang T, Yang W, Shaman J. Substantial undocumented infection facilitates the rapid dissemination of novel coronavirus (SARS-CoV-2). Science [Internet]. 2020 Mar 16 [cited 2021 Jun 27];368(6490):489–93. Available from: https://doi.org/10.1126/science.abb3221

[58] WHO | World Health Organization [Internet]. COVID-19 Clinical management: living guidance; 2021 Jan 25 [cited 2021 Jun 27]. Available from: https://www.who.int/publications/i/item/WHO-2019-nCoV-clinical-2021-1

[59] Workman J. The Proportion Of Covid-19 Cases That Are Asymptomatic In South Korea: Comment On Nishiura Et Al. International Journal of Infectious Diseases [Internet]. 2020 Jul [cited 2021 Jun 27];96:398. Available from: https://doi.org/10.1016/j.ijid.2020.05.037

[60] Médica Sur: Excelencia médica, calidez humana. [Internet]. ¿Quieres saber sobre COVID 19?; [cited 2021 Jun 27]. Available from: https://www.medicasur.com.mx/es_mx/ms/Identifica_COVID_19_leve_moderado_o_grave

[61] Long QX, Tang XJ, Shi QL, Li Q, Deng HJ, Yuan J, Hu JL, Xu W, Zhang Y, Lv FJ, Su K, Zhang F, Gong J, Wu B, Liu XM, Li JJ, Qiu JF, Chen J, Huang AL. Clinical and immunological assessment of asymptomatic SARS-CoV-2 infections. Nature Medicine [Internet]. 2020 Jun 18 [cited 2021 Jun 27];26(8):1200–4. Available from: https://doi.org/10.1038/s41591-020-0965-6

[62] Redacción Médica [Internet]. Coronavirus y estudio de seroprevalencia: cómo se

hace y para qué sirve; 2020 Apr 27 [cited 2021 Jun 28]. Available from: https://www.redaccionmedica.com/secciones/sanidad-hoy/coronavirus-y-estudio-de-seroprevalencia-como-se-hara-y-para-que-sirve-1789

[63] CuidatePlus [Internet]. PCR, IgG, IgM y antígenos: ¿Cómo sé si he pasado el coronavirus?; [cited 2021 Jun 28]. Available from: https://cuidateplus.marca.com/bienestar/2020/07/30/pcr-igg-e-igm-como-se-he-pasado-coronavirus-174147.html

[64] Centers for Disease Control and Prevention [Internet]. El COVID-19 y su salud; 2021 Jul 15 [cited 2021 Aug 28]. Available from: https://espanol.cdc.gov/coronavirus/2019-ncov/testing/serology-overview.html

[65] Centers for Disease Control and Prevention [Internet]. SARS-CoV-2 Testing Strategy: Considerations for Non-Healthcare Workplaces; 2020 Mar 17 [cited 2021 Aug 28]. Available from: https://www.cdc.gov/coronavirus/2019-ncov/community/organizations/testing-non-healthcare-workplaces.html

[66] Pan Y, Zhang D, Yang P, Poon LL, Wang Q. Viral load of SARS-CoV-2 in clinical samples. The Lancet Infectious Diseases [Internet]. 2020 Apr [cited 2021 Aug 28];20(4):411–2. Available from: https://doi.org/10.1016/s1473-3099(20)30113-4

[67] ELMUNDO [Internet]. ¿Qué pasa cuando te contagias de Covid estando vacunado?; 2021 Aug 3 [cited 2021 Aug 4]. Available from: https://www.elmundo.es/ciencia-y-salud/salud/2021/08/03/6108cf92fc6c83ee208b459b.html

[68] Dan JM, Mateus J, Kato Y, Hastie KM, Yu ED, Faliti CE, et al. Immunological memory to SARS-CoV-2 assessed for up to 8 months after infection. Science [Internet].

2021 Jan 6 [cited 2021 Aug 11]:4063. Available from: https://doi.org/10.1126/science.abf4063

[69] Blanco Arbués J, Sarukhan A, Díez Antón J, Bassat Orellana Q, Campins Martí M, Güerri Fernández R, Brotons C, Sans Corrales M, Miró Meda JM, Sanjosé Llongueras SD. What do we know about Immunity to SARS-CoV-2? Implications for Public Health Policies. Barcelona: Institut de Salut Global de Barcelona (ISGlobal); 2021 Feb.

[70] Turner JS, Kim W, Kalaidina E, Goss CW, Rauseo AM, Schmitz AJ, Hansen L, Haile A, Klebert MK, Pusic I, O'Halloran JA, Presti RM, Ellebedy AH. SARS-CoV-2 infection induces long-lived bone marrow plasma cells in humans. Nature [Internet]. 2021 May 24 [cited 2021 Aug 28];595(7867):421–5. Available from: https://doi.org/10.1038/s41586-021-03647-4

[71] RTVE.es [Internet]. Coronavirus | Fase 0: España comienza su desescalada gradual tras 50 días de estricto confinamiento; [cited 2021 Jun 28]. Available from: https://www.rtve.es/noticias/20200504/fase-0-espana-comienza-su-desescalada-gradual-tras-50-dias-estricto-confinamiento/2013250.shtml

[72] Redacción Médica [Internet]. Coronavirus: infectados en España y la evolución del brote desde el origen; [cited 2021 Jun 28]. Available from: https://www.redaccionmedica.com/secciones/sanidad-hoy/coronavirus-infectados-espana-y-evolucion-covid19-desde-origen-4148

[73] Coronavirus – gob.mx [Internet]. Inicia la fase 3 por COVID-19 – Coronavirus; [cited 2021 Jun 28]. Available from: https://coronavirus.gob.mx/2020/04/21/inicia-la-fase-3-por-covid-19-2/

[74] COVID-19 [Internet]. Plan gradual hacia la Nueva Normalidad; [cited 2021 Jun 28]. Available from: https://covid19.cdmx.gob.mx/nuevanormalidad

[75] Coronavirus – gob.mx [Internet]. Semáforo – Coronavirus; [cited 2021 Jun 28]. Available from: https://coronavirus.gob.mx/semaforo/

[76] WHO | World Health Organization [Internet]. Elevating political leadership for Pandemic Preparedness and Response Meeting with the UN General Assembly; [cited 2021 Aug 8]. Available from: https://www.who.int/news/item/28-07-2021-elevating-political-leadership-for-pandemic-preparedness-and-response-meeting-with-the-un-general-assembly

[77] WHO | World Health Organization [Internet]. HE Ellen Johnson Sirleaf and Rt Hon. Helen Clark brief Member States at the United Nations General Assembly on pandemic response; [cited 2021 Sep 23]. Available from: https://www.who.int/news/item/28-07-2021-he-ellen-johnson-sirleaf-and-rt-hon.-helen-clark-brief-member-states-at-the-united-nations-general-assembly-on-pandemic-response

[78] Sachs JD, Abdool Karim S, Aknin L, Allen J, Brosbøl K, Cuevas Barron G, et al. Priorities for the COVID-19 pandemic at the start of 2021: statement of the Lancet COVID-19 Commission. The Lancet [Internet]. 2021 Mar [cited 2021 Aug 8];397(10278):947-50. Available from: https://doi.org/10.1016/s0140-6736(21)00388-3

[79] World Trade Organization - Home page - Global trade [Internet]. World Bank, IMF, WHO, WTO heads call for urgent action to accelerate global vaccine access; [cited 2021 Jun 28]. Available from: https://www.wto.org/spanish/news_s/news21_s/covid_30jun21_s.htm

[80] WHO | World Health Organization [Internet]. Vaccine equity; [cited 2021 Aug 8]. Available from: https://www.who.int/campaigns/vaccine-equity

[81] World Trade Organization - Home page - Global trade [Internet]. WTO receives petition asking for universally accessible and affordable COVID-19 vaccines; [cited 2021 Jun 22]. Available from: https://www.wto.org/english/news_e/news20_e/trip_09dec20_e.htm

[82] Alliance PV. Medium [Internet]. Open Letter: Former Heads of State and Nobel Laureates Call on President Biden To Waive...; 2021 Apr 14 [cited 2021 Aug 28]. Available from: https://peoplesvaccinealliance.medium.com/open-letter-former-heads-of-state-and-nobel-laureates-call-on-president-biden-to-waive-e0589edd5704

[83] UN News [Internet]. WHO chief hails 'monumental moment' in COVID fight, as US throws support behind vaccine patent waiver; [cited 2021 Aug 8]. Available from: https://news.un.org/en/story/2021/05/1091382

[84] Krishtel P, Malpani R. Suspend intellectual property rights for covid-19 vaccines. BMJ [Internet]. 2021 May 28 [cited 2021 Aug 8]:1344. Available from: https://doi.org/10.1136/bmj.n1344

[85] Storz U. The patent maze of COVID 19 vaccines. Expert Opinion on Therapeutic Patents [Internet]. 2021 Jul 26 [cited 2021 Aug 28]:1–12. Available from: https://doi.org/10.1080/13543776.2021.1945581

[86] Home - Consilium [Internet]. Cumbre del G-7, Cornualles (Reino Unido), 11 a 13 de junio de 2021; [cited 2021 Jun 28]. Available from: https://www.consilium.europa.eu/es/meetings/international-summit/2021/06/11-13/

[87] Ramírez DB. France 24 [Internet]. Economía - Cumbre del G7: tanto anuncios como críticas tras el encuentro de los países más poderosos; 2021 Jun 15 [cited 2021 Jun 28]. Available from: https://www.france24.com/es/programas/econom%C3%B3a/20210615-economia-cumbre-paises-g7-anuncios-criticas

[88] Zou D, et al. Epidemic Model Guided Machine Learning for COVID-19 Forecasts in the United States; 2020. 15 p. medRxiv preprint. Available from: https://doi.org/10.1101/2020.05.24.20111989

[89] Tiwari I, Sarin P, Parmananda P. Predictive modeling of disease propagation in a mobile, connected community using cellular automata. Chaos: An Interdisciplinary Journal of Nonlinear Science [Internet]. 2020 Aug [cited 2021 Aug 8];30(8):081103. Available from: https://doi.org/10.1063/5.0021113

[90] Aleta A, Martín-Corral D, Pastore y Piontti A, Ajelli M, Litvinova M, Chinazzi M, Dean NE, Halloran ME, Longini Jr IM, Merler S, Pentland A, Vespignani A, Moro E, Moreno Y. Modelling the impact of testing, contact tracing and household quarantine on second waves of COVID-19. Nature Human Behaviour [Internet]. 2020 Aug 5 [cited 2021 Aug 28];4(9):964–71. Available from: https://doi.org/10.1038/s41562-020-0931-9

[91] Firth JA, Hellewell J, Klepac P, Kissler S, Kucharski AJ, Spurgin LG. Using a real-world network to model localized COVID-19 control strategies. Nature Medicine [Internet]. 2020 Aug 7 [cited 2021 Aug 28];26(10):1616–22. Available from: https://doi.org/10.1038/s41591-020-1036-8

[92] Leng T, White C, Hilton J, Kucharski A, Pellis L, Stage H, Davies NG, Keeling MJ, Flasche S. The effectiveness of social bubbles as part of a Covid-19 lockdown exit strategy, a modelling study. Wellcome Open Research [Internet]. 2021 Mar 29 [cited 2021 Aug 28];5:213. Available from: https://doi.org/10.12688/wellcomeopenres.16164.2

[93] Real Academia de Ciencias Exactas Físicas Naturales. YouTube [Internet]. [Video], Respuesta de la comunidad matemática a la pandemia de COVID-19; 2021 Mar 3 [cited 2021 Aug 28]; [107 min., 28 sec.]. Available from: https://www.youtube.com/watch?v=b2UwpvA6NcY

[94] Hethcote HW. The Mathematics of Infectious Diseases. SIAM Review [Internet]. 2000 Jan [cited 2021 Aug 11];42(4):599–653. Available from: https://doi.org/10.1137/s0036144500371907

[95] Anderson RM. Directly transmitted viral and bacterial infections of man. In: The Population Dynamics of Infectious Diseases: Theory and Applications [Internet]. Boston, MA: Springer US; 1982 [cited 2021 Aug 28]. p. 1–37. Available from: https://doi.org/10.1007/978-1-4899-2901-3_1

[96] May RM, Anderson B, Anderson RM. Infectious Diseases of Humans: Dynamics and Control. Oxford: Oxford University Press, USA; 1992. 766 p.

[97] Brauer F. Compartmental Models in Epidemiology. In: Mathematical Epidemiology [Internet]. Berlin, Heidelberg: Springer Berlin Heidelberg; 2008 [cited 2021 Aug 28]. p. 19–79. Available from: https://doi.org/10.1007/978-3-540-78911-6_2

[98] Diekmann O, Heesterbeek JA. Mathematical Epidemiology of Infectious Diseases: Model Building, Analysis and Interpretation. West Sussex: Wiley; 2000. 303 p.

[99] Castillo-Chavez C, Brauer F. Mathematical Models in Population Biology and Epidemiology. New York: Springer; 2001. 448 p.

[100] Brauer F, Kribs C. Dynamical Systems for Biological Modeling [Internet]. Boca Raton: Chapman and Hall/CRC; 2015 [cited 2021 Sep 23]. Available from: https://doi.org/10.1201/b20687

[101] Brauer F, van den Driessche P, Wu J, editors. Mathematical Epidemiology [Internet]. Berlin, Heidelberg: Springer Berlin Heidelberg; 2008 [cited 2021 Sep 23]. Available from: https://doi.org/10.1007/978-3-540-78911-6

[102] Keeling MJ, Rohani P. Modeling Infectious Diseases in Humans and Animals. Princeton: Princeton University Press; 2007. 408 p.

[103] Martcheva M. An Introduction to Mathematical Epidemiology. New York: Springer; 2015. 467 p.

[104] Vynnycky E, White R. An Introduction To Infectious Disease Modelling. Oxford: Oxford University Press, USA; 2010.

[105] Abbott S, Hellewell J, Thompson RN, Sherratt K, Gibbs HP, Bosse NI, et al. Estimating the time-varying reproduction number of SARS-CoV-2 using national and subnational case counts. Wellcome Open Research [Internet]. 2020 Jun 1 [cited 2021 Aug 8];5:112. Available from: https://doi.org/10.12688/wellcomeopenres.16006.1

[106] Park SW, Bolker BM, Funk S, Metcalf CJ, Weitz JS, Grenfell BT, Dushoff J. Roles of generation-interval distributions in shaping relative epidemic strength, speed, and control of new SARS-CoV-2 variants. MedRxiv. 2021 Mar 5.

[107] Zhao S, Cao P, Gao D, Zhuang Z, Cai Y, Ran J, Chong MK, Wang K, Lou Y, Wang W, Yang L, He D, Wang MH. Serial interval in determining the estimation of reproduction number of the novel coronavirus disease (COVID-19) during the early outbreak. Journal of Travel Medicine [Internet]. 2020 Mar 12 [cited 2021 Aug 8];27(3). Available from: https://doi.org/10.1093/jtm/taaa033

[108] Zhao S, Cao P, Chong MK, Gao D, Lou Y, Ran J, Wang K, Wang W, Yang L, He D, Wang MH. COVID-19 and gender-specific difference: Analysis of public surveillance data in Hong Kong and Shenzhen, China, from January 10 to February 15, 2020. Infection Control &

Hospital Epidemiology [Internet]. 2020 Mar 9 [cited 2021 Aug 18];41(6):750-1. Available from: https://doi.org/10.1017/ice.2020.64

[109] Wong GN, Weiner ZJ, Tkachenko AV, Elbanna A, Maslov S, Goldenfeld N. Modeling COVID-19 Dynamics in Illinois under Nonpharmaceutical Interventions. Physical Review X [Internet]. 2020 Nov 16 [cited 2021 Aug 28];10(4). Available from: https://doi.org/10.1103/physrevx.10.041033

[110] Tkachenko AV, Maslov S, Elbanna A, Wong GN, Weiner ZJ, Goldenfeld N. Time-dependent heterogeneity leads to transient suppression of the COVID-19 epidemic, not herd immunity. Proceedings of the National Academy of Sciences [Internet]. 2021 Apr 8 [cited 2021 Jun 22];118(17):e2015972118. Available from: https://doi.org/10.1073/pnas.2015972118

[111] He D, Dushoff J, Day T, Ma J, Earn DJ. Inferring the causes of the three waves of the 1918 influenza pandemic in England and Wales. Proceedings of the Royal Society B: Biological Sciences [Internet]. 2013 Sep 7 [cited 2021 Aug 23];280(1766):20131345. Available from: https://doi.org/10.1098/rspb.2013.1345

[112] Lin Q, Zhao S, Gao D, Lou Y, Yang S, Musa SS, Wang MH, Cai Y, Wang W, Yang L, He D. A conceptual model for the coronavirus disease 2019 (COVID-19) outbreak in Wuhan, China with individual reaction and governmental action. International Journal of Infectious Diseases [Internet]. 2020 Apr [cited 2021 Aug 8];93:211–6. Available from: https://doi.org/10.1016/j.ijid.2020.02.058

[113] Ritchie H, Mathieu E, Rodés-Guirao L, Appel C, Giattino C, Ortiz-Ospina E, Hasell J, Macdonald B, Beltekian D, Roser M. Our World in Data [Internet]. Coronavirus Pandemic (COVID-19) - Statistics and Research; [cited 2021 Jul 1]. Available from: https://ourworldindata.org/coronavirus

[114] Altizer S, Dobson A, Hosseini P, Hudson P, Pascual M, Rohani P. Seasonality and the dynamics of infectious diseases. Ecology Letters [Internet]. 2006 Mar 31 [cited 2021 Aug 8];9(4):467–84. Available from: `https://doi.org/10.1111/j.1461-0248.2005.00879.x`

[115] Augeraud-Véron E, Sari N. Seasonal dynamics in an SIR epidemic system. Journal of Mathematical Biology [Internet]. 2013 Feb 13 [cited 2021 Aug 18];68(3):701–25. Available from: `https://doi.org/10.1007/s00285-013-0645-y`

[116] Jódar L, Villanueva RJ, Arenas A. Modeling the spread of seasonal epidemiological diseases: Theory and applications. Mathematical and Computer Modelling [Internet]. 2008 Aug [cited 2021 Aug 8];48(3-4):548–57. Available from: `https://doi.org/10.1016/j.mcm.2007.08.017`

[117] Katriel G. Existence of Periodic Solutions for the Periodically Forced Sir Model. Journal of Mathematical Sciences [Internet]. 2014 Aug 2 [cited 2021 Aug 8];201(3):335–42. Available from: `https://doi.org/10.1007/s10958-014-1993-x`

[118] Katriel G, Stone L. Attack rates of seasonal epidemics. Mathematical Biosciences [Internet]. 2012 Jan [cited 2021 Aug 8];235(1):56–65. Available from: `https://doi.org/10.1016/j.mbs.2011.10.007`

[119] Mummert A. Studying the recovery procedure for the time-dependent transmission rate(s) in epidemic models. Journal of Mathematical Biology [Internet]. 2012 Jun 20 [cited 2021 Aug 8];67(3):483–507. Available from: `https://doi.org/10.1007/s00285-012-0558-1`

[120] Mena RH, Velasco-Hernandez JX, Mantilla-Beniers NB, Carranco-Sapiéns GA, Benet L, Boyer D, Castillo IP. Using posterior predictive distributions to analyse epidemic models:

COVID-19 in Mexico City. Physical Biology [Internet]. 2020 Sep 22 [cited 2021 Aug 8];17(6):065001. Available from: https://doi.org/10.1088/1478-3975/abb115

[121] Gu Y. COVID-19 Projections Using Machine Learning | We use artificial intelligence to accurately forecast infections, deaths, and recovery timelines of the COVID-19 / coronavirus pandemic in the US and globally [Internet]. COVID-19 Projections | Mexico; [cited 2021 Aug 8]. Available from: https://covid19-projections.com/mexico

[122] sc-cosmo – Stanford-CIDE COronavirus Simulation MOdel [Internet]. [cited 2021 Aug 18]. Available from: https://www.sc-cosmo.org/wp-content/uploads/2020/05/PADeCI_boletin-2-1.pdf

[123] Holmdahl I, Buckee C. Wrong but Useful – What Covid-19 Epidemiologic Models Can and Cannot Tell Us. New England Journal of Medicine [Internet]. 2020 Jul 23 [cited 2021 Aug 12];383(4):303–5. Available from: https://doi.org/10.1056/nejmp2016822

[124] Montesinos-López OA, Hernández-Suárez CM. Modelos matemáticos para enfermedades infecciosas. Salud Pública de México [Internet]. 2007 Jul [cited 2021 Aug 8];49(3). Available from: https://doi.org/10.1590/s0036-36342007000300007

[125] Blackwood JC, Childs LM. An introduction to compartmental modeling for the budding infectious disease modeler. Letters in Biomathematics [Internet]. 2018 Aug 16 [cited 2021 Aug 28];5(1):195–221. Available from: https://doi.org/10.1080/23737867.2018.1509026

[126] Ridenhour B, Kowalik JM, Shay DK. The basic reproductive number R_0: considerations for its application in public health. American Journal of Public Health. 2018;108(16):455–65.

[127] Diekmann O, Heesterbeek JA, Metz JA. On the definition and the computation of the basic reproduction ratio R_0 in models for infectious diseases in heterogeneous populations. Journal

of Mathematical Biology [Internet]. 1990 Jun [cited 2021 Aug 8];28(4). Available from: https://doi.org/10.1007/bf00178324

[128] Diekmann O, Heesterbeek JA, Roberts MG. The construction of next-generation matrices for compartmental epidemic models. Journal of The Royal Society Interface [Internet]. 2009 Nov 5 [cited 2021 Aug 18];7(47):873–85. Available from: https://doi.org/10.1098/rsif.2009.0386

[129] de-Camino-Beck T, Lewis MA, van den Driessche P. A graph-theoretic method for the basic reproduction number in continuous time epidemiological models. Journal of Mathematical Biology [Internet]. 2008 Dec 2 [cited 2021 Aug 8];59(4):503–16. Available from: https://doi.org/10.1007/s00285-008-0240-9

[130] Bichara D, Castillo-Chavez C. Vector-borne diseases models with residence times – A Lagrangian perspective. Mathematical Biosciences [Internet]. 2016 Nov [cited 2021 Aug 8];281:128–38. Available from: https://doi.org/10.1016/j.mbs.2016.09.006

[131] Conlan AJ, Klepac P, Kucharski AJ, Kissler S, Tang ML, Fry H, Gog JR. Human mobility data from the BBC Pandemic project. medRxiv. 2021 Feb 23:128–38.

[132] Ferguson N, et al. Report 9: Impact of non-pharmaceutical interventions (NPIs) to reduce COVID-19 mortality and healthcare demand. London: Imperial College; 2020 Mar. 20 p.

[133] LANL COVID-19 Cases and Deaths Forecasts [Internet]. LANL COVID-19 Cases and Deaths Forecasts; [cited 2021 Aug 18]. Available from: https://covid-19.bsvgateway.org/

[134] Lu FS, et al. Estimating the Cumulative Incidence of COVID-19 in the United States Using Four Complementary Approaches. medRxiv. 2020 Aug 20:1–4.

[135] Basnarkov L. SEAIR Epidemic spreading model of COVID-19. Chaos, Solitons & Fractals [Internet]. 2020 Oct [cited 2021 Aug 18]:110394. Available from: https://doi.org/10.1016/j.chaos.2020.110394

[136] Ivorra B, Ferrández MR, Vela-Pérez M, Ramos AM. Mathematical modeling of the spread of the coronavirus disease 2019 (COVID-19) taking into account the undetected infections. The case of China. Communications in Nonlinear Science and Numerical Simulation [Internet]. 2020 Sep [cited 2021 Aug 18];88:105303. Available from: https://doi.org/10.1016/j.cnsns.2020.105303

[137] Castro M, et al. Predictability: Can the turning point and end of an expanding epidemic be precisely forecast? [Internet]. Ithaca: arXiv; 2020 Apr [cited 2021 Aug 18]. 20 p. Available from: https://arxiv.org/abs/2004.08842

[138] Karin O, et al. Cyclic exit strategies to suppress COVID-19 and allow economic activity. medRxiv [Internet]. 2020:1-23. Available from: https://www.medrxiv.org/content/10.1101/2020.04.04.20053579v4

[139] Zhao H, Feng Z. Staggered release policies for COVID-19 control: Costs and benefits of relaxing restrictions by age and risk. Mathematical Biosciences [Internet]. 2020 Aug [cited 2021 Aug 18];326:108405. Available from: https://doi.org/10.1016/j.mbs.2020.108405

[140] Hossain MP, Junus A, Zhu X, Jia P, Wen TH, Pfeiffer D, Yuan HY. The effects of border control and quarantine measures on global spread of COVID-19. SSRN Electronic Journal [Internet]. 2020 [cited 2021 Aug 18]. Available from: https://doi.org/10.2139/ssrn.3547219

[141] Epidemic Spreading in Real Networks: An Eigenvalue Viewpoint. In: Proceedings 22nd International Symposium on Reliable Distributed Systems [Internet]; 2003 Oct 8; Florence,

Italy. [place unknown]: IEEE; 2003 [cited 2021 Aug 18]. Available from: https://doi.org/10.1109/reldis.2003.1238049

[142] Prakash BA, et al. Got the Flu (or Mumps)? Check the Eigenvalue! [Internet]. arXiv [Preprint]. 2010 [cited 2021 Aug 18]: 26 p. Available from: https://arxiv.org/abs/1004.0060

[143] Brockmann D, Helbing D. The Hidden Geometry of Complex, Network-Driven Contagion Phenomena. Science [Internet]. 2013 Dec 12 [cited 2022 Mar 12];342(6164):1337–42. Available from: https://doi.org/10.1126/science.1245200

[144] Hens C, Harush U, Haber S, Cohen R, Barzel B. Spatiotemporal signal propagation in complex networks. Nature Physics [Internet]. 2019 Jan 28 [cited 2022 Mar 12];15(4):403–12. Available from: https://doi.org/10.1038/s41567-018-0409-0

[145] Pastor-Satorras R, Castellano C, Van Mieghem P, Vespignani A. Epidemic processes in complex networks. Reviews of Modern Physics [Internet]. 2015 Aug 31 [cited 2022 Mar 12];87(3):925–79. Available from: https://doi.org/10.1103/revmodphys.87.925

[146] Aronna MS, Guglielmi R, Moschen LM. A model for COVID-19 with isolation, quarantine and testing as control measures. Epidemics [Internet]. 2021 Mar [cited 2021 Aug 18];34:100437. Available from: https://doi.org/10.1016/j.epidem.2021.100437

[147] Tkachenko AV, et al. Time-dependent heterogeneity leads to transient suppression of the COVID-19 epidemic, not herd immunity [Internet]. medRxiv [Preprint]. 2021: 9 p. Available from: https://www.medrxiv.org/content/10.1101/2020.07.26.20162420v4

[148] Morciglio A, Zhang B, Chowell G, Hyman JM, Jiang Y. Mask-Ematics: Modeling the Effects of Masks in COVID-19 Transmission in High-Risk Environments. Epidemiologia [Internet]. 2021 May 31 [cited 2021 Sep 23];2(2):207-26. Available from: https://doi.org/10.3390/epidemiologia2020016

[149] Ramos AM, Vela-Pérez M, Ferrández MR, Kubik AB, Ivorra B. Modeling the impact of SARS-CoV-2 variants and vaccines on the spread of COVID-19. Communications in Nonlinear Science and Numerical Simulation [Internet]. 2021 Nov [cited 2021 Aug 18];102:105937. Available from: https://doi.org/10.1016/j.cnsns.2021.105937

[150] Anderson R, May R. Directly transmitted infections diseases: control by vaccination. Science [Internet]. 1982 Feb 26 [cited 2022 Mar 12];215(4536):1053–60. Available from: https://doi.org/10.1126/science.7063839

[151] Wang Z, Bauch CT, Bhattacharyya S, d'Onofrio A, Manfredi P, Perc M, Perra N, Salathé M, Zhao D. Statistical physics of vaccination. Physics Reports [Internet]. 2016 Dec [cited 2022 Mar 12];664:1–113. Available from: https://doi.org/10.1016/j.physrep.2016.10.006

[152] Liu K, Lou Y. Optimizing COVID-19 vaccination programs during vaccine shortages. Infectious Disease Modelling [Internet]. 2022 March [cited 2022 Mar 12];7:286-298. Available from: https://doi.org/10.1016/j.idm.2022.02.002

CHAPTER 2

Epidemiology of COVID-19

María Eugenia Jiménez-Corona[*1], **Manlio F. Márquez-Murillo**[2]

[*] **Corresponding author:** mejimenez777@gmail.com, Phone: +52 555573-2911 ext. 21013

[1] Department of Epidemiology, National Institute of Cardiology, Mexico City, Mexico

[2] Deputy Director Clinical Investigation, National Institute of Cardiology, Mexico City, Mexico

Abstract. In the last days of December 2019, in a seafood market in Wuhan, China, an outbreak of pneumonia of unknown origin was identified and later reported to the World Health Organization (WHO) regional office through the International Health Regulations for its dissemination to WHO member countries. The WHO declared the outbreak of a Public Health Emergency of International Concern (PHEIC) on January 30th, and on March 11th, 2020, the WHO Director-General declared it a pandemic. Today, it has been spread to more than 200 countries. The SARS-CoV-2 pandemic could be considered the health event with the greatest impact worldwide in the last 100 years. As of March 11th, 2021, one year later, more than 17 million cases and 2,615,018 deaths have been registered. The clinical picture caused by SARS-CoV-2 ranges from mild to severe forms. Some require hospitalization and, in some cases, even treatment in Intensive Care Units is needed due to multiorgan disease. Medium and long-term sequelae are still under investigation. The pandemic has affected health services in Mexico and all over the world, not only due to the hospital reconversion for the care of patients with COVID-19 in the face of the emergency, but also because the care of patients with other conditions has been delayed with a negative impact on the physical and mental health of populations. Likewise, it has deranged several social activities such as travel, commerce, and education.

Key words: Severe acute respiratory syndrome, antigens, antibodies, COVID-19, coronavirus, epidemic, epidemiology, fatality, mortality, outbreak, pandemic, PHEIC, population, preventive measures, SARS-CoV-2, spike protein, vaccines, zoonosis.

1 INTRODUCTION

1.1 Importance

It is essential to establish the origin and to follow the evolution of a pandemic to identify the factors that could allow to define health public actions and interventions for the containment and mitigation of such events. This knowledge can also help to prevent or reduce the frequency of new pandemics.

1.2 Preliminaries

Epidemics and pandemics have accompanied man throughout the history of mankind. The Spanish influenza pandemic in 1918, known as "the mother of pandemics" claimed the lives of more than 50 million people. In 1957-1958 and 1968, there were two other major epidemics also due to influenza viruses, the A virus (H2N2) and the influenza A virus (H3N2), respectively. The 1918-1919 pandemic is the benchmark against which all other epidemics and pandemics are compared, due to the unprecedented number of victims [1].

Various factors favor the emergence and reemergence of pathogens, as well as their spread, including population growth, the increase in disorganized urbanization, international travel, human migratory movements, and climate change [2, 3].

In this century, various threats to global public health have occurred, of which 70-80% are related to emerging or reemerging diseases of zoonotic origin (transmitted from animals to humans): SARS-CoV in 2003, influenza A(H5N1) virus in 2004, influenza A(H1N1) virus in 2009, MERS-CoV from the Middle East in 2012, influenza A(H7N9) virus in 2013, Ebola virus and the Zika virus in 2014, among others [4]. In this 21st century, the first virus that triggered the alarm of the World Health Organization (WHO) was the Severe Acute Respiratory Syndrome (SARS) coronavirus in 2003 in China [5]. In 2009, a less deadly pandemic than the 1918 pandemic was the result of a combination of genetic changes in the virus, and was the first pandemic of this century, caused by the influenza A (H1N1) virus, with Mexico as its epicenter. Worldwide, an estimated 151,700 to 575,400 deaths were caused by infection with influenza A(H1N1)pdm09 (2009 H1N1 Pandemic) virus during the first year that the virus circulated [6]. Later, this virus became a seasonal virus and to date circulates globally and is currently part of the composition of seasonal influenza vaccines [7].

2 CORONAVIRUSES OF PUBLIC HEALTH IMPORTANCE

Coronaviruses are an extensive family of viruses, some of which can cause diseases in humans (zoonoses), ranging from the common cold to severe clinical pictures. such as those caused by the Severe Acute Respiratory Syndrome coronavirus (SARS-CoV) identified in 2003. In 2012, another coronavirus of importance to public health that causes the Middle East Respiratory Syndrome (MERS-CoV), was identified in Saudi Arabia. In 2019, the SARS-CoV-2 coronavirus that causes COVID-19 emerged [8–10]. Although the three coronaviruses identified in 2003, 2012, and 2019, have had an impact on public health, there are large differences in the number of cases, deaths, and fatality rates (Fig. 1).

SARS-CoV-2	SARS-CoV	MERS-CoV
Dec 2019 – Mar 2021	2002 – 2003	Apr 2002 – Dec 2019
117,799,584	8,098	2,499
Confirmed cases	Confirmed cases	Confirmed cases
2,615,018	774	861
Deaths4	Deaths	Deaths
> 200	26	27
Countries affected	Countries affected	Countries affected
2.4%	9.6%	34.4%
Case fatality rate	Case fatality rate	Case fatality rate

Figure 1: Comparison of coronavirus of importance in Public Health

Coronaviruses pass from animals to humans, due to an adaptation process of the pathogen to new environments. SARS-CoV passed from civets (a species of cat) to humans and MERS-CoV from camels to humans [11]. The most likely origin of the SARS-CoV-2 virus is in the coronaviruses that infect bats. However, it is not clear whether the virus was spread directly to humans or by an intermediate host, as is the possibility that this virus infects companion animals, livestock, and wildlife that could act as viral reservoirs [12]. There are other known coronaviruses that are circulating in animals and have not yet infected humans [13, 14]. Coronaviruses have pandemic potential and have been shown to cause serious illness. These viruses can cause illnesses ranging from a clinical picture similar to the common cold to serious illnesses such as those caused by SARS-CoV, MERS-CoV, and SARS-CoV-2 [15, 16].

3 THE SARS-COV-2 VIRUS

SARS-CoV-2 belongs to the Orthocoronavirinae subfamily, whose members show characteristic crown-shaped tips on their surface [17]. It has a diameter of 80 to 120 nm, and is single-stranded, lipid-enveloped RNA. Four types of coronaviruses have been described, including α-coronavirus, β-coronavirus, δ-coronavirus, and γ-coronavirus [18–20]. SARS CoV-2 belongs to the group of beta coronaviruses such as the MERS-coronavirus. SARS and SARS-CoV-2 have approximately 79% genome sequence homology, and SARS-CoV-2 has a greater similarity to coronaviruses found in bats, causing SARS [18, 21]. Various studies have shown that SARS-CoV-2 binds to angiotensin-converting enzyme-2 (ACE-2), similar to SARS-CoV. This is due to the similarity of the receptor binding site found in spike proteins [22]. Coronaviruses use the spike protein (S) found on its surface to recognize and bind to specific receptors on the surface of the host cell, allowing the virus to enter it and cause infection or disease [18].

4 ORIGIN AND EVOLUTION OF THE PANDEMIC

Defining a timeline and highlighting the main milestones in the COVID-19 pandemic is not an easy task, since, more than a year after its onset, a series of events have occurred that allow us to see its rapid evolution. In the last days of December 2019, China identified an outbreak of atypical pneumonia of unknown origin in Wuhan, Hubei province. On January 1st, 2020, the WHO requested information from the Chinese authorities on the outbreak of atypical pneumonia cases in Wuhan, which was reported to the WHO in the last days of December 2019 [21]. On January 21, 2020, the United States notified its first confirmed case of infection by the new coronavirus. This was the first case in the WHO Region of the Americas. On January 9th, the announcement of the identification and isolation of the new coronavirus nCoV19 was issued, and three days later the complete sequencing of the virus genome was done [21, 23]. On January 13, Thailand reported the first imported case outside of China. By January 24, China counted 835 cases; on January 30, the WHO Emergency Committee recommended to the Director General that the outbreak of the new coronavirus be declared as a Public Health Emergency of International Concern (PHEIC), given the spread and characteristics of the outbreak [23].

Initially, the virus was called 2019-nCoV, later on February 11th, 2020 it was called

SARS-CoV-2, and the disease it causes was called Coronavirus Disease 2019 (COVID-19). On March 7th, the first 100,000 cases of COVID-19 were already registered and on March 11th, the pandemic of SARS-CoV-2 was declared, the second pandemic of the 21st century, and on that date there were more than 118,000 cases in 114 countries, and 4,291 deaths [23, 24]. On March 18, the Solidarity Clinical Trial began to evaluate the effect of medications, considering three important outcomes in patients with COVID-19: mortality, need for assisted respiration, and length of hospitalization. This large clinical trial involved nearly 12,000 patients, 500 hospitals in more than 30 countries [25].

In April 2020, the "Access to COVID-19 Tools Accelerator" (ACT) initiative is presented, with the purpose of developing treatments and vaccines against COVID-19. The mainstay of the ACT for vaccines is the COVAX initiative created to promote and achieve global equitable access to vaccines [23, 26]. Throughout 2020, the United Kingdom, South Africa and, Brazil reported variants of SARS-CoV 2 [27]. On December 31, the WHO published its first validation for use in emergency of a vaccine against COVID-19 and emphasized the need for equitable global access. As of March 18th, 2021, regulatory authorities from different countries have authorized nine vaccines against COVID-19 for emergency use [23, 28]. By March 19th, there were 121,464,666 confirmed cases, 2,684,093 deaths, and 364,184,603 doses of vaccines had been administered worldwide [29] (Fig. 2).

Some important events at the start of the pandemic are listed below, in chronological order:

- Cluster of cases of pneumonia of unknown origin reported in Wuhan to China National Health Commission 01/01/2020,
- Huanan Seafood Wholesale market closed 07/01/2020,
- Novel coronavirus isolated 01/11/2020,
- First fatal case reported in Japan 01/19/2020,

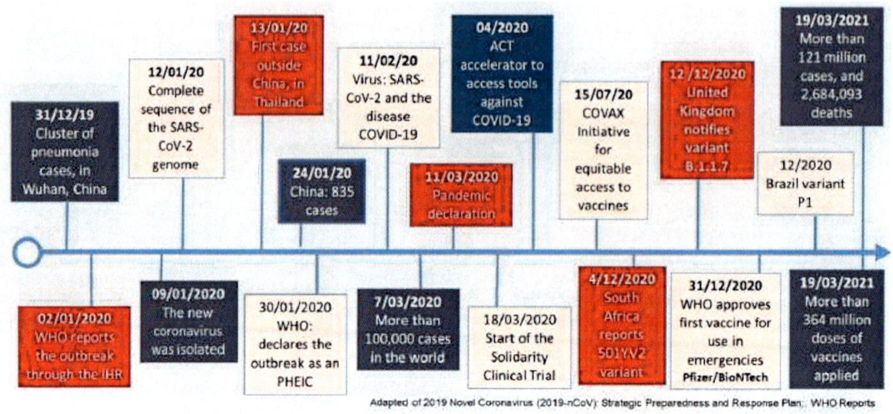

Figure 2: Timeline of early stages of COVID-19, 31/12/2019 to 19/03/2021

- Whole genome sequence shared with WHO and public (virus designated 2019 nCoV) 01/16/2020,
- First case reported in Japan 01/19/2020,
- First case reported in Republic of Korea,
- Two cases in Beijing and one case in Guandong 01/13/2020,
- First case reported from Thailand 01/20/2020,
- First reports of infection in healthcare workers caring for patients with 2019 nCoV.

5 INTERNATIONAL HEALTH REGULATIONS AND MECHANISMS FOR PREPARING AND RESPONDING TO THREATS TO PUBLIC HEALTH

The International Health Regulations (IHR 2005) is a legally binding international agreement signed by 196 countries, including all Member States of the WHO. Its objective is to help the international community prevent and address acute public health risks (Fig. 3) that may cross borders and threaten populations around the world [30].

Figure 3: Main Actions of the International Health Regulations (IHR)

Their actions are aimed at:

- Detecting international public health threats.
- Assessing specific diseases and potential international public health emergencies regardless of origin or source.
- Notifying through an international digital network of National Liaison Centers (CNE) available 24/7, one for each country.
- Complying with the requirements for an internationally organized response. This is a challenge that requires time, commitment and willingness to change.

The IHR was modified in 2005 after the events associated with SARS in 2003. There was a need to update the protocols established by the previous regulation, as well as the expansion of its basic capabilities and objectives. The first country to use the protocols established in the current edition of the 2005 IHR was Mexico during the 2009 influenza A(H1N1) pandemic, which was the first Public Health Emergency of International Concern (PHEIC), that turned out to be the first pandemic of the XXI century [31].

Therefore, six events have been called PHEIC: Influenza A(H1N1) in 2009, Ebola in 2013-2015, Polio in 2014, Zika in 2016, Ebola again in 2018-2020, and COVID-19 in 2020 [32].

6 WHAT IS A PUBLIC HEALTH EMERGENCY OF INTERNATIONAL CONCERN?

A PHEIC is defined in the IHR (2005) as "an extraordinary event that has been determined and constitutes a risk to the public health of other countries due to the international spread of a disease, and it could require a coordinated international response". This definition implies that the situation is serious, sudden, unusual, or unexpected; that it has implications for public health that go beyond the borders of the affected state, and that may require immediate and coordinated international action [30].

Health risks are identified through epidemiological surveillance systems, and international surveillance uses the protocols of the IHR and the National Focal Points, one for each WHO member country that work 24/7 and have an important component of Event-Based Surveillance, to communicate the risks and evolution of diseases that can constitute a PHEIC. (Fig. 4).

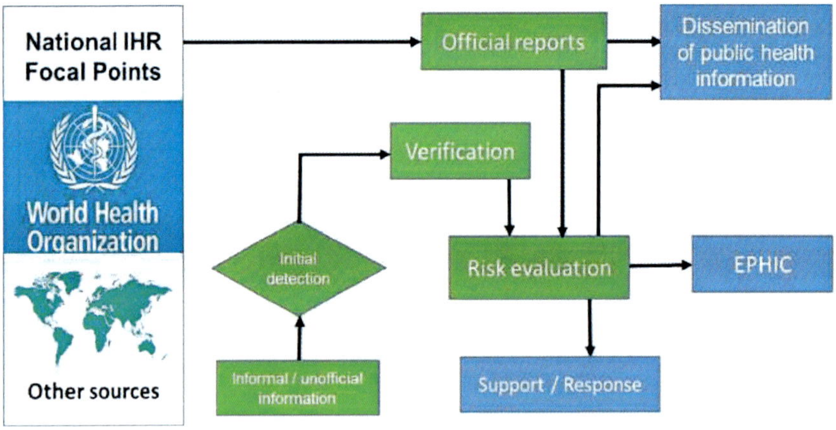

Figure 4: Flowchart for handling events of public health through International Health Regulations (IHR)

At the global level, the strategy and the coordination mechanism to control COVID-19 was established by the WHO through the IHR, and it deals with three main challenges: 1) How to carry out response actions effectively in different countries and in different contexts? 2) How to mobilize resources quickly in a strategic way? and 3) how to proactively and orderly encourage people from different regions of the world to participate in the global strategy to cope with the pandemic?

On February 12, 2020, WHO published a strategic plan that contained guidelines for operational planning in support of country preparedness and response. Its guidelines focused on the following pillars: coordination, planning, and monitoring at the country level with the following actions [33].

1. Risk communication and community participation.
2. Surveillance, rapid response teams and case investigation.
3. Points of entry (ports, airports, and border crossings).
4. National Public Health Laboratories.
5. Infection prevention and control.
6. Case management.
7. Operational and logistical support.

Each country has special conditions and therefore needs its own strategy to respond to threats to public health. In the face of the COVID-19 pandemic, the success of each country also depends on the success of all other countries that suffer from the pandemic. The way in which the pandemic is controlled is fundamental, not only for the worldwide success of finally "eliminating or controlling" SARS-CoV-2. It also affects the freedom to travel, trade and exchange goods in a globalized economy, and influences local and global health due to consequences on morbidity and mortality [34].

Countries need to be prepared and to devise coping strategies and response plans to face the threats to public health represented by epidemics and pandemics. To reduce the impact of an epidemic or pandemic, plans must be intersectoral and involve not only health, but also economy, education, public safety and basic services, tourism, among others. To control the COVID-19 pandemic, various plans have been designed depending on the conditions of each country, and based on previous experiences with intersectoral actions, which include health but are not restricted to that sector. These actions begin with a campaign to flatten the curve of cases and deaths as the first prerequisite to control the pandemic and start by identifying risk or vulnerable groups, including health personnel, due to their high exposure. Here are some key points in response plans for pandemic management: [35–37].

- Define a general coordinator of the strategy. The coordinator commander must have the authority to mobilize all necessary resources at the national level. Each state must also designate a state coordinator with similar state authority. The various stages of the epidemic in different regions require targeting responses to specific places and times.
- Have enough diagnostic tests. Not everyone needs to be tested, but everyone with symptoms does. This was the key to success in South Korea. Any decision about case management depends on sound medical evaluation and the results of diagnostic tests.
- Supply personal protective equipment to healthcare workers and provide the necessary equipment to hospitals. Warrant an extensive supply of personal protective equipment (PPE) to those on the front lines of patient care. Distribute ventilators and other necessary medical equipment to hospitals and healthcare institutions. Crisis care standards should be in place to make unavoidable and ethically sound decisions about the use of available equipment and supplies.
- Differentiate the population into five groups and treat accordingly:
  1. Known to be infected.
  2. Presumed to be infected (i.e., people with signs and symptoms consistent with the infection who initially tested negative).

3. Exposed.
4. Not known to have been exposed nor infected.
5. Recovered from the infection and are sufficiently immune.

- Hospitalize people with serious illnesses or serious risk. Establish centers to care for people with mild or moderate risk illnesses; to reduce transmission. Convert hotels and convention centers into quarantine centers to house those who have been exposed and separate them from the general population for two weeks.
- Mobilize the public. Everyone has a role to play in this effort. Unlike other health events with global repercussions, cooperation between countries, universities, and scientists for the same purpose, the development of new diagnostic methods, treatments, and vaccines has not been seen. Take advantage of tools such as information technology, social networks, artificial intelligence, and maximum speed computing to find innovative solutions.
- Investigation in real time. Clinical care has improved considerably with research results to more precisely define the clinical picture of COVID-19. Research continues to identify drugs that already existed and may be useful and for the development of new drugs including antivirals that can help in the treatment of the disease and its complications.
- Participation of the population in a proactive and orderly manner in the fight against COVID-19. It is important to protect the population from exposure to the virus, which is an effective way to block transmission routes. Define communication strategies that allow the population to be informed of the most frequent signs and symptoms of COVID-19, when they should stay home, when they should request medical attention, identify the warning signs; provide reliable information on vulnerable groups and the evolution of the pandemic with a risk communication approach and with the participation of the population.
- Decisions to shape the public health response to the COVID-19 pandemic and the revival of

the economy must be scientifically based.

In Mexico, the response to pandemics, emerging diseases, or both, is in charge of the National Committee for Health Safety [38], established in 2003; it includes the participation of federal agencies relevant to the response, and works throughout the country and together with the State Committees for Health Safety. As a precedent, there is the National Plan for Preparedness and Response to an Influenza Pandemic, which was presented in 2005 and has subsequently been updated [39]. The timely implementation of coordinated actions to meet the needs of care and reduce the consequences, are essential to contain and mitigate these types of events that affect public health. Some of the fundamental lines of action are: coordination, epidemiological surveillance (including laboratory and genomic surveillance), medical care, creation and support of a strategic reserve, communication, and social mobilization.

7 GLOBAL EPIDEMIOLOGICAL SITUATION AND IN MEXICO OF COVID-19

Worldwide, the COVID-19 pandemic has caused great damage and could be considered the health event with the greatest global impact in the last 100 years. More than 117 million people have been infected by SARS-CoV-2 and more than 2,615,018 deaths have been registered as of March 11, 2021; it has caused severe forms of disease and long-term sequelae. Likewise, an excess of mortality has been observed in various analysis, mainly in vulnerable groups.

The pandemic has negatively affected health services, among other reasons due to the hospital reconversion, necessary for the care of patients with COVID-19, which has delayed the care of patients with other pathologies; likewise travel, commerce, education and other social activities. In general, it has had a negative impact on the physical and mental health of populations [40].

Throughout the world, until March 11, 2021, there have been 117,799,584 confirmed cases, 2,615,018 deaths, with a fatality of 2.22% and 446,872 new cases. (Fig. 5).

At the time this text was written (March 11, 2021), the countries with the highest number of cases are the United States (29,000,561), India (11,333,728), Brazil (11,277,717), the Russian

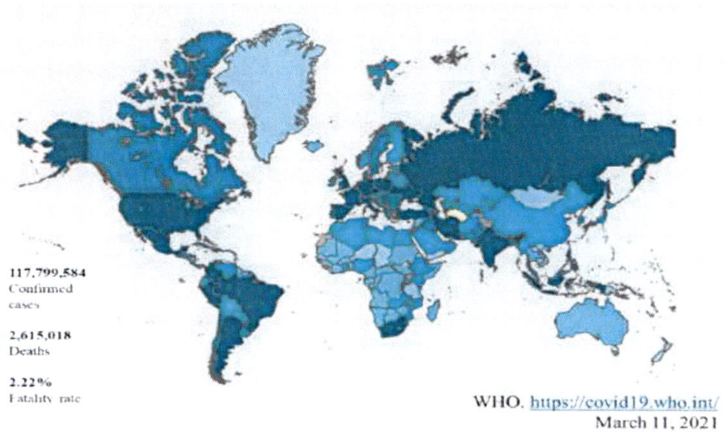

Figure 5: Distribution of confirmed cases and deaths globally

Federation (4,380,525), United Kingdom (4,248,290), France (3,946,733), Spain (3,183,704), Italy (3,175,807), Turkey (2,850,930), Germany (2,558,455), Colombia (2,290,539), Argentina (2,185,747), and Mexico (2,151,028) [41].

According to the six WHO Regions, America concentrates the highest number of cases (52,202,902), followed by Europe (40,438,291), and in the third place Southeast Asia (13,789,730) [41] (Fig. 6). Until March 11, 2021, a total of 2,615,018 deaths have been registered. The countries with the highest number of deaths in descending order are: The United States 527,068 (20.16%) deaths, Brazil 272,889 (10.44%), Mexico 193,142 (7.39%) deaths, India 158,446 (6.06%) and the United Kingdom 125,343 (4.79%) deaths, [41] (Fig. 7).

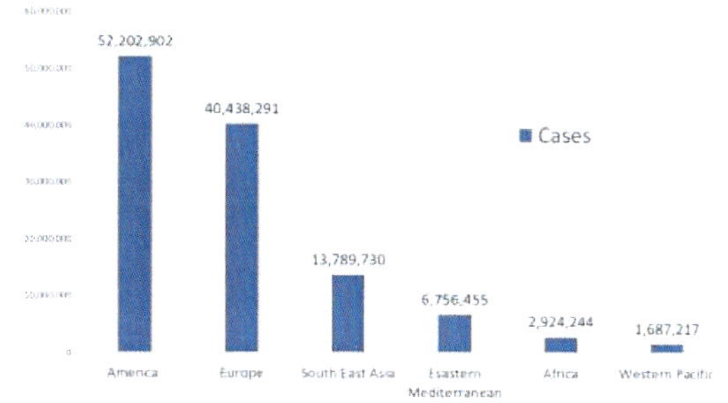

Figure 6: Distribution of accumulated COVID-19 cases by WHO Regions

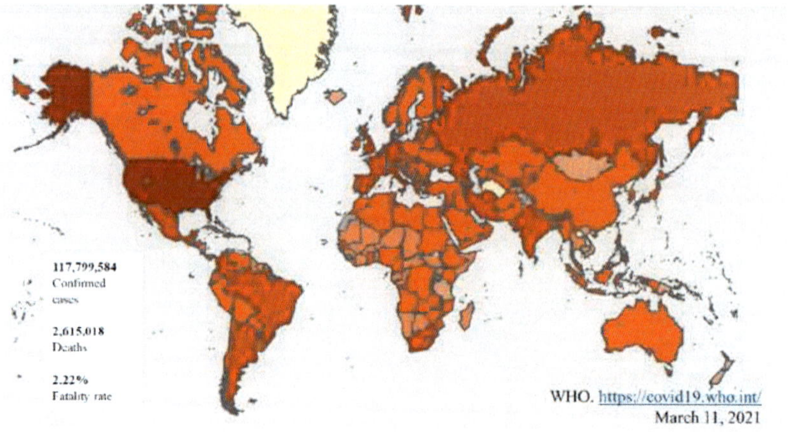

Figure 7: Distribution of deaths from COVID-19 globally

The distribution of WHO Regions during the pandemic allows us to observe the waves that have occurred, currently the American continent is the one with the highest number of accumulated cases [41] (Fig. 8).

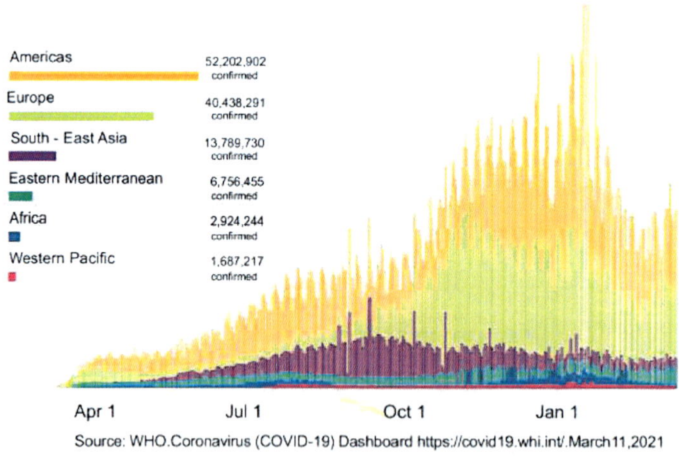

Figure 8: Epidemiological situation by WHO region, March 11, 2021

The notification rate of new cases and deaths from COVID-19 in the last 14 days is an indicator that reveals the evolution of the pandemic in recent days. (Fig. 9). However, these indicators are affected by the local testing strategy, laboratory capacity, and the effectiveness of each country's epidemiological surveillance systems. Therefore, the comparison of the epidemiological situation with respect to COVID-19 between countries should not be based only on these rates. In each country, these indicators are useful to monitor the national situation over time. Testing policies and the number of tests performed per 100,000 people vary markedly between countries. More extensive testing will inevitably lead to more cases being detected [42].

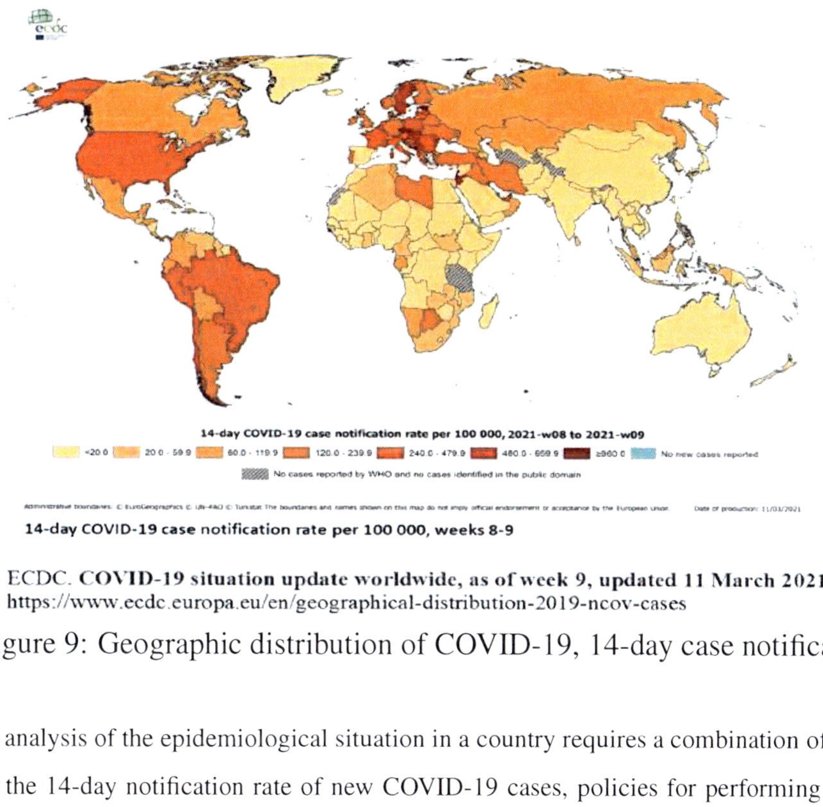

ECDC. **COVID-19 situation update worldwide, as of week 9, updated 11 March 2021**
https://www.ecdc.europa.eu/en/geographical-distribution-2019-ncov-cases

Figure 9: Geographic distribution of COVID-19, 14-day case notification

The analysis of the epidemiological situation in a country requires a combination of indicators such as the 14-day notification rate of new COVID-19 cases, policies for performing diagnostic tests, the number of tests performed, the positivity rate of tests, excess mortality, and hospital admission and discharge rates, as well as in Intensive Care Units (ICU), among others. Even when multiple indicators are used, cross-country comparisons should be made with caution and with relevant epidemiological experience [42, 43].

In the first months of 2020, in some countries, the quarantine helped to prevent a greater number of deaths.

Between March 9-15 2020, an average of 395 deaths were reported per day, between April 10-16 before the peak in 2020, 6,868 deaths were registered on average per day and between March 2-8, 2021, 8,665 deaths were registered. Of these, 3,093 (35.7%) correspond to Europe, 2,855 (32.9%) to Latin America, 1,560 to the United States (18.0%), and the remaining 13.4% to other regions; in the daily percentage distribution of the number of deaths by WHO regions the predominance of Europe and America is observed throughout the entire pandemic [44].

Although in the last weeks of February and the first week of March, 2020 a general decrease in cases and deaths has been observed, prevention measures must still be maintained to avoid infection [45]. Even though there are already approved vaccines for emergency use, their distribution and application are not fast and imply a lengthy process of production, management, conservation, delivery, and distribution for which well-defined logistical aspects are required. Vaccination is far from reaching 70-75% [46], which has been indicated as the minimum population percentage required to resume activities, under the conditions of the new reality that we live in. The emergence of new variants, in addition to those already reported in the United Kingdom, South Africa, and Brazil [27, 47–49], constitutes another element to continue with the measures that have an impact on the prevention of disease.

8 TRANSMISSION MECHANISMS AND "REPRODUCTION NUMBER" (R_0)

The infection by SARS-Cov-2 can be transmitted by asymptomatic, pre-symptomatic, and symptomatic people. SARS-CoV-2 is spread mainly through respiratory droplets during close person-to-person contact, coughing, sneezing, or talking in a confined space; fomites can also be considered in the transmission of this disease. The virus remains on surfaces during three to four days depending on humidity and temperature conditions. SARS-CoV-2 is rapidly inactivated on surfaces in sunlight. Transmission of close contact aerosols through smaller aerosolized particles is likely to combine with respiratory droplets in a confined, crowded, and poorly ventilated indoor environment, thus creating favorable conditions for transmission. On the other hand, there is no conclusive evidence of vertical transmission [50]. An expert panel for COVID-19 in Japan has focused on the "3 Cs", namely "poorly ventilated closed spaces", "crowded spaces" and with "close contact" among people.

The transmission rate of SARS-CoV-2 is higher compared to that of SARS and MERS-CoV. The main difference between the current SARS-CoV-2 pandemic and SARS is the speed with which the first is spreading [51, 52]. A meta-analysis on R_0, carried out by He et al. combined seven studies obtaining an R_0 of 3.15 (95% CI 2.41 - 3.90) with a standard deviation of 0.38 [53] (Fig. 10).

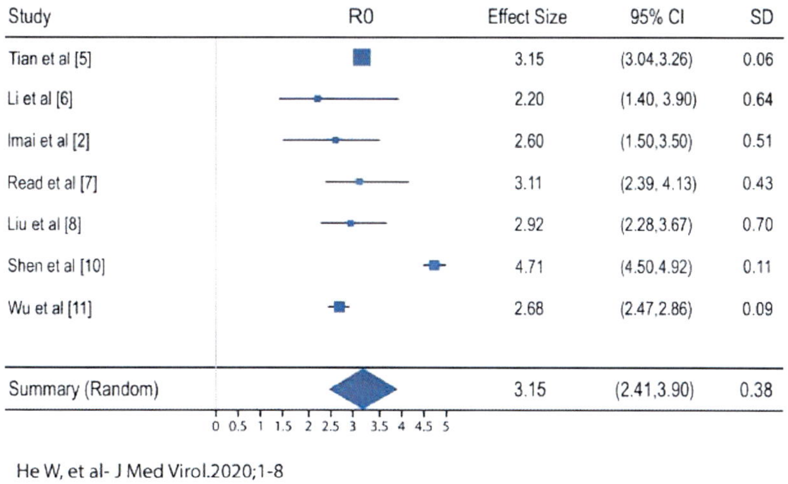

Figure 10: Meta-analysis of the R_0 and reported results in seven different studies

The incubation period for COVID-19 ranges from 2 to 14 days, with an average of 5.2 days (95% confidence interval (95% CI) 4.1 to 7.0) [54]. In a meta-analysis by He et al. which included all people who underwent a diagnostic test even if they were asymptomatic, the mean time of incubation was 5.08 days, the asymptomatic infection rate, 46% with 95% CI (18.48% -73.60%), and the case fatality rate 2.72% with a 95% CI (1.29% - 4.16%) [53, 54].

9 PREVENTIVE MEASURES

In addition to the actions carried out by the health sector, the population itself plays an important role in reducing the probability of exposure and transmission of the virus. Health promotion is the first among a number of other preventive measures. These measures to avoid infection by SARS-CoV-2 are relatively simple but have a great impact on health. They are mainly focused on containing the spread of SARS-CoV-2, and should be implemented and reinforced in the population continuously, with special attention to risk groups, such as the elderly, persons with comorbidities such as diabetes, hypertension, morbid obesity, cardiovascular diseases and cancer, among others, which are more likely to present with complications [55].

The virus can enter the body through the eyes, nose, or mouth. Therefore, preventive measures to avoid infection with SARS-CoV-2 are related to personal and environmental hygiene measures such as ([56, 57]):

- Washing hands frequently with soap and water or use 70% alcohol-based gel solutions for at least 20 seconds.

- Wearing a surgical mask or face mask, both indoors (supermarkets, stores, and public transport) and in busy outdoor situations, in areas with a higher incidence of COVID-19 and when physical distancing cannot be guaranteed.

- Maintaining a physical distance from other people of at least one meter (ideally 2 meters) in public places and indoors (for example: supermarkets, shops, and public transport). Physical distance should also be maintained in busy outdoor settings, in areas with a higher incidence of COVID-19, and when physical distancing cannot be guaranteed.

- Avoiding meetings especially of large groups of people.

- When coughing or sneezing, covering nose and mouth with a tissue or the inner corner of your arm (label sneeze).
- Not touching the face with dirty hands, especially nose, mouth and eyes.
- Cleaning and disinfecting surfaces and objects of common use in houses, offices, closed places, transport, meeting centers, etc.,
- Ventilating areas and allowing the entry of sunlight.
- Staying home when suffering respiratory illnesses and seeing a doctor if any of the symptoms appear (fever over $38°C$, headache, sore throat, runny nose, etc.).
- Avoiding contact with people with respiratory diseases.

WHO gives the following recommendations to enhance the safety of the environment ([58]):

- Avoid the 3 "Cs": spaces that are closed, congested, or involve close contact. Outbreaks have been reported in restaurants, gyms, nightclubs, offices, and places of worship where people gather, often in crowded indoor places where people often talk loudly, shout, or sing.
- The risks of contagion with the COVID-19 virus are highest in crowded and insufficiently ventilated spaces where infected people spend a lot of time together and in close proximity. In these settings, the virus is more easily spread by respiratory droplets or aerosols, making it even more important to take precautions.
- Meet outdoors, these gatherings are safer than indoors, particularly in small indoor spaces that lack outside air circulation.

Updated WHO recommendations on the use of masks or face masks ([59]):

- In areas with community transmission of COVID-19, nonmedical masks should always be used by the general public in closed places such as shops, workplaces, and schools or if a physical distance of at least one meter cannot be maintained.

- Even if the distance can be maintained, if ventilation does not meet the requirements of national institutions regarding SARS-COV2 in terms of temperature and humidity, masks should always be used as a preventive measure.
- In outdoor settings, the WHO maintains its recommendation to use nonmedical, cloth three-layer masks with a filter, specially if interpersonal distance of at least one meter cannot be maintained.
- Experts advise against the use of facial masks with valves. "The risk is that if a person wears a mask with a valve and is infected, he may be expelling infected aerosols. It does not imply a risk for those who use it, but it is a risk for others".
- The use of masks at home is recommended when there is a visitor who is not a member of the household and the ventilation is poor, regardless of whether a physical distance of at least one meter can be maintained.
- Masks should also be used at home with adequate ventilation if a physical distance of at least one meter cannot be maintained.
- The WHO advises that people should not wear masks during vigorous-intensity physical exercise as they can reduce the ability to breathe comfortably. Ensure a physical distance of at least one meter and good ventilation during exercise.
- Children under five years should not use masks, and the decision to use them in children 6-11 years old should be based on a risk approach.
- Special considerations are required for immunosuppressed children or pediatric patients with certain diseases (e.g. cancer) and other health conditions that may interfere with mask use.

To demonstrate the effectiveness of different personal protection measures to prevent infection by SARS-COV-2, Chu et al. [60] carried out a study in which they describe a reduction in the risk of contracting COVID-19 based on the use of personal protective equipment (mask and eye protection) and maintaining distancing between people. Among the people who did not use a mask or face mask, 17.4% were infected compared to 3.1% who used a mask; 16.0% of those who did not use eye protection had infection compared to 5.5% with eye protection; and of the people who had a distance of less than one meter, 12.8% had an infection compared to 2.6% in those who had a distance greater than one meter [60]. It is important to note that none of these measures offers complete protection, so it is necessary to combine them along with other measures. (Fig. 11).

Intervention	**Chance or infection or transmission**	
	Whitout intervention	**With intervention**
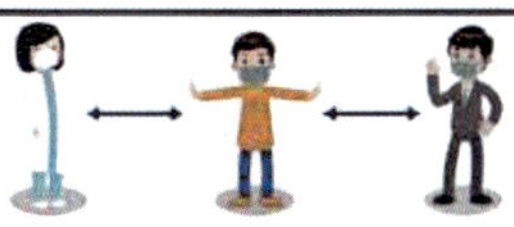 Physical distancing	Less than 1m distancing **12.8%**	1m or more distancing **2.6%**
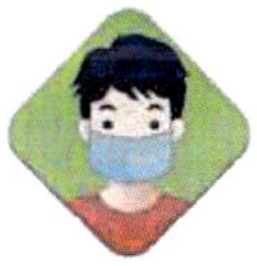 Face mask	Without mask **17.4%**	With mask **3.1%**
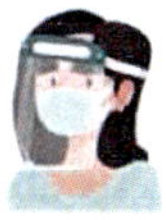 Eye protection	Without eye protection **16.0%**	With eye protection **5.5%**

Adapted from Chu DK et al. Lancet. 020;395(10242):1973-1987. doi: 10.1016/S0140-6736(20)31142-9.

Figure 11: What protects against COVID-19 infection or transmission?

Improving environmental factors such as temperature, humidity, stability of fomites and ventilation and filtering systems in buildings and public places (hospitals, hotels, restaurants, recreation sites) can have a significant impact on the dissemination of the infection. Considering these factors and knowing their dynamics is important in preventing the spread of COVID-19 [61].

It is essential to fully recognize the importance of airborne spread of COVID-19 in regulations to prevent the transmission of infections indoors. Authorities should recognize that the virus is spread through the air and recommend that appropriate control measures be put in place to prevent further spread of the SARS-CoV-2 virus, in particular the removal of virus-laden droplets from indoor air by ventilation [62]. Azuma et al. developed recommendations regarding ventilation and air conditioning to prevent COVID-19 infection, considering closed spaces, as well as spaces that have ventilation or air conditioning systems [50] (Fig. 12).

Spaces	Recommendation
Every indoor space	• Enough ventilation is necessary to prevent COVID-19 infection. • Opening windows is effective for ventilation and opening them wide and for a longer time is desirable. • In summer, air conditioners are necessary to prevent health risks such as heatstroke. • General air conditioners do not function as ventilators, so mechanical ventilation and opening windows are necessary.
Spaces in which air conditioning and ventilation systems are installed	• It is necessary to check the systems and to confirm enough ventilation rates are secured. • It is necessary to limit the number of persons in a room or shorten the time they are inside secure enough ventilation rates per person. • It is necessary to investigate what the building is used for, how often it is used, what kind of airconditioning and ventilation system is used in the building when taking such measures as the better control of air-conditioning and ventilation systems, or the use of air cleaners, and the use of humidifiers in winter.

Source: Azuma K, et al. Enviro mental Health and Preventive Medicine. 2020 25:66.
doi.org/10.1186/s12199-020-00904-2

Figure 12: Recommendations on ventilation and air-conditioning measures to prevent COVID-19 infection

Fig. 13 is a model (so-called "Swiss cheese" for easiness of remembering) that summarizes the combination of personal and environmental measures that provide adequate protection to prevent the transmission of the disease.

10 CONCLUDING REMARKS

For more than one year, since the beginning of the COVID-19 pandemic, the world has faced a global health crisis that has also affected the social, economic, and political sector. The

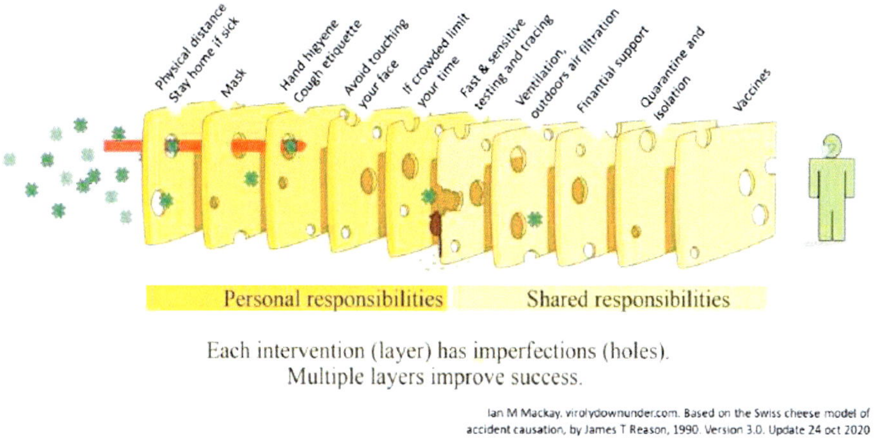

Figure 13: "Swiss cheese" model to represent the sum of preventive measures against SARS-CoV-2

SARS-CoV-2 pandemic constitutes the most important public health event in terms of global impact of the last 100 years, only comparable with the influenza pandemic of 1918.

At the beginning, there were no vaccines and no specific treatment. For the development of vaccines and drugs against SARS-COV-2, an initiative called the ACT accelerator was created, designed to develop vaccines and drugs against COVID-19, with a specific section for vaccines called the COVAX mechanism, whose purpose is to achieve global and equitable access to vaccines. This goal is far from being a reality, but remains as the only hope for the entire world to achieve herd immunity. Vulnerable populations in all countries must be the highest priority for vaccination. Currently, in a time record, vaccines have been developed with different production platforms. As of February 18th, 2021, at least seven different vaccines across the three main platforms have been tested and applied in many countries. This must be viewed as a great scientific achievement.

The eventual end of the pandemic is not in sight. There is also uncertainty as to what the characteristics of that "end" will be. Therefore, we must continue to reinforce the most important non-pharmacological preventive measures that have proven so far to be effective in reducing the transmission of COVID-19. On April 27th, 2021, globally, new COVID-19 cases increased for the ninth consecutive week, with nearly 5.7 million new cases reported. The number of new deaths increased for the sixth consecutive week, with over 87 000 new deaths reported. For the third consecutive week, the South-East Asia region reported the highest relative increases in both case and death incidences, India being a special region of concern. WHO, in collaboration with national authorities, institutions, and researchers, continues to monitor SARS CoV-2 variants of interest and variants of concern. Due to the risk of the appearence of new variants, and as long as there is not a significant proportion of vaccinated people all over the world, we cannot stop the preventive measures that have been used so far, even in those people who have the complete vaccination scheme against SARS-CoV-2.

11 CONSENT FOR PUBLICATION

Not applicable.

12 CONFLICT OF INTEREST

The authors declare no conflict of interest, financial or otherwise.

13 ACKNOWLEDGEMENTS

We want to express our gratitude to all the staff, from all areas of the Ignacio Chávez National Institute of Cardiology, who participated, directly and indirectly, in the care of COVID-19 patients.

References

[1] Jester B, Uyeki TM, Jernigan DB, Tumpey TM. Historical and clinical aspects of the 1918 H1N1 pandemic in the United States. Virology [Internet]. 2019 Jan [cited 2021 Jul 1];527:32–7. Available from: https://doi.org/10.1016/j.virol.2018.10.019

[2] El Zowalaty ME, Järhult JD. From SARS to COVID-19: A previously unknown SARS-related coronavirus (SARS-CoV-2) of pandemic potential infecting humans – Call for a One Health approach. One Health [Internet]. 2020 Jun [cited 2021 Jul 1];9:100124. Available from: https://doi.org/10.1016/j.onehlt.2020.100124

[3] Cruz-Pacheco G, Bustamante-Castañeda JF, Guy Caputo J, Jiménez- Corona ME, Ponce-de-León A. Dispersion of a New Coronavirus SARS-CoV-2 by Airlines in 2020: Temporal Estimates of the Outbreak in Mexico. Revista de investigación Clínica [Internet]. 2020 Jun 23 [cited 2021 Jul 1];72(3). Available from: https://doi.org/10.24875/ric.20000113

[4] Major infectious threats in the 21st and collaboration Century mechanisms against them. [Internet]. Geneva; 2020 May [cited 2021 Jul 1]. 1 p. World Health Organization. Available from: https://www.who.int/docs/default-source/epi-win/timeline-of-major-infectious-threats-in-21st-century-collabobration-machanism.pdf?sfvrsn=73d42d606

[5] Stadler K, Masignani V, Eickmann M, Becker S, Abrignani S, Klenk HD, Rappuoli R. SARS – beginning to understand a new virus. Nature Reviews Microbiology [Internet]. 2003 Dec [cited 2021 Sep 27];1(3):209–18. Available from: https://doi.org/10.1038/nrmicro775

[6] Centers for Disease Control and Prevention [Internet]. 2009 H1N1 Pandemic; 2019 Jun [cited 2021 Sep 27]. Available from: https://espanol.cdc.gov/flu/pandemic-resources/2009-h1n1-pandemic.html

[7] WHO | World Health Organization [Internet]. Recommended composition of influenza virus vaccines for use in the 2021-2022 northern hemisphere influenza season; 2020 [cited 2021 Feb 26]. Available from: https://www.who.int/publications/m/item/recommended-composition-of-influenza-virus-vaccines-for-use-in-the-2021-2022-northern-hemisphere-influenza-season

[8] Hui DS, Wong PC, Wang C. SARS: clinical features and diagnosis. Respirology [Internet]. 2003 Nov [cited 2021 Sep 28];8(s1):S20–S24. Available from: https://doi.org/10.1046/j.1440-1843.2003.00520.x

[9] Rabaan A, et al. SARS-CoV-2, SARS-CoV, and MERS-COV: A comparative overview. Le Infezioni in Medicina. 2020;28(2):174–84.

[10] Li J, He X, Yuan Yuan, Zhang W, Li X, Zhang Y, Li S, Guan C, Gao Z, Dong G. Meta-analysis investigating the relationship between clinical features, outcomes, and severity of severe acute respiratory syndrome coronavirus 2 (SARS-CoV-2) pneumonia. American Journal of Infection Control [Internet]. 2021 Jan [cited 2021 Sep 27];49(1):82–9. Available from: https://doi.org/10.1016/j.ajic.2020.06.008

[11] OpenWHO [Internet]. Introducción a la COVID-19: métodos de detección, prevención,

respuesta y control; [cited 2021 Sep 27]. Available from: https://openwho.org/courses/introduccion-al-ncov?locale=en

[12] Conceicao C, Thakur N, Human S, Kelly JT, Logan L, Bialy D, et al. The SARS-CoV-2 Spike protein has a broad tropism for mammalian ACE2 proteins. PLOS Biology [Internet]. 2020 Dec 21 [cited 2021 Sep 27];18(12):e3001016. Available from: https://doi.org/10.1371/journal.pbio.3001016

[13] Wardeh M, Baylis M, Blagrove MS. Predicting mammalian hosts in which novel coronaviruses can be generated. Nature Communications [Internet]. 2021 Feb 16 [cited 2021 Sep 27];12(1). Available from: https://doi.org/10.1038/s41467-021-21034-5

[14] Alekseev KP, Vlasova AN, Jung K, Hasoksuz M, Zhang X, Halpin R, Wang S, Ghedin E, Spiro D, Saif LJ. Bovine-Like Coronaviruses Isolated from Four Species of Captive Wild Ruminants Are Homologous to Bovine Coronaviruses, Based on Complete Genomic Sequences. Journal of Virology [Internet]. 2006 Oct 8 [cited 2021 Sep 28];82(24):12422–31. Available from: https://doi.org/10.1128/jvi.01586-08

[15] WHO | World Health Organization [Internet]. Coronavirus; [cited 2021 Sep 28]. Available from: https://www.who.int/health-topics/coronavirus

[16] Cui J, Li F, Shi ZL. Origin and evolution of pathogenic coronaviruses. Nature Reviews Microbiology [Internet]. 2018 Dec 10 [cited 2021 Sep 28];17(3):181–92. Available from: https://doi.org/10.1038/s41579-018-0118-9

[17] Rauf A, Abu-Izneid T, Olatunde A, Ahmed Khalil A, Alhumaydhi FA, Tufail T, Shariati MA, Rebezov M, Almarhoon ZM, Mabkhot YN, Alsayari A, Rengasamy KR. COVID-19 Pandemic: Epidemiology, Etiology, Conventional and Non-Conventional Therapies. International Journal of Environmental Research and Public Health [Internet]. 2020 Nov

4 [cited 2021 Sep 28];17(21):8155. Available from: https://doi.org/10.3390/ijerph17218155

[18] Wang W, Tang J, Wei F. Updated understanding of the outbreak of 2019 novel coronavirus (2019-nCoV) in Wuhan, China. Journal of Medical Virology [Internet]. 2020 Feb 12 [cited 2021 Sep 28];92(4):441–7. Available from: https://doi.org/10.1002/jmv.25689

[19] Chan JF, Lau SK, Woo PC. The emerging novel Middle East respiratory syndrome coronavirus: The "knowns" and "unknowns". Journal of the Formosan Medical Association [Internet]. 2013 Jul [cited 2021 Sep 28];112(7):372–81. Available from: https://doi.org/10.1016/j.jfma.2013.05.010

[20] Zhu N, Zhang D, Wang W, Li X, Yang B, Song J, Zhao X, Huang B, Shi W, Lu R, Niu P, Zhan F, Ma X, Wang D, Xu W, Wu G, Gao GF, Tan W. A Novel Coronavirus from Patients with Pneumonia in China, 2019. New England Journal of Medicine [Internet]. 2020 Feb 20 [cited 2021 Sep 28];382(8):727–33. Available from: https://doi.org/10.1056/nejmoa2001017

[21] Wu F, Zhao S, Yu B, Chen YM, Wang W, Song ZG, Hu Y, Tao ZW, Tian JH, Pei YY, Yuan ML, Zhang YL, Dai FH, Liu Y, Wang QM, Zheng JJ, Xu L, Holmes EC, Zhang YZ. A new coronavirus associated with human respiratory disease in China. Nature [Internet]. 2020 Feb 3 [cited 2021 Sep 28];579(7798):265–9. Available from: https://doi.org/10.1038/s41586-020-2008-3

[22] Hoffmann M, Kleine-Weber H, Schroeder S, Krüger N, Herrler T, Erichsen S, Schiergens TS, Herrler G, Wu NH, Nitsche A, Müller MA, Drosten C, Pöhlmann S. SARS-CoV-2 Cell Entry Depends on ACE2 and TMPRSS2 and Is Blocked by a Clinically Proven Protease Inhibitor. Cell [Internet]. 2020 Apr [cited 2021 Sep 28];181(2):271–80. Available from: https://doi.org/10.1016/j.cell.2020.02.052

[23] WHO | World Health Organization [Internet]. Cronología de la respuesta de la OMS a la COVID-19. 2021 Jan 29 [cited 2021 Sep 28]. Available from: https://www.who.int/es/news/item/29-06-2020-covidtimeline

[24] WHO | World Health Organization [Internet]. Alocución de apertura del Director General de la OMS en la rueda de prensa sobre la COVID-19 celebrada el 11 de marzo de 2020; 2021 Mar 11 [cited 2021 Sep 28]. Available from: https://www.who.int/es/director-general/speeches/detail/who-director-general-s-opening-remarks-at-the-media-briefing-on-covid-19---11-march-2020

[25] WHO | World Health Organization [Internet]. Ensayo clínico Solidaridad sobre tratamientos contra la COVID-19; [cited 2021 Sep 28]. Available from: https://www.who.int/es/emergencies/diseases/novel-coronavirus-2019/global-research-on-novel-coronavirus-2019-ncov/solidarity-clinical-trial-for-covid-19-treatments

[26] WHO | World Health Organization [Internet]. El Acelerador del acceso a las herramientas contra la COVID-19; 2020 [cited 2021 Sep 28]. Available from: https://www.who.int/es/initiatives/act-accelerator

[27] WHO | World Health Organization [Internet]. Weekly epidemiological update on COVID-19 – 16 March 2021; 2021 Mar 14 [cited 2021 Sep 28]. Available from: https://www.who.int/publications/m/item/weekly-epidemiological-update---16-march-2021

[28] Zimmer C, Corum J, Wee SL. The New York Times [Internet]. Coronavirus Vaccine Tracker; 2020 Jun 10 [cited 2021 Sep 28]. Available from: https://www.nytimes.com/interactive/2020/science/coronavirus-vaccine-tracker.html

[29] WHO Coronavirus (COVID-19) Dashboard | WHO Coronavirus (COVID-19) Dashboard

With Vaccination Data [Internet]. WHO Coronavirus (COVID-19) Dashboard; 2021 Mar 19 [cited 2021 Sep 28]. Available from: https://covid19.who.int/.

[30] Reglamento Sanitario Internacional 2005. Tercera edición. Ginebra: [publisher unknown]; 2005. 104 p. Informe de la Organización Mundial de la Salud. https://apps.who.int/iris/bitstream/handle/10665/246186/9789243580494-spa.pdf;\jsessionid=B8625629D721249D999CF93EA883B727?sequence=1.

[31] Kerman RS. Enfrentando desafíos en el contexto de la salud pública internacional. Comunidad y Salud. 2016;14(1). http://ve.scielo.org/scielo.php?script=sciarttextpid=S1690-32932016000100001lng=estlng=es.

[32] Wilder-Smith A, Osman S. Public health emergencies of international concern: a historic overview. Journal of Travel Medicine [Internet]. 2020 Dec [cited 2021 Sep 28];27(8). Available from: https://doi.org/10.1093/jtm/taaa227

[33] PAHO/WHO | Pan American Health Organization [Internet]. Plan estratégico de preparación y respuesta para la enfermedad por coronavirus 2019 (COVID-19) - Pautas para la planificación operativa de la preparación y la respuesta de los países. - OPS/OMS | Organización Panamericana de la Salud; [cited 2021 Sep 28]. Available from: https://www.paho.org/es/documentos/plan-estrategico-preparacion-respuesta-para-enfermedad-por-coronavirus-2019-covid-19

[34] Kofler W, Glazachev OS, Lyshol H, Tellnes G. Is fighting against COVID-19 enough? Scandinavian Journal of Public Health [Internet]. 2020 Nov 12 [cited 2021 Sep 28]:140349482096953. Available from: https://doi.org/10.1177/1403494820969539

[35] Fineberg HV. Ten Weeks to Crush the Curve. New England Journal of Medicine [Internet].

2020 Apr 23 [cited 2021 Sep 28];382(17):e37. Available from: https://doi.org/10.1056/nejme2007263

[36] Qian X, Ren R, Wang Y, Guo Y, Fang J, Wu ZD, Liu PL, Han TR. Fighting against the common enemy of COVID-19: a practice of building a community with a shared future for mankind. Infectious Diseases of Poverty [Internet]. 2020 Apr 7 [cited 2021 Sep 28];9(1). Available from: https://doi.org/10.1186/s40249-020-00650-1

[37] OMS. Preparación y respuesta ante emergencias. https/www.who.int/csr/don/31-december-2020-sras-cov2-variants/es/

[38] Secretaría de Salud. Acuerdo por el que se crea el Comité Nacional para la Seguridad en Salud.(Sep 2003) http://www.salud.gob.mx/unidades/cdi/nom/compi/a220903.html

[39] Secretaría de Salud. Plan nacional para la preparación y respuesta ante la intensificación de la influenza estacional o ante una pandemia de influenza. https://www.gob.mx/cms/uploads/attachment/file/356290/Plan_Nacional_Influenza.pdf

[40] Santi RL, Lopez Santi R, Márquez MF, Piskorz D, Saldarriaga C, Lorenzatti A, Wyss F, Martín AV, Perales JS, Arcela JC, De Lourdes Rojas Gimon E, Sambadaro G, Perez GE, Mendoza I, Lanas F, Flores R, Liprandi AS, Alexander B, Baranchuk A. Ambulatory Patients with Cardiometabolic Disease and Without Evidence of COVID-19 During the Pandemic. The CorCOVID LATAM Study. Global Heart [Internet]. 2021 Feb 17 [cited 2021 Sep 28];16(1):15. Available from: https://doi.org/10.5334/gh.932

[41] WHO Coronavirus (COVID-19) Dashboard | WHO Coronavirus (COVID-19) Dashboard With Vaccination Data [Internet]. WHO Coronavirus (COVID-19) Dashboard; [cited 2021 Sep 28]. Available from: https://covid19.who.int/.

[42] European Centre for Disease Prevention and Control [Internet]. Interpretation of COVID-19 data presented on this website; [cited 2021 Sep 28]. Available from: https://www.ecdc.europa.eu/en/interpretation-covid-19-data

[43] Coronavirus – gob.mx [Internet]. Coronavirus – gob.mx; [cited 2021 Sep 28]. Available from: https://coronavirus.gob.mx/.

[44] H WK. Medium [Internet]. Data Analysis using JHU CSSE COVID-19 Daily Report Dataset; 2020 Aug 12 [cited 2021 March 11]. Available from: https://towardsdatascience.com/data-analysis-using-jhu-csse-covid-19-daily-report-dataset-c8a9120ed23

[45] Noticias ONU [Internet]. Una noticia alentadora: bajan los casos de COVID-19 a nivel mundial; [cited 2021 Sep 28]. Available from: https://news.un.org/es/story/2021/02/1487412

[46] Frederiksen LS, Zhang Y, Foged C, Thakur A. The Long Road Toward COVID-19 Herd Immunity: Vaccine Platform Technologies and Mass Immunization Strategies. Frontiers in Immunology [Internet]. 2020 Jul 21 [cited 2021 Sep 28];11. Available from: https://doi.org/10.3389/fimmu.2020.01817

[47] Worl Health Organization; WHO. (2020) SARS-CoV-2 Variants. Disease Outbreak News.31 December 2020. https://www.who.int/csr/don/31-december-2020-sars-cov2-variants/en/

[48] Arif TB. The 501.V2 and B.1.1.7 variants of coronavirus disease 2019 (COVID-19): A new time-bomb in the making? Infection Control & Hospital Epidemiology [Internet]. 2021 Jan 11 [cited 2021 Sep 28]:1-2. Available from: https://doi.org/10.1017/ice.2020.1434

[49] Callaway E. Fast-spreading COVID variant can elude immune responses. Nature [Internet]. 2021 Jan 21 [cited 2021 Sep 28];589(7843):500–1. Available from: https://doi.org/10.1038/d41586-021-00121-z

[50] Azuma K, Yanagi U, Kagi N, Kim H, Ogata M, Hayashi M. Environmental factors involved in SARS-CoV-2 transmission: effect and role of indoor environmental quality in the strategy for COVID-19 infection control. Environmental Health and Preventive Medicine [Internet]. 2020 Nov 3 [cited 2021 Sep 28];25(1). Available from: https://doi.org/10.1186/s12199-020-00904-2

[51] Chen TM, Rui J, Wang QP, Zhao ZY, Cui JA, Yin L. A mathematical model for simulating the phase-based transmissibility of a novel coronavirus. Infectious Diseases of Poverty [Internet]. 2020 Feb 28 [cited 2021 Sep 28];9(1). Available from: https://doi.org/10.1186/s40249-020-00640-3

[52] Liu Y, Gayle AA, Wilder-Smith A, Rocklöv J. The reproductive number of COVID-19 is higher compared to SARS coronavirus. Journal of Travel Medicine [Internet]. 2020 Feb 13 [cited 2021 Sep 28];27(2). Available from: https://doi.org/10.1093/jtm/taaa021

[53] He W, Yi GY, Zhu Y. Estimation of the basic reproduction number, average incubation time, asymptomatic infection rate, and case fatality rate for COVID-19: Meta-analysis and sensitivity analysis. Journal of Medical Virology [Internet]. 2020 Jun 9 [cited 2021 Sep 28];92(11):2543–50. Available from: https://doi.org/10.1002/jmv.26041

[54] Li P, Fu JB, Li KF, Liu JN, Wang HL, Liu LJ, Chen Y, Zhang YL, Liu SL, Tang A, Tong ZD, Yan JB. Transmission of COVID-19 in the terminal stages of the incubation period: A familial cluster. International Journal of Infectious Diseases [Internet]. 2020 Jul [cited 2021 Sep 28];96:452–3. Available from: https://doi.org/10.1016/j.ijid.2020.03.027

[55] WHO | World Health Organization [Internet]. Información básica sobre la COVID-19; [cited 2021 Sep 28]. Available from: https://www.who.int/es/emergencies/diseases/novel-coronavirus-2019/question-and-answers-hub/q-a-detail/coronavirus-disease-covid-19

[56] European Centre for Disease Prevention and Control [Internet]. Questions and answers on COVID-19: Prevention; [cited 2021 Sep 28]. Available from: https://www.ecdc.europa.eu/en/covid-19/questions-answers/questions-answers-prevention

[57] gob.mx [Internet]. Recomendaciones para la población (COVID-19); [cited 2021 Sep 28]. Available from: https://www.gob.mx/salud/documentos/covid19-recomendaciones-para-la-poblacion

[58] WHO | World Health Organization [Internet]. Brote de enfermedad por coronavirus (COVID-19): Orientaciones para el público; [cited 2021 Sep 28]. Available from: https://www.who.int/es/emergencies/diseases/novel-coronavirus-2019/advice-for-public

[59] Noticias ONU [Internet]. La nueva guía de la OMS sobre el uso de mascarillas contra el COVID-19; [cited 2021 Sep 28]. Available from: https://news.un.org/es/story/2020/12/1485002

[60] Chu DK, Akl EA, Duda S, Solo K, Yaacoub S, Schünemann HJ, et al. Physical distancing, face masks, and eye protection to prevent person-to-person transmission of SARS-CoV-2 and COVID-19: a systematic review and meta-analysis. The Lancet [Internet]. 2020 Jun [cited 2021 Sep 28];395(10242):1973–87. Available from: https://doi.org/10.1016/s0140-6736(20)31142-9

[61] Azuma K, Kagi N, Kim H, Hayashi M. Impact of climate and ambient air pollution

on the epidemic growth during COVID-19 outbreak in Japan. Environmental Research [Internet]. 2020 Nov [cited 2021 Sep 28];190:110042. Available from: https://doi.org/10.1016/j.envres.2020.110042

[62] Morawska L, Cao J. Airborne transmission of SARS-CoV-2: The world should face the reality. Environment International [Internet]. 2020 Jun [cited 2021 Sep 28];139:105730. Available from: https://doi.org/10.1016/j.envint.2020.105730

CHAPTER 3

COVID-19 Pathophysiology, Clinical Manifestations, and Drug Treatment

Daniel Manzur Sandoval[*,1], Gustavo Rojas-Velasco[1], Efrén Melano Carranza[1], Camelia Cruz Rodríguez[1], Arturo Arzate Ramírez[1], Francisco Javier González Ruiz[1], Gerardo Arteaga Cárdenas[1], María Alexandra López Polanco[1], Eduardo Alberto González Escudero[1], Edgar García Cruz[1], Luis Augusto Baeza Herrera[1], Luis Efrén Santos Martínez[1]

[*] **Corresponding author:** drdanielmanzur@gmail.com, Phone: +52 555573-2911 ext. 24506

[1] Cardiovascular Intensive Care Unit, National Institute of Cardiology, Mexico City, Mexico

Abstract. COVID-19 is caused by a single-stranded RNA encapsulated betacoronavirus, known as SARS-CoV-2, implicated in the pandemic that started in China in 2019. Viral replication consists of five stages that culminate in the release of the new virion. The exaggerated inflammatory response of COVID-19 is characterized by an elevation of acute phase reactants such as C-reactive protein and ferritin. It is associated with an unfavorable clinical course, intensified

Andrés Fraguela-Collar (Ed.)

by abnormal activation of the protein complex called the inflammasome. When the immune response does not control the virus, lung tissue damage occurs that leads to the massive release of proinflammatory cytokines, producing acute respiratory failure syndrome. Vascular permeability is increased; interaction with coagulation factors develops disseminated intravascular coagulation and multiorgan failure. Up to 33% of cases can be asymptomatic. Clinical manifestations can be mild or severe and involve various organs and systems. Among the most commonly affected are: respiratory, cardiovascular, renal, and hematological and coagulation systems. Among the most representative laboratory data are: elevation of inflammatory markers (CRP, inflammatory cytokines, tumor necrosis factor), high levels of D-Dimer, elevation of troponin I, lymphopenia, thrombocytopenia, alteration of liver enzymes and kidney function. There are risk factors and comorbidities that contribute to the severity of the clinical picture (mainly cardiovascular and metabolic diseases): diabetes mellitus, high blood pressure, obesity, chronic lung diseases, cancer, and chronic kidney failure. There are also other genetic factors associated with the host's immunopathogenesis and response to SARS COV-2 infection. There are various imaging methods that allow adequate identification and involvement of the pulmonary and cardiovascular systems with great sensitivity and specificity (computed tomography and echocardiography). The pandemic imposed decisions with very little information regarding what may be useful as a therapeutic strategy. This uncertainty applies to the treatment indicated in the prevention phase, as well as to the different stages of severity of the disease. In many cases, treatments were applied without having gone through a trial phase but only with the theoretical support of its probable benefit. However, over time, controlled studies showed that they did not provide any benefit and that they could even have a deleterious effect. Other therapies still in use have shown contradictory results in the different clinical trials where they were tested. Very few therapeutic options have shown undisputable benefit so far. The only ones that can modify the presentation or course of the disease are vaccines, which have also been developed in record time and in controlled trials, and all those that have been approved showed a decrease in the risk of infection and in the risk of presenting a severe manifestation of the disease.

Key words: Angiotensin-converting enzyme, acute respiratory distress syndrome, asymptomatic infection, Beta-coronavirus, cardiovascular system, clinical manifestations, Caspase 1, Coronavirus, COVID-19, cytokine storm, dyspnea, echocardiography, Ferritin, hemo-phagocytosis, hypoxia, inflammation immune system, inflammasome, inflammatory response, Interleukin 6, lympho-histiocytosis, micro-angiopathy, Procaspase, Protein C, RNA, SARS-CoV-2, thrombosis, T lymphocytes, viral replication, respiratory failure.

1 INTRODUCTION

1.1 Importance

This chapter provides a comprehensive overview of three crucial aspects related to COVID-19 and its causal agent SARS-CoV-2. In the first place, it exposes the mechanisms of viral damage of SARS-CoV-2, its biochemical components, the inflammatory response it triggers, as well as the thrombotic phenomena it causes, all of which are essential to understand the pathophysiology of COVID-19. It also reviews the clinical manifestations of COVID-19 across a wide spectrum of clinical conditions, including both asymptomatic and mild and severe symptomatic forms. This is of great importance to provide early and adequate medical care and to achieve the highest possible reduction in mortality. Finally, it summarizes the scientific evidence supporting the therapeutic options available so far, all of them aimed at mitigating the systemic inflammation produced by cytotoxic damage and preventing related complications.

1.2 Preliminaries

COVID-19 is caused by the SARS-CoV-2 virus and until July 2021 it has caused more than 3.8 million deaths worldwide. Although the majority of patients do not require hospitalization, a minority present with severe illness with acute respiratory distress syndrome. Currently, more information is known about the transmission and clinical presentation of patients with SARS-CoV2 but less about the pathophysiology of the disease.

Coronaviruses are RNA viruses with a wide distribution among humans, other mammals, and birds that cause respiratory, enteric, liver, or neurological diseases. Until now, six species of coronavirus are known to cause disease in humans [1].

SARS-CoV-2 is a member of the Coronaviridae family of the order Nidovirales. The family consists of two subfamilies, Coronavirinae and Torovirinae, and the members of the Coronavirinae subfamily are subdivided into four genera: a) Alphacoronavirus contains human coronavirus (HCoV) -229E and HCoV-NL63; b) Betacoronavirus includes HCoV-OC43, human severe acute respiratory syndrome coronavirus (SARS-HCoV), HCoV-HKU1, and Middle East respiratory syndrome coronavirus (MERS-CoV); c) Gammacoronavirus includes whale and bird viruses; d) Deltacoronavirus includes viruses isolated from pigs and birds [2–7]. SARS-CoV-2 is an enveloped, positive-sense, single-stranded RNA (+ serna) virus. It belongs to Betacoronavirus along with two other highly pathogenic viruses, SARS-CoV and MERS-CoV.

Three stages of COVID-19 disease have been described. The first is the early stage, the first days of symptoms, when the administration of antiviral regimes is considered effective even when it has not been possible to find a drug or a combination of antivirals that clearly modify the course of the disease. The regime with Lopinavir/ritonavir that were considered a therapeutic option, did not show any benefit in patients with SARS-CoV-2 infection in controlled studies, with no difference in mortality at 28 days compared to placebo. Other drugs such as Hydroxychloroquine or Chloroquine that, theoretically prevent the virus from entering the cell, did not show any benefit when they were administered in prophylaxis to health personnel who cared for patients infected by SARS-CoV-2, but were associated with a significant increase in adverse events, so that its use is not currently recommended. In this early stage, plasma of convalescent patients has been used, on the assumption that it would provide antibodies to the patient in the initial stage that could improve their immune response to viral infection, but with less than encouraging results. In the next stage (pulmonary stage), when the patient develops greater lung damage, the usefulness of the use of steroids and anticoagulants have been demonstrated, but there is still doubt about the benefit of immunomodulatory, anti-inflammatory drugs. Therefore, the beneficial effect of these therapies has only been observed in patients with severe disease requiring supplemental oxygen support, but none in mildly affected COVID-19 patients for whom they could be harmful. The different therapeutic options are examined one by one in the following sections.

This chapter has been divided into three related parts. The first one examines the most updated information about the pathophysiology of the disease, and it includes the characterization of the virus and the description of the inflammatory process and the thrombotic cascade of events that accompany it. The second one describes the most salient clinical manifestations of the disease, with especial emphasis on cardiovascular and pulmonary specific organ damage. The third part reviews the different therapeutic options that have been used and studied so far, and critically examines the amount and quality of evidence supporting each option.

2 PATHOPHYSIOLOGY OF THE DISEASE

2.1 Virology

The SARS-CoV2 virus is a member of the coronavirus family, with single-stranded and encapsulated RNA, the size of the virion is 80-120 nm in diameter, it has an 87.6 - 89% similarity of its nucleotides with the coronaviruses originating from the bat. Within its arrangement, it has four structural proteins: spike protein (S), nucleocapsid (N), membrane protein (M), and coat proteins (E); this virus uses the lipid membrane of host cells to complete the envelope of its new virion [8].

Coronaviruses are divided into four genera: α, β, γ, and δ, of which only the α and β genera are human pathogens. The pathogenic coronaviruses (MERS-CoV, SARS-CoV, and SARS-CoV-2) belong to the genus of beta coronaviruses. The length of its genome is 26-32 kilobases in which 24-27 genes are encoded: two-thirds of the 5'ends encode the polyproteins pp1a and pp1ab, cleaved into 16 nonstructural proteins, the structural proteins (S, N, M, E) are encoded in the terminal third of the genome, the 3'2 end [9].

The viral replication cycle in host cells is divided into five stages: a) cell attachment and entry,

b) viral replicase transcription, c) genomic transcription and replication, d) translation of structural proteins, and e) assembly and release of the new virion [9]. The viral entry is determined by the S protein, which binds to the receptor for angiotensin-converting enzyme 2 (ACE2); the binding of these two structures promotes the viral entry. The high affinity between these two proteins is probably related to the severity and high transmissibility of COVID-19. Once attached, proteolytic cleavage is carried out by the transmembrane serine protease (TMPRSS2), which allows both the viral fusion to cellular membranes and release of the viral genome into the host. Once the viral RNA is free, the translation of its genome begins, generating pp1ab polyproteins, of which the pp1a and pp1ab portions are cleaved, generating 15-16 nonstructural proteins, the latter having inhibitory functions in the initial immune response and as transcription cofactors and replication (RNA-dependent RNA polymerase [RdRp], helicase, and RNA-modifying enzymes). Structural proteins are translated in the endoplasmic reticulum and receive posttranslational modifications to be fully functional. These proteins are formed in the intermediate compartment between the Golgi apparatus and the endoplasmic reticulum; they are transported to the cell membrane and finally released by exocytosis [9, 10].

2.2 Inflammatory Response

The current pandemic caused by SARS-CoV-2 represents a good example of a viral infection associated with a generalized inflammatory response and activation of coagulation in symptomatic patients. The immune system becomes the body's main defender against foreign agents, this system combines a range of cells and mediators to offer protective immunity against infectious agents [11]. The response to infection must be quick and effective. However, this response may be exaggerated and cause direct harm to the host. The exaggerated inflammatory response in COVID-19 is characterized by an elevation of acute-phase reactants, such as C-reactive protein and ferritin, and the development of lymphopenia, and is associated with an unfavorable clinical course. Therefore, anti-inflammatory therapy has shown favorable results in specific contexts.

[12, 13].

The inflammatory process in patients with SARS-CoV-2 is perpetuated by the abnormal activation of the protein complex called the inflammasome. It consists of a sensing protein, an adapter protein, and an effector protein, which is a cysteine protease called procaspase-1. The sensor protein includes NLRs [Nucleotide-binding Oligomerization Domain (NOD) and Leucine Rich-Repeat (LRR) receptors, and the adapter molecule ASC (Apoptosis-Associated Speck-like protein). There are several types of inflammasome, and one that is related to inflammatory processes and expression in cells of the innate immune system such as monocytes, macrophages, dendritic cells, neutrophils, lymphocytes, endothelial cells, epithelial cells that recognize pathogen-associated molecular patterns (PAMPs) or associated with damage (DAMPs) is present in SARS-CoV-2. When these stimuli are present, the inflammasome forms a complex and procaspase-1 becomes caspase-1 and this, in turn, is converted into interleukin 1 beta (IL 1β) and IL18 responsible for promoting inflammation [13].

The innate response is initiated by activating caspases that favor pyrocytosis. For this reason, the virus is considered a cytopathic virus, since it not only induces cell injury but also stimulates their death. They are generated from proinflammatory cytokines and chemokines (including IL-6, IP-10, macrophage inflammatory protein 1α (MIP1α), MIP1β, and MCP1). These proteins attract monocytes, macrophages, and T cells to the site of infection, promoting further inflammation (with the addition of IFNγ produced by T cells) and establishing a proinflammatory feedback loop that eventually damages the lung infrastructure. The adaptive response is activated by T lymphocytes through Toll-like receptors (TLRs) and the nuclear transcription factor NFkB, proinflammatory cytokines are released, effecting a cytokine storm, and by activation, of B lymphocytes, both T and B infiltrate the lungs and various organs. This could partially explain the observed lymphopenia. CD4 + T and CD8 + T cells in particular play a significant antiviral role by balancing the fight against pathogens with the risk of autoimmunity or overwhelming inflammation [11–14].

The activation of the nuclear factors KB, NF-kB induces the expression of type 1 interferon, and it is the first line of defense against viral infection at the site of entry [11–15].

During virus infection, PAMPs and DAMPs are recognized by lung epithelial cells and macrophages, and a higher production of proinflammatory cytokines is generated, in particular IL-6, INF-g, CXCL-10, monocyte chemoattractant protein-1 (MCP-1), among others, and a lower production of antiinflammatory cytokines, such as IL-17. When the immune response does not adequately control the virus, it spreads more aggressively by damaging the lung tissue, activating macrophages and granulocytes that lead to this massive release of proinflammatory cytokines, and cause respiratory failure syndrome. Other severe effects are the increment of vascular permeability and the interaction with coagulation factors that produce disseminated intravascular coagulation and multiple organ failure [14–16].

Ferritin-like C-reactive protein is an acute-phase reactant. That is, they are proteins in the presence of inflammation. H-ferritin has immunomodulatory effects, in addition to being an acute phase protein during systemic infection after its activation by the innate immune system. This ferritin modulates and delays the production of antibodies by B lymphocytes, decreases phagocytosis, and acts in the regulation of granule and monocytopoiesis. Ferritin can suppress the immune response by inducing antiinflammatory cytokines such as IL-10 [17].

Finally, inflammation in COVID-19 presents as a multisystemic inflammatory syndrome, which has been best described in children, as Kawasaki type, which, in turn, is associated with thrombotic microangiopathy. In this situation, the main clinical manifestation is lung and skin damage induced by complement activation via lectins. Similarly, a series of cases of the multisystemic inflammatory syndrome have been reported in adults [18].

Macrophage activation syndrome, also called secondary hemophagocytic lymphohistiocytosis (sHLH), is a poorly recognized inflammatory syndrome characterized by fulminant and fatal hypercytokinemia with multiple organ failure. It is most often triggered by viral infections. It is characterized by constant fever, cytopenias, and hyperferritinemia. Pulmonary involvement (including acute respiratory distress syndrome or ARDS) occurs in approximately 50% of patients, and leads to pulmonary edema and damage to the liver, heart, and kidneys. These symptoms are associated with the cytokine storm. The sustained elevation of IL-6 and IL-1, in addition to very high C-reactive protein (CRP) and hyperferritinemia, is decisive for the diagnosis of SAM / HLH. IL-6 can generate this process through two signaling pathways known as "cis", or classical and "trans". In the cis pathway, IL-6 binds to the membrane IL-6 receptor (mIL-6R) in a gp130 complex. Subsequent signal transduction is mediated by JAK (Janus kinase) and STAT3 (signal transducer and activator of transcription) [19].

2.3 Thrombotic Phenomena

The inflammatory system acts in conjunction with the hemostatic system, creating a continuum between both systems in which the activation of one of them activates the other. This response is given by cytokines and mediators that intervene in the hemostatic system by increasing platelet reactivity, endothelial dysfunction, activation of the coagulation cascade, reduction of natural anticoagulants, and suppression of fibrinolytic activity. This concept is known as thromboinflammation.

SARS-CoV-2 infection has been associated with the complications of venous and arterial thrombosis, which include myocardial infarction, cerebral vascular events, and venous thromboembolism. Other prothrombotic abnormalities have been identified in patients with COVID-19. Viral infection of endothelial cell conditions perivascular infiltration of T lymphocytes with activation of aberrant macrophages, causing the death of endothelial and inflammatory cells and thrombotic microangiopathy, [20].

The hemostatic disorders observed in COVID-19 can be due to hypoxia, thrombus inflammation, endotheliopathy and hypercoagulable state Hypoxia resulting in vasoconstriction and reduced blood flow that contributes to endothelial dysfunction transforming the endothelium into a procoagulant and proinflammatory phenotype, altering factors transcription, COVID-19 releases proinflammatory cytokines resulting in the release of large amounts of Von Willebrand Factor and overexpression of tissue factor, [21].

The pathophysiology of thromboembolism in COVID-19 is more dependent on platelets and is related to endothelial inflammation in addition to hypercoagulability associated with an increase in the concentration of coagulation factors, acquired antiphospholipid antibodies, and a decrease in endogenous anticoagulant proteins. Platelet-rich thrombi and the abundant number of megakaryocytes in the microvasculature have been observed in diffuse damage, especially in the alveoli in severe cases of COVID-19, in addition to an increase in viscosity, which contributes to endothelial damage, [22].

Thrombosis can occur via angiotensin, which promotes the release of the glycoprotein tissue factor, a receptor for coagulation, in response to endothelial cells, alveolar epithelial cells, fibroblasts, and cells of innate immunity express tissue factor, which in combination with Factor VIII / VIIa activate the extrinsic coagulation pathway, contributing to thrombin formation. Thrombin a proteinase initiates platelet activation, promotes prolonged aggregation and release of a substance (thromboxane A2), cells express PAR-1, a receptor-coupled G protein, thrombin is dose-dependent, high concentrations with inflammation and tissue damage. PAR-1 promotes a profibrotic phenotype in fibroblasts, alveolar inflammation, and apoptosis [20, 21].

Platelet activation also promotes the aggregation of monocytes and neutrophils. These neutrophils release factors such as cathelicidin, which can activate platelets, which in turn release proinflammatory factors such as IL 1B, thromboxane, platelet-activating factor PAF as well as ADP. The activation of protein C modulates thrombin signaling and activates coagulation by inhibiting thrombin. The decrease in protein C, protein S, and thrombomodulin are risk factors for thrombotic disorders. Platelets are also activated by the adhesion of proteins to the extracellular matrix, in particular, Von Willebrand factor, collagen, fibronectin, and thrombospondin. The multiple platelet membrane glycoproteins and integrins are receptors for extracellular matrix proteins to facilitate platelet adhesion and as an initial step in thrombus formation. These extracellular matrix proteins are characteristic of COVID-19 pathophysiology.

3 CLINICAL MANIFESTATIONS OF SARS-COV-2 INFECTION

The COVID-19 is emerging and evolving disease, the clinical manifestations known to date are mentioned below.

3.1 Asymptomatic Infection

Asymptomatic infection is estimated to be so common that 33% . This data was based on various studies and surveys showing that 46% of people at the time of a positive screening test had no symptoms. Other studies have shown that up to 73% of asymptomatic individuals remain so during follow-up [22, 23].

Nevertheless, patients with asymptomatic infection may have specific abnormalities. For instance, up to 50% showed typical ground-glass imaging [24].

3.2 Symptomatic Infection

Most infections are not serious. Eighty-one percent evolve with mild pneumonia, 14% with severe disease or pulmonary involvement > 50% on imaging, and 5% have a critical illness with respiratory failure, shock, or multiple organ dysfunction with an overall fatality rate of 2.3%, [25–27].

The case fatality rate only indicates the death rate among documented cases. Since many severe acute respiratory syndrome coronavirus 2 infections are asymptomatic, the death rate from infection is considerably lower, and some studies have estimated that it ranges between 0.5 and 1%, [28–30].

There are risk factors that may favor the development of serious disease, this adverse evolution occurs predominantly in older adults or in persons with certain underlying medical comorbidities.

SARS-CoV-2 infection can be contracted at any age. However, adults and older adults are most affected and are more likely to have a serious illness.

The Chinese Center for Disease Control and Prevention reported that the fatality rates were 8% and 15% percent among people aged 70-79 and $\geq$ 80, respectively. Mortality up to 20 times higher reported in people over 80 years of age [29–31].

Other reports mention that 80 percent of deaths occurred in people 65 years of age or older. In contrast, 18- to 34-year-olds accounted for only 5 percent of adults hospitalized for COVID-19 in a large healthcare database study and had a death rate of 2.7%. Morbid obesity, hypertension, and male sex were associated with mortality in this age group [32, 33]. Comorbidities and other conditions that have been associated with serious illness and mortality include:

- Cardiovascular disease,
- Diabetes mellitus,
- Hypertension,
- Chronic lung disease,
- Cancer (particularly hematologic malignancies, lung cancer, and metastatic disease),
- Chronic kidney disease,
- Obesity,
- Smoking.

The United States Centers for Disease Control and Prevention (CDC) has created a list of certain comorbidities that have been associated with serious illness (defined as infections resulting in hospitalization, admission to the intensive care unit [ICU], intubation or mechanical ventilation, and death) and notes the variation in the strength of associations. The male gender has accounted for a disproportionately high number of critical cases and deaths in multiple cohorts around the world [34–36].

Particular characteristics of the laboratory data have also been associated with poorer results. These include:

- High elevated inflammatory markers (e.g., C-reactive protein [CRP], ferritin) and inflammatory cytokines (i.e., interleukin 6 [IL-6] and tumor necrosis factor [TNF] -alpha),
- High D-dimer (> 1 mcg / mL),
- High prothrombin time (PT),
- High troponin,
- High creatine phosphokinase (CPK),
- Lymphopenia,
- Thrombocytopenia,
- High liver enzymes,
- High lactate dehydrogenase (LDH).

Patients with severe disease have higher viral RNA concentrations in respiratory samples than those with milder disease. Detection of viral RNA in the blood has been associated with severe conditions, including organ damage (e.g., lung, heart, kidney), coagulopathy, and mortality [37–42].

The association of host genetic factors with severe disease is also under study. As an example, a genome-wide association study identified a relationship between polymorphisms in genes encoding ABO blood group and COVID-19 respiratory failure. Type A was associated with an increased risk and type O with a lower risk for both infection and severe disease [43].

3.3 Clinical Manifestations

The incubation period for COVID-19 is generally within 14 days after exposure. Most cases occur approximately 4 to 7 days after exposure with a median incubation period of four days [20, 44].

In a systematic review that included 152 studies with > 40,000 patients, at least 26 different clinical manifestations were described: The most frequent were: fever (144 studies), cough (139 studies), dyspnea (99 studies), diarrhea (85 studies), fatigue (78 studies), headache (76 studies), and myalgia (69 studies). Six symptoms had a general prevalence greater than 25%, considering studies that reported specific clinical manifestations: fever (58.66%), cough (54.52%), dyspnea (30.82%), malaise (29,75%), fatigue (28.16%), and sputum / discharge (25.33%). Neurological symptoms (20.82%), dermatological manifestations (20.45%), anorexia (20.26%), myalgia (16.9%), sneezing (14.71%), sore throat (14.41%), rhinitis (14.29%), piloerection (13.49%), headache (12.17%), chest pain (11.49%), and diarrhea (9.59%) were other frequent symptoms. Only one study reported dermatological manifestations. Hemoptysis (1.65%) was the least frequent clinical manifestation [45].

Associated symptoms described in a report of more than 370,000 confirmed COVID-19 cases with known symptoms reported to the CDC are as follows:

- Cough in 50%,
- Fever (> 38°C) in 43%,
- Myalgia in 36%,
- Headache in 34%,
- Dyspnea in 29 percent,
- Sore throat by 20%,
- Diarrhea in 19%,

- Nausea / vomiting in 12%,
- Loss of smell or taste and rhinorrhea in less than 10% each.

Gastrointestinal symptoms (e.g., diarrhea, abdominal pain, vomiting, and nausea) are reported as the initial symptoms . The combined prevalence was 18% overall .

Cognitive manifestations have also been described, in addition to nonspecific signs and symptoms, such as falls, general deterioration, and delirium.

Dermatological findings in COVID-19 patients are not well characterized. Maculopapular, vesicular/urticarial eruptions, and transient livedo reticularis have been reported mainly in children and young adults with documented or suspected COVID-19, although no association has been established, [46–51].

3.3.1 Complications of COVID-19

The main complication is acute respiratory distress syndrome (ARDS) in patients with severe disease and it can appear shortly after the onset of dyspnea; 20% of ARDS develop an average of eight days after the onset of symptoms. The need for mechanical ventilation in hospitalized patients ranges from 12% to 24% [32, 52–54].

Other complications include those of the cardiovascular system: arrhythmias, acute cardiac injury, and shock. Up to one-third of severely ill patients admitted to the ICU develop cardiomyopathy [55, 56].

Thrombotic and embolic complications have been described such as, pulmonary embolism and acute stroke [57, 58].

Neurological complications include encephalopathy, particularly among critically ill patients, in up to 1/3 of cases. Strokes, movement disorders, motor and sensory deficits, ataxia, and seizures occur less frequently [59–61].

Other inflammatory complications and manifestations mediated by autoantibodies have also been described. Guillain-Barré syndrome can occur 5-10 days after the initial symptoms. A multisystem inflammatory syndrome with clinical characteristics like Kawasaki disease and toxic shock syndrome has also been described in children with COVID-19 [19, 62, 63].

Secondary infections do not appear to be common overall complications of COVID-19. The reported rate of bacterial or fungal coinfections is 8%; however, aspergillosis based on elevated serum galactomannan levels or bronchoalveolar lavage (BAL) has been reported [64, 65].

Autopsy studies have detected SARS-CoV-2 RNA (and in some cases antigen) in kidneys, liver, heart, brain, and blood, in addition to respiratory tract samples, suggesting that the virus spreads systemically in some cases. It is not known with certainty whether direct viral cytopathic effects at these sites contribute to the observed complications [38, 66–68], (Fig. 1).

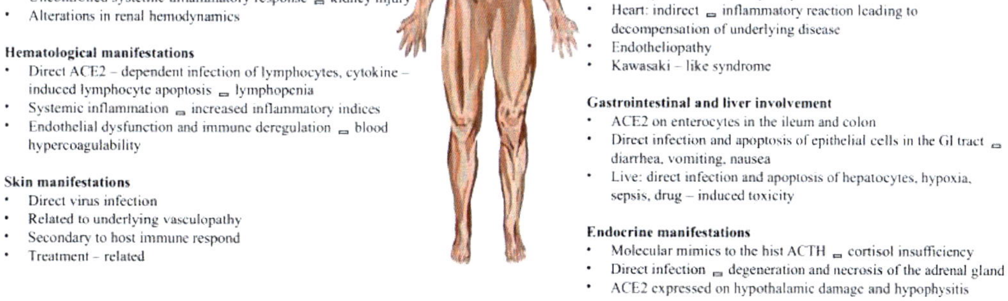

Figure 1: Overview of the systemic manifestations of COVID-19 infection

3.3.2 Damage and Manifestations to a Specific Organ of Infection by SARS-CoV-2

Although COVID-19 primarily presents as pulmonary infection transmitted by airborne droplets of saliva, the data suggest multiple organ involvement. This systemic involvement is mainly related to the binding of the SARS-CoV-2 virus to the angiotensin-converting enzyme 2 (ACE2) receptors located in different organs cells [69]. Pulmonary involvement ranges from asymptomatic disease or mild pneumonia to severe disease associated with hypoxia and critical respiratory failure. Cardiovascular complications, including, heart failure, arrhythmias, and myocardial injury were associated with a low survival rate [25, 34].

Gastrointestinal manifestations are frequent and persist for days [46]. Neurological symptoms develop a broad spectrum affecting the central nervous system, including anosmia and ageusia, peripheral nervous system, and skeletal muscles. Likewise, the liver, kidneys, skin, eyes, and endocrine organs are affected by COVID-19 infection [48, 50, 70].

3.3.3 Pulmonary Manifestations and Specific Organ Damage by SARS-CoV-2 Infection

The severity of pulmonary damage associated with SARS-CoV-2 infection ranges from no symptoms or mild pneumonia (81%) to severe hypoxia (14%), and critical respiratory failure (5%) or death (2.3%) [29]. Among those hospitalized 20 to $>$ 40% developed acute respiratory distress syndrome (ARDS). The SARS-CoV-2 binding to ACE2 receptor [71]. The ACE2 receptor is expressed on type II alveolar epithelial cells. This explains the viral tropism and pulmonary vulnerability. SARS-CoV-2 infection induces alveolar inflammatory lesions. Proinflammatory cytokines and chemokine concentrations, and tumor necrosis factor (TNF)-α, interleukin 1β (IL-1β), IL-6 are increased [72]. It has been hypothesized that the cytokine storm plays a central role in COVID-19 disease [19, 62]. The macrophage activation syndrome (MAS) share similar characteristics extensive hemophagocytosis. After the proinflammatory stage it follows a immunosuppression stage characterized by lymphopenia and low CD4 and CD8 T cell counts [15, 73]. Autopsy data demonstrate acute interstitial pneumonia and diffuse alveolar damage

(DAD) with macrophage infiltration, formation of hyaline membranes and edema and thickening of the alveolar wall as well as damage of the microvasculature with hyaline thrombosis (intra and extra) of the pulmonary vessels, hemorrhage, edema of the vascular wall, intravascular entrapment of neutrophils and infiltration of immune cells [74–77]. The term diffuse pulmonary intravascular coagulopathy (CIP) describes this vascular immunopathology located to the lungs [37, 78]. Microthrombus formation within the pulmonary vascular bed causes pulmonary infarction, pulmonary hemorrhage, pulmonary hypertension, and secondary right ventricular failure [79, 80]. (Fig. 2).

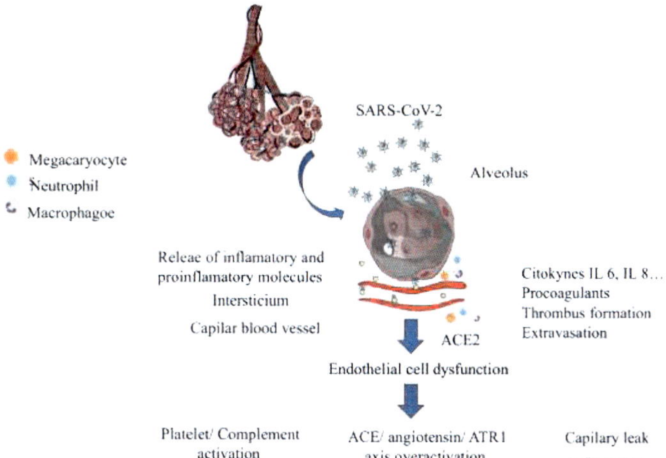

Figure 2: Vascular injury related to SARS-CoV-2

Hypoxia is common in COVID-19 pneumonia, is often insidious and paradoxically well tolerated [81]. However, the typical ARDS, pulmonary compliance, and hypoxia-driven tachypnea allow considerable volume and hypocapnia, without stimulating the sensation of dyspnea. Recently, a model has been proposed that includes two time-related phenotypes that contribute to the severity of the infection, the patient's comorbidities and physiological reserve, the period between disease onset and hospitalization, and the host's immune response. The L phenotype is seen in the early stages of the disease; there is significant lung compliance and the ventilation / perfusion ratio (Va / Q ratio) is low, but there is dysfunctional regulation of perfusion with hypoxic vasoconstriction. At this stage, both lung weight and lung recruitment capacity are low with a minimal amount of non-ventilated lung tissue. This becomes the H phenotype with decreased lung compliance due to edema, and an increase in the fraction of cardiac output that perfuses non-ventilated tissue.

Type L patients tend to remain stable for some time and then may improve or worsen and transform into type H, as a consequence of the evolution of COVID-19 pneumonia, but also of the injury induced by excessive stress ventilation, [82].

The fatal ARDS in COVID-19 patients is the increase in circulating proinflammatory cytokines, IL-1, IL-6 , interferon, and TNF-α. This is called "cytokine storm" due response to SARS-CoV-2 infection that leads to endothelial cell dysfunction, vascular barrier , capillary leak, and alveolar damage [83]. Anti-IL-6 inhibitors, and corticosteroids, especially dexamethasone, have been evaluated in patients with severe COVID-19 [84, 85].

3.3.4 Cardiovascular Involvement

In the cardiovascular system, SARS-CoV-2 infection occurs after the binding of the viral protein peak to the human ACE2 receptor . Viral entry occurs by endocytosis after the interaction of glycoprotein S1 (viral peak protein) with the receptor-binding domain of ACE2 receptors. This is followed by the release of the viral genome, synthesis of viral structural protein, and genome accumulation of mature virions, and then release by exocytosis (Fig. 3). The immune response triggered by SARS-CoV-2 is responsible for both the resolution of the disease and its pathogenesis when this response is out of control. The involvement of multiple systems in COVID-19 occurs as a result of cytokine storm and damage mediated by these inflammatory cytokines [83, 86, 87], (Fig. 3).

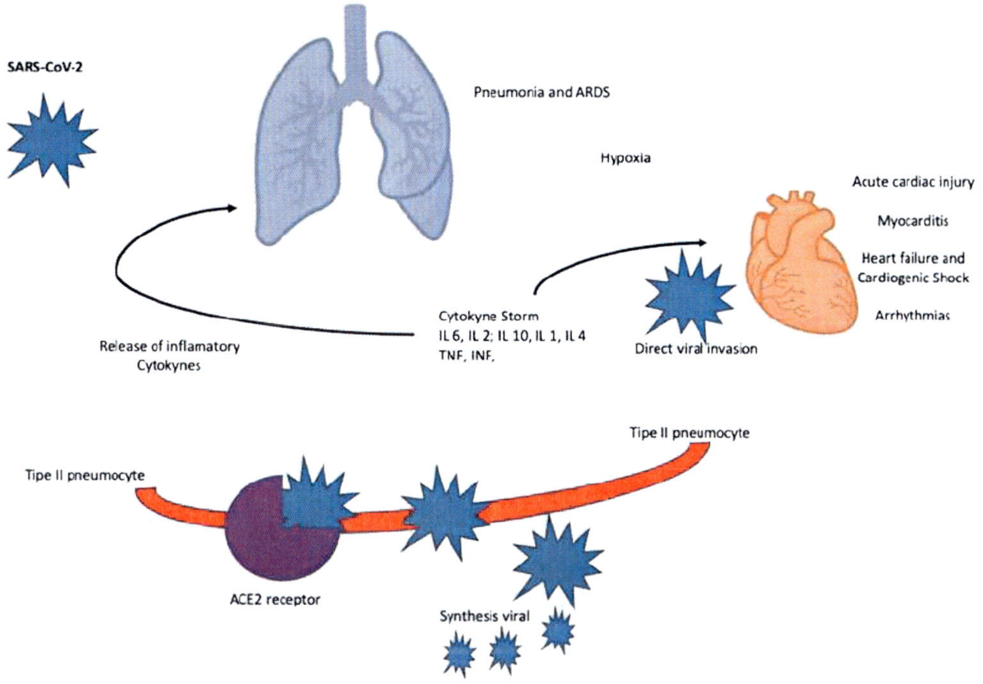

Figure 3: Mechanism of viral invasion, replication, and pathogenesis

In patients with COVID-19 infection, underlying comorbidities, such as cardiovascular diseases have been associated with [poor] outcomes and survival [20, 34, 53], while the appearance of cardiovascular complications, heart failure, arrhythmias, and myocardial injury [24, 87]. Evidence of myocardial injury in COVID-19 patients has been found [88]. ACE2 expression is high in cardiac tissue and can potentially facilitate direct myocardial damage induced by viral infection. Isolated cases of COVID-19 induced myocarditis have also been reported, supporting the hypothesis of direct myocardial injury by SARS-CoV-2. ACE2 plays an important role in the renin-angiotensin system by catalyzing the conversion of angiotensin II to angiotensin protective effect on the cardiovascular system [89–91]. Importantly, the binding of SARS-CoV-2 to ACE2 results in the loss of the external catalytic effect of ACE2, [58, 76–79]. Subsequently, the theoretical negative regulation of ACE2 and the decrease of angiotensin levels [92] in patients with COVID-19 can compromise cardiac function [56, 93, 94]. Systemic cytokines can also activate the microvascular endothelium and induce dysfunction of the coronary microvasculature, which can lead to myocardial ischemia and myocardial injury [55, 95–97].

Inflammation and subsequent dysfunction of the endothelium in various organs are the results of both the direct effect of SARS-CoV-2 infection on endothelial cells and the indirect effects of the host's inflammatory response. Severe respiratory complications and associated hypoxia have been common findings in COVID-19 patients. Besides, hypotension, as a common clinical feature in both sepsis and cytokine storm syndrome, can also reduce myocardial oxygen supply [95]. Myocarditis mild or fulminant can be a clinical manifestation of COVID-19 and can lead to systolic dysfunction of the left ventricle or even cardiogenic shock [55, 98, 99].

Heart failure has been reported as a complication in $> 20\%$ of cases [94, 100–102]. The incidence of lethal arrhythmias such as sustained ventricular tachycardia or ventricular fibrillation were 5.9% in the first reports from China [103, 104]. It is important to note that arrhythmias also can be induced by medical treatment of COVID-19, some agents and their combinations may prolong the QTc interval and predispose to helical tachyarrhythmia or other ventricular arrhythmias [98, 105–107]. Recently, a Kawasaki-like syndrome was reported, characterized by circulatory dysfunction and syndrome of macrophage activation [108, 109]. Other reports in Italy, showed a 30-fold increase in the incidence of Kawasaki-like disease during the COVID-19 pandemic [110].

3.3.5 Image Results

Chest X-rays can be normal in early or mild disease. Common abnormal radiographic findings were consolidation and ground-glass opacities, with bilateral peripheral and lower lung distributions. Lung involvement increases during the disease, peaking in severity 10 to 12 days after the onset of symptoms. Spontaneous pneumothorax has also been described, although it is relatively uncommon (0.56%) [111–114].

Chest computed tomography (CT) may be more sensitive than the chest x-ray and some chest CT findings may be characteristic of COVID-19. No finding can completely rule out the possibility of COVID-19. If a CT scan is done, the Radiological Society of North America has categorized the features as typical, indeterminate, or atypical of COVID-19. Chest CT in patients with COVID-19 more frequently demonstrates ground-glass opacities with or without consolidation abnormalities, consistent with viral pneumonia. The following findings are the most frequent:

- Ground glass opacities: $> 80\%$,
- Ground glass opacity with mixed consolidation: $> 50\%$,
- Adjacent pleural thickening: $> 50\%$,
- Thickening of the interlobular septum: $> 40\%$,
- Air bronchograms: $> 40\%$.

Other less common findings were a crazy paving pattern (ground glass opacities with overlapping septal thickening), bronchiectasis, pleural effusion, pericardial effusion, and lymphadenopathy. Chest CT abnormalities in COVID-19 are often bilateral, have a peripheral distribution, and involve the lower lobes [115–117]. Pulmonary ultrasonography has been used to evaluate lung involvement in patients with suspected COVID-19 when other imaging resources are not readily available. Lung ultrasound findings in patients with documented COVID-19 include thickening, suspension, and interruption of the pleural line, visible B lines under the pleura that appear discrete, multifocal, or confluent; patchy, striped, and nodular consolidation; and air bronchogram signs [118–120].

4 DRUG TREATMENT

4.1 Convalescent Patient Plasma

Recovered patients' plasma has been used for years to treat patients with inflammatory diseases, with the theory that antibodies contained in convalescent patients' plasma will be useful in helping patients to recover. It has been used in diseases such as Ebola, influenza, SARS 1 virus, among others, with diverse outcomes [121]. The COVID-19 pandemic has stimulated a lot of studies in the search for an effective treatment against SARS-CoV-2. The use of Convalescent Plasma (CP) of recovered patients has been a subject of research.

The greatest experience with the use of CP in COVID-19 is reported by the Mayo Clinic of the United States [122], where its uncontrolled, open, and generalized use limits the value of the results obtained. However, in this study, it was suggested that the use of convalescent plasma reduced mortality at 7 and 30 days in those patients under 80 years of age, not intubated, and in whom the administration of plasma was within the first 72 hours after diagnosis.

Three randomized, double-blind, placebo-controlled studies from Argentina, China, and India contradict the results of the Mayo Clinic observational study. None of these studies demonstrated a benefit in mortality or clinical recovery with the use of convalescent plasma. However, the onset of clinical manifestations when using plasma was longer than 72 hours, with a minimum of 8 days [122–125].

More recently, a randomized clinical trial demonstrated that CP reduces the risk of progression to severe disease in patients older than 64 years, and with the administration of therapy in the first 72 hours of the onset of symptoms [126].

In general, it is considered a safe therapy with the same risks involved in the transfusion of plasma. The potential benefits are a reduction in mortality, a decrease in the need for mechanical ventilation, a decrease in viral load reflected in a shorter time until obtaining a negative PCR in nasopharyngeal material, and a reduction in the time to recovery. Multiplies studies and clinical observation show benefit from the use of plasma but this evidence is low to very low quality to draw absolute conclusions [122, 127].

In theory and with the currently existing evidence, the higher the antibody titers in the Convalescent Plasma, the greater the benefit. The criticism of the use of PC is the absence of measurement of antibody titers in transfusion recipients, and in studies where antibody measurement was done in recipients, its value was similar to that found in donors. Slightly under

20% of donors are considered to contain enough antibodies in their plasma to produce a benefit from its use [128].

In conclusion, convalescent plasma therapy is safe and could be useful and improve the prognosis in noncritical patients, if it is administered ideally in the first 72 hours after diagnosis, hospitalization, or onset of symptoms, and with sufficient antibody titers. Despite approval by the Food and Drug Association (FDA) for the use of convalescent plasma in the treatment of COVID-19, some international organizations such as the National Institutes of Health (NIH) and the Infectious Diseases Society of America (IDSA) of the United States consider the current evidence insufficient to be in favor or against its use. This could change in the future as new evidence is added. There is still a need for standardization in the processes for evaluating antibody titers in convalescent plasma, defining the value of useful antibodies and the dose of plasma to be administered.

4.2 Remdesivir

The use of antivirals could not be lacking in the search for an effective treatment with COVID-19. Remdesivir is an adenosine nucleoside analog prodrug that, when activated, inhibits the RNA-dependent RNA polymerase of SARS-CoV-2, essentially inhibiting its replication. It has been effective in in vitro studies and animal models to prevent and treat the disease. It was the first drug authorized by the Food and Drug Administration (FDA) for the treatment of COVID-19 in adult and pediatric populations over 12 years of age, weighting over 40 kilograms [129].

The ACTT study is a randomized clinical trial that evaluated the efficacy and safety of Remdesivir in just over a thousand adult patients with confirmed COVID-19 and a severe condition defined by the need for oxygen support or saturation less than or equal to 94% in room air. The main objective was the evaluation of the time to clinical recovery measured on an ordinal scale of 8 ascending items in a nonhospitalized patient without limitation to death by COVID-19. The study demonstrated a significant decrease in time to recovery in the Remdesivir group, with a non-significant trend of lower mortality without being associated with adverse events compared to placebo [130].

The World Health Organization Solidarity study included hospitals in 30 different countries evaluating more than eleven thousand hospitalized patients for the use of Remdesivir, hydroxychloroquine, lopinavir, and interferon. Unlike the ACTT study, no benefit in mortality, mechanical ventilation requirement, or length of hospitalization was demonstrated with any of the drugs compared to placebo [131]. This led the WHO to not recommend the use of Remdesivir as a treatment for COVID-19. The potential benefits that have been evaluated are a decrease in mortality, decrease in the need for mechanical ventilation or extracorporeal circulation, reduction of time to improvement, and viral load in the upper or lower respiratory tract. For most of these outcomes, the results have been negative, except for the recovery time. Clinical improvement was evaluated by different ordinal clinical scales. Most of the trials evaluated moderate to severe COVID-19 patients and even critically ill patients [131].

Remdesivir must be administered in an in-patient setting. The dose is 200 mg intravenously initially, followed by 4 or 9 days of 100 mg intravenous daily [129]. Two studies have evaluated the difference between both regimens, the first of which [132] also compared them with standard disease care in patients with moderate COVID-19 (SpO2 $\geq$ 94% at room air with pulmonary infiltrates), and found that the 5-day scheme had the best results in terms of clinical improvement [132]. The second study directly compared both schemes in patients with severe forms of the disease (SpO2 $\leq$ 94% on room air or use of supplemental oxygen), and found no differences between the two doses [133].

The possibility of providing the same benefit with a shorter duration scheme improves the cost-benefit ratio and reduces the possibility of adverse drug reactions. The most common adverse reactions are gastrointestinal symptoms with nausea or vomiting, elevated transaminases, increased prothrombin time, and hypersensitivity reactions.

Monitoring of kidney and liver function should be done before treatment and whenever deemed necessary by medical judgment. In general, it is a safe treatment. In clinical trials the frequency of reported adverse events was even higher in the placebo group. Treatment should be suspended in the event of an increase in the transaminase level above 10 times the normal value or a reduction in the glomerular filtration rate below 30 ml/min.

Recently, it has been shown that its use in conjunction with Baricitinib enhances the benefits of both drugs without increasing adverse effects. An improvement in recovery time was demonstrated especially in patients with oxygen use through high-flow nasal tips or noninvasive mechanical ventilation and a trend to decrease mortality compared to Remdesivir alone [134]. Co-administration with dexamethasone is expected to produce a null or slight decrease in the levels of the antiviral.

In conclusion, Remdesivir is perhaps the drug with the best evidence of potential benefit in COVID-19 infection in patients with moderate to severe disease, in reducing mortality, but particularly in reducing the time to clinical improvement. Subsidiary analyses of studies have shown that the benefit is greater if it is used in the early stages of the disease. Information on the safety and efficacy of its use in pregnant women and children under 12 years of age is scarce, therefore its use should be avoided in these population groups. One of the most important drawbacks for its generalized indication is the high cost of the drug and the limited availability in the world market.

4.3 Baricitinib

Until before the COVID-19 epidemic, Baricitinib was used in patients with rheumatoid arthritis. In addition to the blocking effect of Janus kinase, Baricitinib inhibits the intracellular protein AP2-related protein kinase 1 (AAK1) and binds to the G protein-associated kinase, which allows it to alter the endocytosis mechanisms of some viruses like Ebola, Hepatitis C, and SARS-CoV-2 [135]. However, the clinical use of this molecule for this purpose is limited.

The first clinical evidence of the potential benefit of Baricitinib as a treatment for COVID-19 pneumonia arised from a non-randomized, observational study of 15 patients with moderate infection who received a combination treatment based on Hydroxychloroquine and Baricitinib. In this study, clinical improvement was observed in 13 patients, and 2 cases of fungal or bacterial infection associated with prolonged ICU stay were reported [136]. The level of association was low and the cause could not be established to suggest routine Baricitinib treatment.

As part of the treatment strategies targeting the virus, the Adaptive COVID-19 Treatment Trial (ACTT-1), a controlled clinical trial, was designed to evaluate the clinical efficacy and safety of Remdesivir. The results of this study were encouraging, as it found a decrease in the recovery time which was 10 days in the Remdesivir group (95% CI 9-11) compared to 15 days in the placebo group (95% CI 13-18). The difference was statistically significant ($p < 0.05$). Albeit not statistically significant, other results were a reduction in mortality at day 15 of disease evolution, 6.7% in the Remdesivir group and 11.9% in the control group, and no increase in the number of adverse events [130].

Despite the promising findings of Remdesivir as a treatment for COVID-19, patients continued to suffer from a high burden of disease and it was proposed that, in addition to the mechanism of cellular damage, there is damage related to cytokine release; therefore, different research groups postulated the role of different target blockers.

Therefore, a second phase of the Adaptive COVID-19 Treatment Trial (ACTT-2), was designed, which aimed to evaluate the superiority of the combination of Remdesivir and Baricitinib compared to Remdesivir alone [30]. To date, this is the only randomized clinical trial that evaluated the role of Baricitinib during the disease. The results of this RCT were a decreasing trend in mortality in the combined group compared to Remdesivir alone (4.7% vs 7.1%), higher clinical recovery (69.3% vs 59.7%), and a lower probability of requiring invasive mechanical ventilation or the use of extracorporeal oxygenation membrane (10% vs 15.2%, RR 0.66; 95% CI 0.46-0.93). Patients who, at randomization, had supplemental oxygen or noninvasive mechanical ventilation also drew more advantages from the combination therapy. This benefit was not found in mechanically ventilated patients. In ACTT-2, patients assigned to the combined treatment arm of the trial had a lower rate of respiratory infections compared to Remdesivir (5.9% vs 11.2%) [134].

Based on the evidence presented, the existence of therapeutic alternatives with proven efficacy (Dexamethasone), and the biases of the patients assigned to the Baricitinib study, the expert panel of the Infectious Diseases Society of America [137] suggests the use of Baricitinib in combination with Remdesivir in the following clinical settings:

1. In patients hospitalized for severe COVID-19 (defined by SpO2 $<$ 94% in room air, on supplemental oxygen or noninvasive mechanical ventilation), and who cannot receive glucocorticoids due to some contraindications.

2. In patients hospitalized for COVID-19 who are planned to be included in a randomized clinical trial in combination with dexamethasone.

The role of Baricitinib in combination with dexamethasone has not been clear, but there are some clinical trials aimed at answering this question with results pending publication.

4.4 Anticoagulation and COVID-19

During the advance in the knowledge of the clinical effects associated with COVID-19, it has become clear that the inflammatory component is essential in the pathogenesis of the disease, but vascular dysfunction and venous and arterial thrombosis also play an important role. The mechanisms associated with these processes are hypoxemia, excessive inflammation, immobilization, platelet activation, microvascular thrombosis, and immunological mechanisms that are yet not well clarified [138].

Around the world, hematological alterations such as leukopenia, leukocytosis, lymphopenia, and thrombocytopenia have been found in different cohorts of patients, which are associated with a poor prognosis. Furthermore, the elevation of D-Dimer ($>$ 1000 ng/ml), creatine kinase, C-reactive protein, lactic dehydrogenase, troponin, and ferritin are associated with disease severity [139].

Of particular interest is the elevation of D-dimer, since it is used in risk stratification in patients with suspected deep venous thromboembolism and/or pulmonary thromboembolism. In a series of 184 cases of patients hospitalized for COVID-19 in the ICU, an incidence of 34% of diagnoses of venous and arterial thrombosis was found (95% CI: 20-41%) [57]. Predictors associated with embolic events were age, PT prolongation, and partial tromboplastine time (PTT). It is striking that this group of patients received thromboprophylaxis according to current clinical practice guidelines.

The current treatment of COVID-19 is aimed at managing its main manifestations: inflammation and thrombosis, the latter being of particular interest since there is no standardized prophylactic protocol, but there are alternatives for the study and risk stratification of these patients.

At the time of hospital admission, it is suggested that all patients have a determination of D-dimer concentration, PT, and platelet count.

Treatment alternatives include thromboembolic prophylaxis with low molecular weight heparin (LMWH), such as enoxaparin. Both the International Society of Thrombosis and Hemostasis and the WHO suggest that some LMWH-based prophylaxis regimens can be used in critically ill patients with constant monitoring of fibrinogen levels, kidney function, and platelets. The recommended dose of LMWH is 40 mg of subcutaneous enoxaparin every 24 hours, in case the glomerular filtration rate (GFR) is greater than 30 ml/min, or 30 mg a day in case the GFR is less than the cut-off point. Its use is not suggested in cases of GFR less than 15 ml/min or renal replacement therapy. Therefore, there is no scientific evidence on the use of D-dimers to guide the decision to increase anticoagulant doses [140].

The duration of therapy has not been established on a scientific basis, but based on pathophysiological knowledge which suggests that the inflammation can extend up to 90 days after the onset of the condition, the current recommendation is to maintain antithrombotic prophylaxis for this period [141].

4.5 Steroid Use in COVID-19

Steroids have been used before the COVID-19 pandemic in patients with pneumonia of viral or bacterial origin, as well as in primary or secondary ARDS, with controversial results in clinical trials, meta-analyses, even with limited recommendations in diagnostic guidelines, and treatment [142–144].

One of the clinical trials with the best methodology was that of Dr. Del Villar published in February 2020 that included 277 patients with mechanical ventilation secondary to moderate and severe ARDS, in which the intervention group received 20mg of dexamethasone from day 1 to day 5, and 10mg from day 6 to day 10. The study was stopped after 88% of the population had been recruited to demonstrate a clear benefit in the primary outcome, which was a decrease in the days of mechanical ventilation by 4.9 days (95% CI 2.5 to 7.03) when administered early, and a reduction of 12.5% (2.3% to 22.4%) in in-hospital mortality, with no difference in adverse events such as hyperglycemia or new infections [145].

Due to the lack of a specific etiological treatment against SARS-CoV-2, and the use of steroids in COVID-19 to reduce the inflammatory response it causes, it has been implemented in cross-sectional and prospective studies. Table 1 compiles the main studies on the use of steroids in COVID-19 disease.

A meta-analysis was recently conducted by the World Health Organization, published in The Lancet that included clinical trials with Dexamethasone, Hydrocortisone, and Methylprednisolone. It accords a benefit to the use of any steroid to reduce mortality from COVID-19, although with significant heterogeneity among groups of patients [144].

The current recommendations of the American Society of Infectious Diseases (IDSA) include, with a moderate level of evidence:

1. In critically ill hospitalized patients (patients requiring invasive or noninvasive mechanical ventilation): a strong recommendation with a moderate level of evidence of Dexamethasone 6mg, IV, or PO every 24 hours for 10 days or until home discharge or when it is not available,

Study	Steroid Dose	Population	Outcome	Conclusion
CODEX LANCET 2020 [144]	Dexamethasone 20mg day 1-5 v 10mg day 6-10	299 patients Moderate to Severe ARDS	Day of Mechanical ventilation 6.6 (CI 95% 5.0 a 8.2) Without difference in mortality or adverse effects	High dose steroids reduce days of mechanical ventilation in patient with ARDS by COVID-19
RECOVERY NEJM 2020 [145]	Dexamethasone 6mg (1 to 10 days)	Hospitalization 2104 patients with dexamethasone 4321 Usual care	Mortality at 28 days Dexamethasone 0.83% (CI 95% 0.75 a 0.93) IMV 0.64% (CI 95% 0.51 a 0.81%) O2 0.82 (CI 95% 0.72 a 0.94%)	Less mortality at 28 days in mechanical ventilated, patients with O2 requirements No benefit in patients without oxygen need
Nelson IDSA 2020 [146]	Methylprednisolone	117 patients 1mg/kg/day at least 5 days	Days free for IMV 6.21 ± 7.45 vs 3.14 ± 6.22 $p = 0.44$ Weaning from IMV 45 vs 21% $p = 0.021$ Without significant difference in infections	Use of steroids decrease days of mechanical ventilation and the average of weaning from mechanical ventilation
Prado IDSA 2020 [147]	Methylprednisolone 0.5 mg/kg two times a day up to 5 days	41 patients with ARDS	Without difference in mechanical ventilation or infection rate	No benefit
Passenn Critical Care 2020 [148]	Steroids	20197 patients with steroids systematic review and meta-analysis	Mortality reduction 0.73 (CI 0.57 a 0.87)	Beneficial effect when use, lower risk for mortality and need for IMV

Table 1: Summary of clinical trials of steroid use on COVID-19 infection

its equivalent in some other steroids such as Methylprednisolone 32mg every 24 hours or prednisone 40mg every 24 hours.

2. In severe but not critically ill hospitalized patients (patients with saturation less than 94% or who require supplemental oxygen administration): a conditional recommendation with a moderate level of evidence of 6mg of Dexamethasone IV or PO for 10 days or until discharge or when it is not available, or its equivalent in another steroid such as Methylprednisolone 32mg every 24 hours or prednisone 40mg every 24 hours.
3. In patients with mild disease (patients without hypoxemia, saturation > 94%, the use of steroids is not recommended due to their greater risk.

Concerning steroid use, the National Institutes of Health recommend:

1. The use of steroids in a certain group of patients with or without the associated use of Remdesivir in hospitalized patients, based on the administration of Dexamethasone 6mg PO every 24 hours, or :
    - Prednisone 40mg every 24 hours in a single dose or divided into two doses.
    - Methylprednisolone 32mg every 24 hours in a single dose or divided into two doses.
    - Hydrocortisone: 160mg every 24 hours divided into two to four doses.
2. Monitoring hyperglycemia, infections, and special care in patients with HIV or hepatitis C.

The WHO issued a strong recommendation for the use of corticosteroids (ex. Dexamethasone 6mg orally or intravenously every 24 hours or 50mg of hydrocortisone every 8 hours) for 7 to 10 days in patients with severe or critical COVID-19, and a conditional recommendation not to administer steroids in patients with nonsevere COVID-19.

The administration of steroids at least 6mg of Dexamethasone or its equivalent of another steroid for a period of 5 to 10 days in patients who require oxygen is recommended, especially in those who require mechanical ventilation.

Based on the CODEX study, patients with moderate to severe ARDS, with a dose of Dexamethasone of 20mg for 5 days and then 10mg for another 5 days could have a greater benefit in reducing the days of mechanical ventilation [145].

Patients with COVID-19 who do not have an oxygen saturation lower than 94%, do not require supplemental oxygen, and the use of steroids can be harmful, so it is not recommended.

4.6 Tocilizumab

Within the pathophysiology of COVID-19, there is an important systemic inflammatory response called cytokine storm, characterized by a severe inflammatory response where high levels of interleukin 6 have been documented, hence, the inhibition of this proinflammatory cytokine may provide a therapeutic option, and Tocilizumab being the most widely used drug (Table 2).

In patients with severe progressive or critical disease with elevated inflammatory biomarkers, Tocilizumab is conditionally recommended on the support of a low level of evidence [152].

In observational studies where Tocilizumab has been used with risk propensity analysis, its effectiveness has been demonstrated with a decrease in mortality and an improvement in symptoms in patients with COVID-19. However, this benefit has not shown up in clinical trials with patients with severe or critical COVID-19. In clinical trials, it does not seem to have adverse effects or increase superinfections [153].

Selective inhibitors have not been shown to decrease mortality in COVID-19 patients, but they could decrease the probability of requiring mechanical ventilation in patients when administered before requiring admission to the intensive care unit, without increasing adverse effects [146, 147].

5 CONCLUDING REMARKS

SARS-CoV-2 is a beta coronavirus with four structural proteins involved in viral replication, triggering a systemic inflammatory response and activation of coagulation in symptomatic patients. It is associated with elevation of acute phase reactants as well as lymphopenia. This

Study	Tocilizumab Dose	Population	Outcome	Conclusion
COVACTA [149]	8 mg/kg	438 patients 294 Tocilizumab 144 Placebo	Without difference	The use of tocilizumab was not associated with any benefit and no adverse effects were found
	Maximum dose 800 mg			
EMPACTA [150]	8mg/kg	389 patients	Mechanical ventilation or mortality (0.56 IC 95% 0.33 a 0.97)	May decrease likelihood of IOT
		249 Tocilizumab	Mortality (-5.2 a 7.8%)	
			No difference in adverse events	
		128 Placebo		
Somer IDSA [151]	8mg/kg	Patients with mechanical ventilation	HR mortality adjusted (0.55 IC 0.33 a 0.90) in Tocilizumab group	Super Infections
		Cohort study of 154 patients 78 Tocilizumab Younger group fewer comorbidities		Tocilizumab 54% vs 15% control group
		76 without Tocilizumab		Without associated mortality 22% vs 15%

Table 2: Summary of clinical trials of Tocilizumab

process is perpetuated by abnormal activation of the protein complex called inflammasome. Thromboinflammation and abnormal activation of the coagulation cascade and fibrinolytic activity will promote venous and arterial thrombotic phenomena.

Current knowledge of SARS-CoV-2 is constantly evolving. An early diagnosis of the infectious process to assess the magnitude of the inflammatory response and of the organic damage is essential in supportive treatment. The susceptibility and severity were determined by multiple factors in each individual.

Dexamethasone, based on the RECOVERY clinical trial protocol, is the drug with the best support by the most solid scientific evidence, but it should be used only in patients with Spo2 less than 92% to reduce mortality. The clinical trials in which Tocilizumab, Baricitinib, Remdesivir, and Convalescent Plasma were used had heterogeneous selection criteria and the generalization of the results is complex and risky. In hospitals where these treatment alternatives are available and the use of any of these drugs is recommended, it should always be administered according to the inclusion and exclusion criteria of randomized clinical trials already published.

6 CONSENT FOR PUBLICATION

Not applicable.

7 CONFLICT OF INTEREST

The authors declare no conflict of interest, financial or otherwise.

8 ACKNOWLEDGEMENTS

We want to express our gratitude to all the staff, from all areas of the Ignacio Chávez National Institute of Cardiology, who participated, directly and indirectly, in the care of COVID-19 patients.

References

[1] WHO | World Health Organization [Internet]. WHO Director-General's remarks at the media briefing on 2019-nCoV on 11 February 2020; 2021 Feb 11 [cited 2021 Apr 4]. Available from: https://www.who.int/director-general/speeches/detail/who-director-general-s-remarks-at-the-media-briefing-on-2019-ncov-on-11-february-2020

[2] Zhu N, Zhang D, Wang W, Li X, Yang B, Song J, Zhao X, Huang B, Shi W, Lu R, Niu P, Zhan F, Ma X, Wang D, Xu W, Wu G, Gao GF, Tan W. A Novel Coronavirus from Patients with Pneumonia in China, 2019. New England Journal of Medicine [Internet]. 2020 Feb 20 [cited 2021 Sep 29];382(8):727–33. Available from: https://doi.org/10.1056/nejmoa2001017

[3] Weiss SR, Leibowitz JL. Coronavirus Pathogenesis. In: Advances in Virus Research [Internet]. Elsevier; 2011 [cited 2021 Sep 29]. p. 85–164. Available from: https://doi.org/10.1016/b978-0-12-385885-6.00009-2

[4] Harapan H, Itoh N, Yufika A, Winardi W, Keam S, Te H, Megawati D, Hayati Z, Wagner AL, Mudatsir M. Coronavirus disease 2019 (COVID-19): A literature review. Journal of Infection and Public Health [Internet]. 2020 May [cited 2021 Sep 29];13(5):667–73. Available from: https://doi.org/10.1016/j.jiph.2020.03.019

[5] The species Severe acute respiratory syndrome-related coronavirus: classifying 2019-nCoV and naming it SARS-CoV-2. Nature Microbiology [Internet]. 2020 Mar 2 [cited 2021 Sep 29];5(4):536–44. Available from: https://doi.org/10.1038/s41564-020-0695-z

[6] Huang C, Wang Y, Li X, Ren L, Zhao J, Hu Y, et al. Clinical features of patients infected with 2019 novel coronavirus in Wuhan, China. The Lancet [Internet]. 2020 Feb [cited 2021 Sep 29];395(10223):497–506. Available from: https://doi.org/10.1016/s0140-6736(20)30183-55

[7] Oran DP, Topol EJ. Prevalence of Asymptomatic SARS-CoV-2 Infection. Annals of Internal Medicine [Internet]. 2020 Sep 1 [cited 2021 Sep 29];173(5):362–7. Available from: https://doi.org/10.7326/m20-3012

[8] Machhi J, Herskovitz J, Senan AM, Dutta D, Nath B, Oleynikov MD, Blomberg WR, Meigs DD, Hasan M, Patel M, Kline P, Chang RC, Chang L, Gendelman HE, Kevadiya BD. The Natural History, Pathobiology, and Clinical Manifestations of SARS-CoV-2 Infections. Journal of Neuroimmune Pharmacology [Internet]. 2020 Jul 21 [cited 2021 Sep 29];15(3):359–86. Available from: https://doi.org/10.1007/s11481-020-09944-5

[9] Nishiga M, Wang DW, Han Y, Lewis DB, Wu JC. COVID-19 and cardiovascular disease: from basic mechanisms to clinical perspectives. Nature Reviews Cardiology [Internet]. 2020 Jul 20 [cited 2021 Sep 29];17(9):543–58. Available from: https://doi.org/10.1038/s41569-020-0413-9

[10] Hartenian E, Nandakumar D, Lari A, Ly M, Tucker JM, Glaunsinger BA. The molecular virology of coronaviruses. Journal of Biological Chemistry [Internet]. 2020 Jul 13 [cited 2021 Sep 29];295(37):12910–34. Available from: https://doi.org/10.1074/jbc.rev120.013930

[11] López G, Ramírez M, Torres M. Pathophysiology of multi-organ damage in SARS-CoV-2 infection. Acta Pediátrica de México. 2020;1(41):27–41.

[12] Cervera R, Espinosa G, Hernández J, Prieto S, Espigol G, Cid M. Respuesta Inmunoinflamatoria en la COVID-19. In: Respuesta inflamatoria en la Covid-19. Panamericana; 2020. p. 1–17.

[13] Páramo JA. Respuesta inflamatoria en relación con COVID-19 y otros fenotipos protrombóticos. Reumatología Clínica [Internet]. 2020 Jun [cited 2021 Sep 29]. Available from: https://doi.org/10.1016/j.reuma.2020.06.004

[14] Rodríguez F, Rodríguez M, Nava C. Immunity, inflammation and thrombosis. Trying to understand the infection due to COVID-19. Medicina Interna de México. 2020;4(36):557–561.

[15] Channappanavar R, Zhao J, Perlman S. T cell-mediated immune response to respiratory coronaviruses. Immunologic Research [Internet]. 2014 May 21 [cited 2021 Sep 29];59(1-3):118–28. Available from: https://doi.org/10.1007/s12026-014-8534-z

[16] Liu Y, Yang Y, Zhang C, Huang F, Wang F, Yuan J, et al. Clinical and biochemical indexes from 2019-nCoV infected patients linked to viral loads and lung injury. Science China Life Sciences [Internet]. 2020 Feb 9 [cited 2021 Sep 29];63(3):364–74. Available from: https://doi.org/10.1007/s11427-020-1643-8

[17] Morikawa K, Oseko F, Morikawa S. H- and L-rich ferritins suppress antibody production, but not proliferation, of human B lymphocytes in vitro. Blood [Internet]. 1994 Feb 1 [cited 2021 Sep 29];83(3):737–43. Availablefrom:https://doi.org/10.1182/blood.v83.3.737.737

[18] Morris SB, Schwartz NG, Patel P, Abbo L, Beauchamps L, Balan S et al. Case series of multisystem inflammatory syndrome in adults associated with SARS-CoV-2 infection – united kingdom and united states, march–august 2020. MMWR. Morbidity and Mortality Weekly Report [Internet]. 9 de octubre de 2020 [cited 2021 Sep 29];69(40):1450–6. Available from: https://doi.org/10.15585/mmwr.mm6940e1

[19] Mehta P, McAuley DF, Brown M, Sanchez E, Tattersall RS, Manson JJ. COVID-19: consider cytokine storm syndromes and immunosuppression. The Lancet [Internet]. 2020 Mar [cited 2021 Sep 29];395(10229):1033–4. Available from: https://doi.org/10.1016/s0140-6736(20)30628-0

[20] Piazza G, Morrow DA. Diagnosis, Management, and Pathophysiology of Arterial and Venous Thrombosis in COVID-19. JAMA [Internet]. 2020 Dec 22 [cited 2021 Sep 29];324(24):2548–9. Available from: https://doi.org/10.1001/jama.2020.23422

[21] Joly BS, Siguret V, Veyradier A. Understanding pathophysiology of hemostasis disorders in critically ill patients with COVID-19. Intensive Care Medicine [Internet]. 2020 May 15 [cited 2021 Sep 29];46(8):1603–6. Available from: https://doi.org/10.1007/s00134-020-06088-1

[22] Hu Z, Song C, Xu C, Jin G, Chen Y, Xu X, Ma H, Chen W, Lin Y, Zheng Y, Wang J, Hu Z, Yi Y, Shen H. Clinical characteristics of 24 asymptomatic infections with COVID-19 screened among close contacts in Nanjing, China. Science China Life Sciences [Internet]. 2020 Mar 4 [cited 2021 Sep 29];63(5):706–11. Available from: https://doi.org/10.1007/s11427-020-1661-4

[23] Wang D, Hu B, Hu C, Zhu F, Liu X, Zhang J, Wang B, Xiang H, Cheng Z, Xiong Y, Zhao Y, Li Y, Wang X, Peng Z. Clinical Characteristics of 138 Hospitalized Patients With 2019 Novel Coronavirus–Infected Pneumonia in Wuhan, China. JAMA [Internet]. 2020 Mar

17 [cited 2021 Sep 29];323(11):1061–9. Available from: https://doi.org/10.1001/jama.2020.1585

[24] Liu K, Fang YY, Deng Y, Liu W, Wang MF, Ma JP, Xiao W, Wang YN, Zhong MH, Li CH, Li GC, Liu HG. Clinical characteristics of novel coronavirus cases in tertiary hospitals in Hubei Province. Chinese Medical Journal [Internet]. 2020 May [cited 2021 Sep 29];133(9):1025–31. Available from: https://doi.org/10.1097/cm9.0000000000000744

[25] Yang X, Yu Y, Xu J, Shu H, Xia J, Liu H, Wu Y, Zhang L, Yu Z, Fang M, Yu T, Wang Y, Pan S, Zou X, Yuan S, Shang Y. Clinical course and outcomes of critically ill patients with SARS-CoV-2 pneumonia in Wuhan, China: a single-centered, retrospective, observational study. The Lancet Respiratory Medicine [Internet]. 2020 May [cited 2021 Sep 29];8(5):475–81. Available from: https://doi.org/10.1016/s2213-2600(20)30079-5

[26] Centers for Disease Control and Prevention [Internet]. Healthcare Workers; [cited 2021 Apr 4]. Available from: https://www.cdc.gov/coronavirus/2019-ncov/hcp/planning-scenarios.html

[27] WHO | World Health Organization [Internet]. Estimating mortality from COVID-19: Scientific brief, 4 August 2020; 2020 Aug 20 [cited 2021 Apr 4]. Available from: https://www.who.int/publications/i/item/WHO-2019-nCoV-Sci-Brief-Mortality-2020.1

[28] Meyerowitz-Katz G, Merone L. A systematic review and meta-analysis of published research data on COVID-19 infection fatality rates. International Journal of Infectious Diseases [Internet]. 2020 Dec [cited 2021 Sep 29];101:138–48. Available from: https://doi.org/10.1016/j.ijid.2020.09.1464

[29] Wu Z, McGoogan JM. Characteristics of and Important Lessons From the Coronavirus Disease 2019 (COVID-19) Outbreak in China. JAMA [Internet]. 2020 Apr 7 [cited 2021 Sep 29];323(13):1239–42. Available from: https://doi.org/10.1001/jama.2020.2648

[30] Wynants L, Van Calster B, Collins GS, Riley RD, Heinze G, Schuit E, et al. Prediction models for diagnosis and prognosis of covid-19: systematic review and critical appraisal. BMJ [Internet]. 2020 Apr 7 [cited 2021 Oct 4]:m1328. Available from: https://doi.org/10.1136/bmj.m1328

[31] Williamson EJ, Walker AJ, Bhaskaran K, Bacon S, Bates C, Morton CE, et al. Factors associated with COVID-19-related death using OpenSAFELY. Nature [Internet]. 2020 Jul 8 [cited 2021 Oct 4];584(7821):430–6. Available from: https://doi.org/10.1038/s41586-020-2521-4

[32] Wu C, Chen X, Cai Y, Xia J, Zhou X, Xu S et al. Risk factors associated with acute respiratory distress syndrome and death in patients with coronavirus disease 2019 pneumonia in wuhan, china. JAMA Internal Medicine [Internet]. July 1, 2020 [cited 2021 Oct 4];180(7):934. Available from: https://doi.org/10.1001/jamainternmed.2020.0994

[33] Chen N, Zhou M, Dong X, Qu J, Gong F, Han Y, Qiu Y, Wang J, Liu Y, Wei Y, Xia J, Yu T, Zhang X, Zhang L. Epidemiological and clinical characteristics of 99 cases of 2019 novel coronavirus pneumonia in Wuhan, China: a descriptive study. The Lancet [Internet]. Feb 2020 [cited 2021 Oct 4];395(10223):507–13. Available from: https://doi.org/10.1016/s0140-6736(20)30211-7

[34] Harrison SL, Fazio-Eynullayeva E, Lane DA, Underhill P, Lip GY. Comorbidities associated with mortality in 31,461 adults with COVID-19 in the United States: a federated electronic medical record analysis. PLOS Medicine [Internet]. 2020 Sep 10 [cited 2021 Oct 5];17(9):e1003321. Available from: https://doi.org/10.1371/journal.pmed.1003321

[35] Lowe KE, Zein J, Hatipoglu U, Attaway A. Association of smoking and cumulative pack-year exposure with COVID-19 outcomes in the cleveland clinic COVID-19 registry. JAMA Internal Medicine [Internet]. 2021 May 1 [cited 2021 Oct 5];181(5):709. Available from: https://doi.org/10.1001/jamainternmed.2020.8360

[36] Yu T, Cai S, Zheng Z, Cai X, Liu Y, Yin S, Peng J, Xu X. Association between clinical manifestations and prognosis in patients with COVID-19. Clinical Therapeutics [Internet]. 2020 Jun [cited 2021 Oct 5];42(6):964–72. Available from: https://doi.org/10.1016/j.clinthera.2020.04.009

[37] Liao D, Zhou F, Luo L, Xu M, Wang H, Xia J, Gao Y, Cai L, Wang Z, Yin P, Wang Y, Tang L, Deng J, Mei H, Hu Y. Haematological characteristics and risk factors in the classification and prognosis evaluation of COVID-19: a retrospective cohort study. The Lancet Haematology [Internet]. 2020 Sep [cited 2021 Oct 4];7(9):e671–e678. Available from: https://doi.org/10.1016/s2352-3026(20)30217-9

[38] Gavriatopoulou M, Korompoki E, Fotiou D, Ntanasis-Stathopoulos I, Psaltopoulou T, Kastritis E, Terpos E, Dimopoulos MA. Organ-specific manifestations of COVID-19 infection. Clinical and Experimental Medicine [Internet]. 2020 Jul 27 [cited 2021 Oct 4];20(4):493–506. Available from: https://doi.org/10.1007/s10238-020-00648-x

[39] Bermejo-Martin JF, González-Rivera M, Almansa R, Micheloud D, Tedim AP, Domínguez-Gil M, et al. Viral RNA load in plasma is associated with critical illness and a dysregulated host response in COVID-19. Critical Care [Internet]. 2020 Dec [cited 2021 Oct 4];24(1). Available from: https://doi.org/10.1186/s13054-020-03398-0

[40] Järhult JD, Hultström M, Bergqvist A, Frithiof R, Lipcsey M. The impact of viremia on organ failure, biomarkers and mortality in a Swedish cohort of critically ill COVID-19 patients.

Scientific Reports [Internet]. 2021 Mar 30 [cited 2021 Oct 4];11(1). Available from: https://doi.org/10.1038/s41598-021-86500-y

[41] Xu D, Zhou F, Sun W, Chen L, Lan L, Li H, Xiao F, Li Y, Kolachalama VB, Li Y, Wang X, Xu H. Relationship between serum severe acute respiratory syndrome coronavirus 2 nucleic acid and organ damage in coronavirus 2019 patients: a cohort study. Clinical Infectious Diseases [Internet]. 2020 Jul 28 [cited 2021 Oct 5]. Available from: https://doi.org/10.1093/cid/ciaa1085

[42] Chu KH, Tsang WK, Tang CS, Lam MF, Lai FM, To KF, Fung KS, Tang HL, Yan WW, Chan HW, Lai TS, Tong KL, Lai KN. Acute renal impairment in coronavirus-associated severe acute respiratory syndrome. Kidney International [Internet]. 2005 Feb [cited 2021 Oct 4];67(2):698–705. Available from: https://doi.org/10.1111/j.1523-1755.2005.67130.x

[43] Ray JG, Schull MJ, Vermeulen MJ, Park AL. Association between ABO and rh blood groups and SARS-CoV-2 infection or severe COVID-19 illness. Annals of Internal Medicine [Internet]. 2020 Nov 24 [cited 2021 Oct 5]. Available from: https://doi.org/10.7326/m20-4511

[44] Guan WJ, Ni ZY, Hu Y, Liang WH, Ou CQ, He JX, et al. Clinical characteristics of coronavirus disease 2019 in china. New England Journal of Medicine [Internet]. 2020 Apr 30 [cited 2021 Oct 5];382(18):1708–20. Available from: https://doi.org/10.1056/nejmoa2002032

[45] da Rosa Mesquita R, Francelino Silva Junior LC, Santos Santana FM, Farias de Oliveira T, Campos Alcântara R, Monteiro Arnozo G, Rodrigues da Silva Filho E, Galdino dos Santos AG, Oliveira da Cunha EJ, Salgueiro de Aquino SH, Freire de Souza CD. Clinical manifestations of COVID-19 in the general population: systematic review. Wiener klinische

Wochenschrift [Internet]. 2020 Nov 26 [cited 2021 Oct 4]. Available from: https://doi.org/10.1007/s00508-020-01760-4

[46] Cheung KS, Hung IF, Chan PP, Lung KC, Tso E, Liu R, et al. Gastrointestinal manifestations of SARS-CoV-2 infection and virus load in fecal samples from a Hong Kong cohort: systematic review and meta-analysis. Gastroenterology [Internet]. 2020 Jul [cited 2021 Oct 5];159(1):81–95. Available from: https://doi.org/10.1053/j.gastro.2020.03.065

[47] Ma N, Li P, Wang X, Yu Y, Tan X, Chen P, Li S, Jiang F. Ocular manifestations and clinical characteristics of children with laboratory-confirmed COVID-19 in wuhan, china. JAMA Ophthalmology [Internet]. 2020 Oct 1 [cited 2021 Oct 5];138(10):1079–86. Available from: https://doi.org/10.1001/jamaophthalmol.2020.3690

[48] Seah I, Agrawal R. Can the coronavirus disease 2019 (COVID-19) affect the eyes? A review of coronaviruses and ocular implications in humans and animals. Ocular Immunology and Inflammation [Internet]. 2020 Mar 16 [cited 2021 Oct 5];28(3):391–5. Available from: https://doi.org/10.1080/09273948.2020.1738501

[49] Colavita F, Lapa D, Carletti F, Lalle E, Bordi L, Marsella P, Nicastri E, Bevilacqua N, Giancola ML, Corpolongo A, Ippolito G, Capobianchi MR, Castilletti C. SARS-CoV-2 isolation from ocular secretions of a patient with COVID-19 in Italy with prolonged viral RNA detection. Annals of Internal Medicine [Internet]. 2020 Aug 4 [cited 2021 Oct 5];173(3):242–3. Available from: https://doi.org/10.7326/m20-1176

[50] Recalcati S. Cutaneous manifestations in COVID-19: a first perspective. Journal of the European Academy of Dermatology and Venereology [Internet]. 2020 May [cited 2021 Oct 4];34(5). Available from: https://doi.org/10.1111/jdv.16387

[51] Behzad S, Aghaghazvini L, Radmard AR, Gholamrezanezhad A. Extrapulmonary

manifestations of COVID-19: radiologic and clinical overview. Clinical Imaging [Internet]. 2020 Oct [cited 2021 Oct 5];66:35–41. Available from: https://doi.org/10.1016/j.clinimag.2020.05.013

[52] Yang M, Zhao J, Zhang Z. More than pneumonia, the potential occurrence of multiple organ failure in 2019 novel coronavirus infection. SSRN Electronic Journal [Internet]. 2020 [cited 2021 Oct 5]. Available from: https://doi.org/10.2139/ssrn.3532272

[53] Cao J, Tu WJ, Cheng W, Yu L, Liu YK, Hu X, Liu Q. Clinical features and short-term outcomes of 102 patients with coronavirus disease 2019 in wuhan, china. Clinical Infectious Diseases [Internet]. 2020 Mar 13 [cited 2021 Oct 5];71(15):748–55. Available from: https://doi.org/10.1093/cid/ciaa243

[54] Cohen PA, Hall LE, John JN, Rapoport AB. The early natural history of SARS-CoV-2 infection. Mayo Clinic Proceedings [Internet]. 2020 Jun [cited 2021 Oct 5];95(6):1124–6. Available from: https://doi.org/10.1016/j.mayocp.2020.04.010

[55] Irabien-Ortiz Á, Carreras-Mora J, Sionis A, Pàmies J, Montiel J, Tauron M. Miocarditis fulminante por COVID-19. Revista Española de Cardiología [Internet]. 2020 Jun [cited 2021 Oct 4];73(6):503–4. Available from: https://doi.org/10.1016/j.recesp.2020.04.001

[56] Babapoor-Farrokhran S, Gill D, Walker J, Rasekhi RT, Bozorgnia B, Amanullah A. Myocardial injury and COVID-19: possible mechanisms. Life Sciences [Internet]. 2020 Jul [cited 2021 Oct 5];253:117723. Available from: https://doi.org/10.1016/j.lfs.2020.117723

[57] Klok FA, Kruip MJ, van der Meer NJ, Arbous MS, Gommers DA, Kant KM, Kaptein FH, van Paassen J, Stals MA, Huisman MV, Endeman H. Incidence of thrombotic complications in critically ill ICU patients with COVID-19. Thrombosis Research [Internet].

2020 Jul [cited 2021 Oct 4];191:145–7. Available from: https://doi.org/10.1016/j.thromres.2020.04.013

[58] Torres-Machorro A, Anguiano-Álvarez VM, Grimaldo-Gómez FA, Rodríguez-Zanella H, Cortina de la Rosa E, Mora-Canela S, Lerma C, García-Cruz E, Ramos-Enriquez Á, Ramirez-Marroquin S, Izaguirre-Ávila R, Rojas-Velasco G. Asymptomatic deep vein thrombosis in critically ill COVID-19 patients despite therapeutic levels of anti-Xa activity. Thrombosis Research [Internet]. 2020 Dec [cited 2021 Oct 4];196:268–71. Available from: https://doi.org/10.1016/j.thromres.2020.08.043

[59] Romero-Sánchez CM, Díaz-Maroto I, Fernández-Díaz E, Sánchez-Larsen Á, Layos-Romero A, García-García J, et al. Neurologic manifestations in hospitalized patients with COVID-19. Neurology [Internet]. 2020 Jun 1 [cited 2021 Oct 4];95(8):e1060–e1070. Available from: https://doi.org/10.1212/wnl.0000000000009937

[60] Mao L, Jin H, Wang M, Hu Y, Chen S, He Q, Chang J, Hong C, Zhou Y, Wang D, Miao X, Li Y, Hu B. Neurologic manifestations of hospitalized patients with coronavirus disease 2019 in Wuhan, China. JAMA Neurology [Internet]. 2020 Jun 1 [cited 2021 Oct 5];77(6):683–90. Available from: https://doi.org/10.1001/jamaneurol.2020.1127

[61] Mahalakshmi AM, Ray B, Tuladhar S, Bhat A, Paneyala S, Patteswari D, Sakharkar MK, Hamdan H, Ojcius DM, Bolla SR, Essa MM, Chidambaram SB, Qoronfleh MW. Does COVID-19 contribute to development of neurological disease? Immunity, Inflammation and Disease [Internet]. 2020 Dec 17 [cited 2021 Oct 4]. Available from: https://doi.org/10.1002/iid3.387

[62] Leisman DE, Ronner L, Pinotti R, Taylor MD, Sinha P, Calfee CS, Hirayama AV, Mastroiani F, Turtle CJ, Harhay MO, Legrand M, Deutschman CS. Cytokine elevation in severe and critical COVID-19: a rapid systematic review, meta-analysis, and comparison with other inflammatory syndromes. The Lancet Respiratory Medicine [Internet]. 2020 Dec [cited

2021 Oct 4];8(12):1233–44. Available from: https://doi.org/10.1016/s2213-2600(20)30404-5

[63] Del Valle DM, Kim-Schulze S, Huang HH, Beckmann ND, Nirenberg S, Wang B, et al. An inflammatory cytokine signature predicts COVID-19 severity and survival. Nature Medicine [Internet]. 2020 Aug 24 [cited 2021 Oct 4];26(10):1636–43. Available from: https://doi.org/10.1038/s41591-020-1051-9

[64] Chauhdary WA, Chong PL, Mani BI, Asli R, Momin RN, Abdullah MS, Chong VH. Primary respiratory bacterial coinfections in patients with COVID-19. The American Journal of Tropical Medicine and Hygiene [Internet]. 2020 Aug 5 [cited 2021 Oct 5];103(2):917–9. Available from: https://doi.org/10.4269/ajtmh.20-0498

[65] Lai CC, Yu WL. COVID-19 associated with pulmonary aspergillosis: a literature review. Journal of Microbiology, Immunology and Infection [Internet]. 2020 Sep [cited 2021 Oct 5]. Available from: https://doi.org/10.1016/j.jmii.2020.09.004

[66] Puelles VG, Lütgehetmann M, Lindenmeyer MT, Sperhake JP, Wong MN, Allweiss L, et al. Multiorgan and renal tropism of SARS-CoV-2. New England Journal of Medicine [Internet]. 2020 Aug 6 [cited 2021 Oct 5];383(6):590–2. Available from: https://doi.org/10.1056/nejmc2011400

[67] Siddiqi HK, Libby P, Ridker PM. COVID-19 – A vascular disease. Trends in Cardiovascular Medicine [Internet]. 2021 Jan [cited 2021 Oct 4];31(1):1–5. Available from: https://doi.org/10.1016/j.tcm.2020.10.005

[68] The Lancet Neurology. Long COVID: understanding the neurological effects. The Lancet Neurology [Internet]. 2021 Apr [cited 2021 Oct 4];20(4):247. Available from: https://doi.org/10.1016/s1474-4422(21)00059-4

[69] Yan R, Zhang Y, Li Y, Xia L, Guo Y, Zhou Q. Structural basis for the recognition of SARS-CoV-2 by full-length human ACE2. Science [Internet]. 2020 Mar 4 [cited 2021 Oct 4];367(6485):1444–8. Available from: https://doi.org/10.1126/science.abb2762

[70] Kordzadeh-Kermani E, Khalili H, Karimzadeh I. Pathogenesis, clinical manifestations and complications of coronavirus disease 2019 (COVID-19). Future Microbiology [Internet]. 2020 Sep [cited 2021 Oct 4];15(13):1287–305. Available from: https://doi.org/10.2217/fmb-2020-0110

[71] Choi HM, Moon SY, Yang HI, Kim KS. Understanding viral infection mechanisms and patient symptoms for the development of COVID-19 therapeutics. International Journal of Molecular Sciences [Internet]. 2021 Feb 9 [cited 2021 Oct 5];22(4):1737. Available from: https://doi.org/10.3390/ijms22041737

[72] McGonagle D, Sharif K, O'Regan A, Bridgewood C. The role of cytokines including interleukin-6 in COVID-19 induced pneumonia and macrophage activation syndrome-like disease. Autoimmunity Reviews [Internet]. 2020 Jun [cited 2021 Oct 5];19(6):102537. Available from: https://doi.org/10.1016/j.autrev.2020.102537

[73] Xu B, Fan CY, Wang AL, Zou YL, Yu YH, He C, Xia WG, Zhang JX, Miao Q. Suppressed T cell-mediated immunity in patients with COVID-19: A clinical retrospective study in Wuhan, China. Journal of Infection [Internet]. 2020 Jul [cited 2021 Oct 5];81(1):e51–e60. Available from: https://doi.org/10.1016/j.jinf.2020.04.012

[74] Calabrese F, Pezzuto F, Fortarezza F, Hofman P, Kern I, Panizo A, von der Thüsen J, Timofeev S, Gorkiewicz G, Lunardi F. Pulmonary pathology and COVID-19: lessons from autopsy. the experience of european pulmonary pathologists. Virchows Archiv [Internet]. 2020 Jul 9 [cited 2021 Oct 5];477(3):359–72. Available from: https://doi.org/10.1007/s00428-020-02886-6

[75] Barth RF, Buja LM, Parwani AV. The spectrum of pathological findings in coronavirus disease (COVID-19) and the pathogenesis of SARS-CoV-2. Diagnostic Pathology [Internet]. 2020 Jul 14 [cited 2021 Oct 4];15(1). Available from: https://doi.org/10.1186/s13000-020-00999-9

[76] Xu Z, Shi L, Wang Y, Zhang J, Huang L, Zhang C, Liu S, Zhao P, Liu H, Zhu L, Tai Y, Bai C, Gao T, Song J, Xia P, Dong J, Zhao J, Wang FS. Pathological findings of COVID-19 associated with acute respiratory distress syndrome. The Lancet Respiratory Medicine [Internet]. 2020 Apr [cited 2021 Oct 4];8(4):420–2. Available from: https://doi.org/10.1016/s2213-2600(20)30076-x

[77] Menter T, Haslbauer JD, Nienhold R, Savic S, Hopfer H, Deigendesch N, Frank S, Turek D, Willi N, Pargger H, Bassetti S, Leuppi JD, Cathomas G, Tolnay M, Mertz KD, Tzankov A. Postmortem examination of COVID-19 patients reveals diffuse alveolar damage with severe capillary congestion and variegated findings in lungs and other organs suggesting vascular dysfunction. Histopathology [Internet]. 2020 Jul 5 [cited 2021 Oct 4];77(2):198–209. Available from: https://doi.org/10.1111/his.14134

[78] Tang N, Li D, Wang X, Sun Z. Abnormal coagulation parameters are associated with poor prognosis in patients with novel coronavirus pneumonia. Journal of Thrombosis and Haemostasis [Internet]. 2020 Apr [cited 2021 Oct 4];18(4):844–7. Available from: https://doi.org/10.1111/jth.14768

[79] García-Cruz E, Manzur-Sandoval D, Baeza-Herrera LA, Díaz-Méndez A, López-Zamora A, González-Ruiz F, Ramos-Enríquez Á, Melano-Carranza E, Rojas-Velasco G, Álvarez-Álvarez RJ, Baranda-Tovar FM. Acute right ventricular failure in COVID-19 infection: a case series. Journal of Cardiology Cases [Internet]. 2021 Jul [cited 2021 Oct 5];24(1):45–8. Available from: https://doi.org/10.1016/j.jccase.2021.01.001

[80] González-Ruiz FJ, Lazcano-Díaz EA, Vásquez-Ortiz ZY, Bernal-Ceballos F, Gopar-Nieto R, Orihuela-Sandoval C, Hernández-Reyes JP, García-Cruz E, Bucio-Reta E, Ramos-Enríquez Á, Cota-Apodaca LA, Efren-Santos L, Broca-García BE, Manzur-Sandoval D, Melano-Carranza E, de la Reguera Guillermo F, Rojas-Velasco G, Baranda-Tovar F. Comprehensive left ventricular mechanics analysis by speckle tracking echocardiography in COVID-19. World Journal of Cardiovascular Diseases [Internet]. 2021 [cited 2021 Oct 5];11(02):113–25. Available from: https://doi.org/10.4236/wjcd.2021.112013

[81] Ottestad W, Seim M, Mæhlen JO. Covid-19 med stille hypoksemi. Tidsskrift for Den norske legeforening [Internet]. 2020 [cited 2021 Oct 4]. Available from: https://doi.org/10.4045/tidsskr.20.0299

[82] Gattinoni L, Chiumello D, Caironi P, Busana M, Romitti F, Brazzi L, Camporota L. COVID-19 pneumonia: different respiratory treatments for different phenotypes? Intensive Care Medicine [Internet]. 2020 Apr 14 [cited 2021 Oct 4];46(6):1099–102. Available from: https://doi.org/10.1007/s00134-020-06033-2

[83] Ragab D, Salah Eldin H, Taeimah M, Khattab R, Salem R. The COVID-19 cytokine storm; what we know so far. Frontiers in Immunology [Internet]. 2020 Jun 16 [cited 2021 Oct 5];11. Available from: https://doi.org/10.3389/fimmu.2020.01446

[84] Ky B, Mann DL. COVID-19 clinical trials. JACC: CardioOncology [Internet]. 2020 Jun [cited 2021 Oct 5];2(2):254–69. Available from: https://doi.org/10.1016/j.jaccao.2020.04.002

[85] Ye Q, Wang B, Mao J. The pathogenesis and treatment of the "Cytokine Storm" in COVID-19. Journal of Infection [Internet]. 2020 Jun [cited 2021 Oct 4];80(6):607–13. Available from: https://doi.org/10.1016/j.jinf.2020.03.037

[86] Kunal S, Gupta K, Sharma SM, Pathak V, Mittal S, Tarke C. Cardiovascular system and

COVID-19: perspectives from a developing country. Monaldi Archives for Chest Disease [Internet]. 2020 May 7 [cited 2021 Oct 4];90(2). Available from: https://doi.org/10.4081/monaldi.2020.1305

[87] Topol EJ. COVID-19 can affect the heart. Science [Internet]. 2020 Sep 23 [cited 2021 Oct 4];370(6515):408–9. Available from: https://doi.org/10.1126/science.abe2813

[88] Puntmann VO, Carerj ML, Wieters I, Fahim M, Arendt C, Hoffmann J, Shchendrygina A, Escher F, Vasa-Nicotera M, Zeiher AM, Vehreschild M, Nagel E. Outcomes of cardiovascular magnetic resonance imaging in patients recently recovered from coronavirus disease 2019 (COVID-19). JAMA Cardiology [Internet]. 2020 Nov 1 [cited 2021 Oct 5];5(11):1265–73. Available from: https://doi.org/10.1001/jamacardio.2020.3557

[89] Ky B, Mann DL. COVID-19 clinical trials. JACC: Basic to Translational Science [Internet]. 2020 May [cited 2021 Oct 5];5(5):501–17. Available from: https://doi.org/10.1016/j.jacbts.2020.04.003

[90] Zhang G, Wu Y, Xu R, Du X. Effects of renin-angiotensin-aldosterone system inhibitors on disease severity and mortality in patients with COVID-19: a meta-analysis. Journal of Medical Virology [Internet]. 2020 Dec 17 [cited 2021 Oct 5]. Available from: https://doi.org/10.1002/jmv.26695

[91] Del Turco S, Vianello A, Ragusa R, Caselli C, Basta G. COVID-19 and cardiovascular consequences: is the endothelial dysfunction the hardest challenge? Thrombosis Research [Internet]. 2020 Dec [cited 2021 Oct 5];196:143–51. Available from: https://doi.org/10.1016/j.thromres.2020.08.039

[92] Li W, Moore MJ, Vasilieva N, Sui J, Wong SK, Berne MA, Somasundaran M, Sullivan JL, Luzuriaga K, Greenough TC, Choe H, Farzan M. Angiotensin-converting enzyme 2 is

a functional receptor for the SARS coronavirus. Nature [Internet]. 2003 Nov [cited 2021 Oct 4];426(6965):450–4. Available from: https://doi.org/10.1038/nature02145

[93] Gupta A, Madhavan MV, Sehgal K, Nair N, Mahajan S, Sehrawat TS, et al. Extrapulmonary manifestations of COVID-19. Nature Medicine [Internet]. 2020 Jul [cited 2021 Oct 4];26(7):1017–32. Available from: https://doi.org/10.1038/s41591-020-0968-3

[94] Bader F, Manla Y, Atallah B, Starling RC. Heart failure and COVID-19. Heart Failure Reviews [Internet]. 2020 Jul 27 [cited 2021 Oct 4];26(1):1–10. Available from: https://doi.org/10.1007/s10741-020-10008-2

[95] Bavishi C, Bonow RO, Trivedi V, Abbott JD, Messerli FH, Bhatt DL. Special Article - Acute myocardial injury in patients hospitalized with COVID-19 infection: a review. Progress in Cardiovascular Diseases [Internet]. 2020 Sep [cited 2021 Oct 5];63(5):682–9. Available from: https://doi.org/10.1016/j.pcad.2020.05.013

[96] Xiong TY, Redwood S, Prendergast B, Chen M. Coronaviruses and the cardiovascular system: acute and long-term implications. European Heart Journal [Internet]. 2020 Mar 18 [cited 2021 Oct 4];41(19):1798–800. Available from: https://doi.org/10.1093/eurheartj/ehaa231

[97] Fox SE, Akmatbekov A, Harbert JL, Li G, Quincy Brown J, Vander Heide RS. Pulmonary and cardiac pathology in African American patients with COVID-19: an autopsy series from New Orleans. The Lancet Respiratory Medicine [Internet]. 2020 Jul [cited 2021 Oct 4];8(7):681–6. Available from: https://doi.org/10.1016/s2213-2600(20)30243-5

[98] Haseeb S, Gul EE, Çinier G, Bazoukis G, Alvarez-Garcia J, Garcia-Zamora S, Lee S, Yeung C, Liu T, Tse G, Baranchuk A. Value of electrocardiography in coronavirus disease 2019

(COVID-19). Journal of Electrocardiology [Internet]. 2020 Sep [cited 2021 Oct 4];62:39–45. Available from: https://doi.org/10.1016/j.jelectrocard.2020.08.007

[99] Manolis AS, Manolis AA, Manolis TA, Apostolopoulos EJ, Papatheou D, Melita H. COVID-19 infection and cardiac arrhythmias. Trends in Cardiovascular Medicine [Internet]. 2020 Nov [cited 2021 Oct 4];30(8):451–60. Available from: https://doi.org/10.1016/j.tcm.2020.08.002

[100] Liu Y, Liu D, Song H, et al. Clinical features and outcomes of 2019 novel coronavirus-infected patients with high plasma BNP levels. MedRxiv. 2020.

[101] Guo T, Fan Y, Chen M, Wu X, Zhang L, He T, Wang H, Wan J, Wang X, Lu Z. Cardiovascular implications of fatal outcomes of patients with coronavirus disease 2019 (COVID-19). JAMA Cardiology [Internet]. 2020 Jul 1 [cited 2021 Oct 5];5(7):811–8. Available from: https://doi.org/10.1001/jamacardio.2020.1017

[102] Agdamag AC, Edmiston JB, Charpentier V, Chowdhury M, Fraser M, Maharaj VR, Francis GS, Alexy T. Update on COVID-19 Myocarditis. Medicina [Internet]. 2020 Dec 9 [cited 2021 Oct 4];56(12):678. Available from: https://doi.org/10.3390/medicina56120678

[103] Bhatla A, Mayer MM, Adusumalli S, Hyman MC, Oh E, Tierney A, et al. COVID-19 and cardiac arrhythmias. Heart Rhythm [Internet]. 2020 Sep [cited 2021 Oct 4];17(9):1439–44. Available from: https://doi.org/10.1016/j.hrthm.2020.06.016

[104] Chang WT, Toh HS, Liao CT, Yu WL. Cardiac involvement of COVID-19: a comprehensive review. The American Journal of the Medical Sciences [Internet]. 2021 Jan [cited 2021 Oct 5];361(1):14–22. Available from: https://doi.org/10.1016/j.amjms.2020.10.002

[105] Mishra AK, Sahu KK, Sargent J. Cardiac drugs and outcome in COVID-19. QJM: An International Journal of Medicine [Internet]. 2020 Apr 14 [cited 2021 Oct 4];113(7):523–4. Available from: https://doi.org/10.1093/qjmed/hcaa127

[106] Long B, Brady WJ, Bridwell RE, Ramzy M, Montrief T, Singh M, Gottlieb M. Electrocardiographic manifestations of COVID-19. The American Journal of Emergency Medicine [Internet]. 2021 Mar [cited 2021 Oct 4];41:96–103. Available from: https://doi.org/10.1016/j.ajem.2020.12.060

[107] Shchedrygina A, Nagel E, Puntmann VO, Valbuena-Lopez S. COVID-19 myocarditis and prospective heart failure burden. Expert Review of Cardiovascular Therapy [Internet]. 2020 Nov 27 [cited 2021 Oct 4]:1–10. Available from: https://doi.org/10.1080/14779072.2021.1844005

[108] Viner RM, Whittaker E. Kawasaki-like disease: emerging complication during the COVID-19 pandemic. The Lancet [Internet]. 2020 Jun [cited 2021 Oct 4];395(10239):1741–3. Available from: https://doi.org/10.1016/s0140-6736(20)31129-6

[109] Shaigany S, Gnirke M, Guttmann A, Chong H, Meehan S, Raabe V, Louie E, Solitar B, Femia A. An adult with Kawasaki-like multisystem inflammatory syndrome associated with COVID-19. The Lancet [Internet]. 2020 Jul [cited 2021 Oct 4];396(10246):e8–e10. Available from: https://doi.org/10.1016/s0140-6736(20)31526-9

[110] Verdoni L, Mazza A, Gervasoni A, Martelli L, Ruggeri M, Ciuffreda M, Bonanomi E, D'Antiga L. An outbreak of severe Kawasaki-like disease at the Italian epicentre of the SARS-CoV-2 epidemic: an observational cohort study. The Lancet [Internet]. 2020 Jun [cited 2021 Oct 4];395(10239):1771–8. Available from: https://doi.org/10.1016/s0140-6736(20)31103-x

[111] Wong HY, Lam HY, Fong AH, Leung ST, Chin TW, Lo CS, Lui MM, Lee JC, Chiu KW, Chung TW, Lee EY, Wan EY, Hung IF, Lam TP, Kuo MD, Ng MY. Frequency and distribution of chest radiographic findings in patients positive for COVID-19. Radiology [Internet]. 2020 Aug [cited 2021 Oct 5];296(2):E72–E78. Available from: https://doi.org/10.1148/radiol.2020201160

[112] Smith DL, Grenier JP, Batte C, Spieler B. A characteristic chest radiographic pattern in the setting of COVID-19 pandemic. Radiology: Cardiothoracic Imaging [Internet]. 2020 Oct 1 [cited 2021 Oct 5];2(5):e200280. Available from: https://doi.org/10.1148/ryct.2020200280

[113] Martinelli AW, Ingle T, Newman J, Nadeem I, Jackson K, Lane ND, et al. COVID-19 and pneumothorax: a multicentre retrospective case series. European Respiratory Journal [Internet]. 2020 Sep 9 [cited 2021 Oct 4];56(5):2002697. Available from: https://doi.org/10.1183/13993003.02697-2020

[114] Zhou C, Gao C, Xie Y, Xu M. COVID-19 with spontaneous pneumomediastinum. The Lancet Infectious Diseases [Internet]. 2020 Apr [cited 2021 Oct 4];20(4):510. Available from: https://doi.org/10.1016/s1473-3099(20)30156-0

[115] Zhao W, Zhong Z, Xie X, Yu Q, Liu J. Relation between chest CT findings and clinical conditions of coronavirus disease (COVID-19) pneumonia: a multicenter study. American Journal of Roentgenology [Internet]. 2020 May [cited 2021 Oct 5];214(5):1072–7. Available from: https://doi.org/10.2214/ajr.20.22976

[116] Ojha V, Mani A, Pandey NN, Sharma S, Kumar S. CT in coronavirus disease 2019 (COVID-19): a systematic review of chest CT findings in 4410 adult patients. European Radiology [Internet]. 2020 May 30 [cited 2021 Oct 4];30(11):6129–38. Available from: https://doi.org/10.1007/s00330-020-06975-7

[117] Fischer AM, Varga-Szemes A, van Assen M, Griffith LP, Sahbaee P, Sperl JI, Nance JW, Schoepf UJ. Comparison of artificial intelligence–based fully automatic chest CT emphysema quantification to pulmonary function testing. American Journal of Roentgenology [Internet]. 2020 May [cited 2021 Oct 5];214(5):1065–71. Available from: https://doi.org/10.2214/ajr.19.21572

[118] Abrams ER, Rose G, Fields JM, Esener D. Point-of-Care ultrasound in the evaluation of COVID-19. The Journal of Emergency Medicine [Internet]. 2020 Sep [cited 2021 Oct 5];59(3):403–8. Available from: https://doi.org/10.1016/j.jemermed.2020.06.032

[119] Peng QY, Wang XT, Zhang LN. Findings of lung ultrasonography of novel corona virus pneumonia during the 2019–2020 epidemic. Intensive Care Medicine [Internet]. 2020 Mar 12 [cited 2021 Oct 4];46(5):849–50. Available from: https://doi.org/10.1007/s00134-020-05996-6

[120] García-Cruz E, Manzur-Sandoval D, Rascón-Sabido R, Gopar-Nieto R, Barajas-Campos RL, Jordán-Ríos A, et al. Critical care ultrasonography during COVID-19 pandemic: The ORACLE protocol. Echocardiography [Internet]. 2020 Aug 29 [cited 2021 Oct 4];37(9):1353–61. Available from: https://doi.org/10.1111/echo.14837

[121] Sun M, Xu Y, He H, Zhang L, Wang X, Qiu Q, Sun C, Guo Y, Qiu S, Ma K. A potentially effective treatment for COVID-19: a systematic review and meta-analysis of convalescent plasma therapy in treating severe infectious disease. International Journal of Infectious Diseases [Internet]. 2020 Sep [cited 2021 Oct 4];98:334–46. Available from: https://doi.org/10.1016/j.ijid.2020.06.107

[122] Klassen SA, Senefeld JW, Johnson PW, Carter RE, Wiggins CC, Shoham S et al. The effect of convalescent plasma therapy on mortality among patients with COVID-19: systematic review and meta-analysis. Mayo Clinic Proceedings [Internet]. May 2021

[cited 2021 Oct 4];96(5):1262–75. Available from: https://doi.org/10.1016/j.mayocp.2021.02.008

[123] Agarwal A, Mukherjee A, Kumar G, Chatterjee P, Bhatnagar T, Malhotra P. Convalescent plasma in the management of moderate covid-19 in adults in India: open label phase II multicentre randomised controlled trial (PLACID Trial). BMJ [Internet]. 2020 Oct 22 [cited 2021 Oct 4]:m3939. Available from: https://doi.org/10.1136/bmj.m3939

[124] Simonovich VA, Burgos Pratx LD, Scibona P, Beruto MV, Vallone MG, Vázquez C, et al. A randomized trial of convalescent plasma in covid-19 severe pneumonia. New England Journal of Medicine [Internet]. 2020 Nov 24 [cited 2021 Oct 5]. Available from: https://doi.org/10.1056/nejmoa2031304

[125] Li L, Zhang W, Hu Y, Tong X, Zheng S, Yang J, et al. Effect of convalescent plasma therapy on time to clinical improvement in patients with severe and life-threatening COVID-19. Jama [Internet]. 2020 Aug 4 [cited 2021 Oct 5];324(5):460–70. Available from: https://doi.org/10.1001/jama.2020.10044

[126] Libster R, Pérez Marc G, Wappner D, Coviello S, Bianchi A, Braem V, et al. Early high-titer plasma therapy to prevent severe covid-19 in older adults. New England Journal of Medicine [Internet]. 2021 Jan 6 [cited 2021 Oct 5]. Available from: https://doi.org/10.1056/nejmoa2033700

[127] Prasad M, Seth T, Elavarasi A. Efficacy and safety of convalescent plasma for COVID-19: a systematic review and meta-analysis. Indian Journal of Hematology and Blood Transfusion [Internet]. 2021 Mar 16 [cited 2021 Oct 5];37(3):347–65. Available from: https://doi.org/10.1007/s12288-021-01417-w

[128] Katz LM. (A little) clarity on convalescent plasma for COVID-19. New England Journal of

Medicine [Internet]. 2021 Feb 18 [cited 2021 Oct 5];384(7):666–8. Available from: https://doi.org/10.1056/nejme2035678

[129] IDSA Home [Internet]. COVID-19 guideline, part 1: treatment and management; 2021 [cited 2021 May 15]. Available from: https://www.idsociety.org/practice-guideline/covid-19-guideline-treatment-and-management/

[130] Beigel JH, Tomashek KM, Dodd LE, Mehta AK, Zingman BS, Kalil AC, et al. Remdesivir for the treatment of covid-19 – final report. New England Journal of Medicine [Internet]. 2020 Nov 5 [cited 2021 Oct 5];383(19):1813–26. Available from: https://doi.org/10.1056/nejmoa2007764

[131] Repurposed antiviral drugs for COVID-19 – interim WHO solidarity trial results. New England Journal of Medicine [Internet]. 2020 Dec 2 [cited 2021 Oct 5]. Available from: https://doi.org/10.1056/nejmoa2023184

[132] Spinner CD, Gottlieb RL, Criner GJ, Arribas López JR, Cattelan AM, Soriano Viladomiu A, et al. Effect of remdesivir vs standard care on clinical status at 11 days in patients with moderate COVID-19. Jama [Internet]. 2020 Sep 15 [cited 2021 Oct 5];324(11):1048–57. Available from: https://doi.org/10.1001/jama.2020.16349

[133] Goldman JD, Lye DC, Hui DS, Marks KM, Bruno R, Montejano R, et al. Remdesivir for 5 or 10 days in patients with severe covid-19. New England Journal of Medicine [Internet]. 2020 Nov 5 [cited 2021 Oct 5];383(19):1827–37. Available from: https://doi.org/10.1056/nejmoa2015301

[134] Kalil AC, Patterson TF, Mehta AK, Tomashek KM, Wolfe CR, Ghazaryan V, et al. Baricitinib plus remdesivir for hospitalized adults with covid-19. New England Journal of Medicine [Internet]. 2020 Dec 11 [cited 2021 Oct 5]. Available from: https://doi.org/10.1056/nejmoa2031994

[135] Bekerman E, Neveu G, Shulla A, Brannan J, Pu SY, Wang S, Xiao F, Barouch-Bentov R, Bakken RR, Mateo R, Govero J, Nagamine CM, Diamond MS, De Jonghe S, Herdewijn P, Dye JM, Randall G, Einav S. Anticancer kinase inhibitors impair intracellular viral trafficking and exert broad-spectrum antiviral effects. Journal of Clinical Investigation [Internet]. 2017 Feb 27 [cited 2021 Oct 4];127(4):1338–52. Available from: `https://doi.org/10.1172/jci89857`

[136] Titanji BK, Farley MM, Mehta A, Connor-Schuler R, Moanna A, Cribbs SK, O'Shea J, DeSilva K, Chan B, Edwards A, Gavegnano C, Schinazi RF, Marconi VC. Use of baricitinib in patients with moderate to severe coronavirus disease 2019. Clinical Infectious Diseases [Internet]. 2020 Jun 29 [cited 2021 Oct 5]. Available from: `https://doi.org/10.1093/cid/ciaa879`

[137] IDSA Home [Internet]. COVID-19 guideline, part 1: treatment and management; [cited 2021 Apr 10]. Available from: `https://www.idsociety.org/practice-guideline/covid-19-guideline-treatment-and-management/`

[138] Bikdeli B, Madhavan MV, Jimenez D, Chuich T, Dreyfus I, Driggin E, et al. COVID-19 and thrombotic or thromboembolic disease: implications for prevention, antithrombotic therapy, and follow-up. Journal of the American College of Cardiology [Internet]. 2020 Jun [cited 2021 Oct 5];75(23):2950–73. Available from: `https://doi.org/10.1016/j.jacc.2020.04.031`

[139] Wang J, Hajizadeh N, Moore EE, McIntyre RC, Moore PK, Veress LA, Yaffe MB, Moore HB, Barrett CD. Tissue plasminogen activator (tPA) treatment for COVID-19 associated acute respiratory distress syndrome (ARDS): a case series. Journal of Thrombosis and Haemostasis [Internet]. 2020 May 11 [cited 2021 Oct 5];18(7):1752–5. Available from: `https://doi.org/10.1111/jth.14828`

[140] Jiménez-Soto R, Montiel-Romero S, Neme-Yunes Y, Demichelis-Gómez MR, Inclán-Alarcón S. Estrategias de anticoagulación en pacientes con COVID-19. Revista de Hematología Mexicana. 2020;21(4):210–24. https://doi.org/10.24245/rev_hematol.v21i4.4727

[141] Menk M, Estenssoro E, Sahetya SK, Neto AS, Sinha P, Slutsky AS, Summers C, Yoshida T, Bein T, Ferguson ND. Current and evolving standards of care for patients with ARDS. Intensive Care Medicine [Internet]. 2020 Nov 6 [cited 2021 Oct 4];46(12):2157–67. Available from: https://doi.org/10.1007/s00134-020-06299-6

[142] Meduri GU, Annane D, Confalonieri M, Chrousos GP, Rochwerg B, Busby A, Ruaro B, Meibohm B. Pharmacological principles guiding prolonged glucocorticoid treatment in ARDS. Intensive Care Medicine [Internet]. 2020 Nov 4 [cited 2021 Oct 4];46(12):2284–96. Available from: https://doi.org/10.1007/s00134-020-06289-8

[143] Sterne JA, Murthy S, Diaz JV, Slutsky AS, Villar J, Angus DC, et al. Association between administration of systemic corticosteroids and mortality among critically ill patients with COVID-19. Jama [Internet]. 2020 Oct 6 [cited 2021 Oct 4];324(13):1330–41. Available from: https://doi.org/10.1001/jama.2020.17023

[144] Tomazini BM, Maia IS, Cavalcanti AB, Berwanger O, Rosa RG, Veiga VC, et al. Effect of dexamethasone on days alive and ventilator-free in patients with moderate or severe acute respiratory distress syndrome and COVID-19. Jama [Internet]. 2020 Oct 6 [cited 2021 Oct 5];324(13):1307–16. Available from: https://doi.org/10.1001/jama.2020.17021

[145] Dexamethasone in hospitalized patients with covid-19 – preliminary report. New England Journal of Medicine [Internet]. 2020 Jul 17 [cited 2021 Oct 5]. Available from: https://doi.org/10.1056/nejmoa2021436

[146] Nelson BC, Laracy J, Shoucri S, Dietz D, Zucker J, Patel N, Sobieszczyk ME, Kubin CJ, Gomez-Simmonds A. Clinical outcomes associated with methylprednisolone in mechanically ventilated patients with COVID-19. Clinical Infectious Diseases [Internet]. 2020 Aug 9 [cited 2021 Oct 5]. Available from: https://doi.org/10.1093/cid/ciaa1163

[147] Jeronimo CM, Farias ME, Val FF, Sampaio VS, Alexandre MA, Melo GC, et al. Methylprednisolone as adjunctive therapy for patients hospitalized with coronavirus disease 2019 (COVID-19; metcovid): a randomized, double-blind, phase iib, placebo-controlled trial. Clinical Infectious Diseases [Internet]. 2020 Aug 12 [cited 2021 Oct 5]. Available from: https://doi.org/10.1093/cid/ciaa1177

[148] van Paassen J, Vos JS, Hoekstra EM, Neumann KM, Boot PC, Arbous SM. Corticosteroid use in COVID-19 patients: a systematic review and meta-analysis on clinical outcomes. Critical Care [Internet]. 2020 Dec [cited 2021 Oct 4];24(1). Available from: https://doi.org/10.1186/s13054-020-03400-9

[149] Rosas IO, Bräu N, Waters M, Go RC, Hunter BD, Bhagani S, et al. Tocilizumab in hospitalized patients with severe covid-19 pneumonia. New England Journal of Medicine [Internet]. 2021 Apr 22 [cited 2021 Oct 5];384(16):1503–16. Available from: https://doi.org/10.1056/nejmoa2028700

[150] Salama C, Han J, Yau L, Reiss WG, Kramer B, Neidhart JD, Criner GJ, Kaplan-Lewis E, Baden R, Pandit L, Cameron ML, Garcia-Diaz J, Chávez V, Mekebeb-Reuter M, Lima de Menezes F, Shah R, González-Lara MF, Assman B, Freedman J, Mohan SV. Tocilizumab in patients hospitalized with covid-19 pneumonia. New England Journal of Medicine [Internet]. 2021 Jan 7 [cited 2021 Oct 5];384(1):20–30. Available from: https://doi.org/10.1056/nejmoa2030340

[151] Somers EC, Eschenauer GA, Troost JP, Golob JL, Gandhi TN, Wang L, et al. Tocilizumab for treatment of mechanically ventilated patients with COVID-19. Clinical Infectious

Diseases [Internet]. 2020 Jul 11 [cited 2021 Oct 5]. Available from: https://doi.org/10.1093/cid/ciaa954

[152] COVID-19 Treatment Guidelines [Internet]. Information on COVID-19 treatment, prevention and research; [cited 2021 Oct 4]. Available from: https://covid19treatmentguidelines.nih.gov/

[153] Tleyjeh IM, Kashour Z, Damlaj M, Riaz M, Tlayjeh H, Altannir M, et al. Since January 2020 Elsevier has created a COVID-19 resource centre with free information in English and Mandarin on the novel coronavirus COVID-19.

CHAPTER 4

Modelling Epidemics: a Perspective on Mathematical Models and Their Use

Jorge X. Velasco-Hernández[*1]

[*] **Corresponding author:** jx.velasco@im.unam.mx, Phone: +52 562-34389 ext. 320

[1] Institute of Mathematics of National Autonomous University of Mexico, Juriquilla, Querétaro-76230

Abstract. In this text, we look at several mathematical models that have been constructed during the present pandemic to address different issues of importance to public health policies about epidemic scenarios and their causes. We start by briefly reviewing the most basic properties of the classic Kermack-McKendrick model and then proceed to look at some generalizations and their applications to contact structures, co-circulation of viral infections, growth patterns of epidemic curves, characterization of probability distributions and passage times necessary to parametrize the compartments that are added to the basic Kermack-McKendrick model. All of these examples revolve around the idea that a system of differential equations is constructed from a specific epidemiological problem, has as a central and main theoretical and conceptual support the epidemiological, medical, and biological context that motivates its construction and analysis.

Key words: Mathematical models, COVID-19, Mathematical epidemiology, COVID population dynamics

1 INTRODUCTION

1.1 Importance

Here, we argue on the importance of theoretical and conceptual perspectives in modelling the COVID-19 pandemic. Fitting equations to data without a sound perspective on the biological feasibility of the model will provide a statistically significant fit but will also fall short of providing useful information for the management, mitigation, and eventual control of the epidemic.

1.2 Preliminaries

The epidemic of SARS-CoV-2 that started in late December 2019 in Wuhan, China, and became a pandemic by late January 2020, is still with us. Mathematical models have been used since the very early days to forecast and inform public health strategies and decisions geared to control or, at least, mitigate the impact of the epidemic. Epidemic models became a notoriety both in the academic, public health and popular realms. The epidemics of infectious diseases are social phenomena whose dynamics are strongly influenced by the inherent heterogeneity of human populations regarding age, gender, genetic profiles, physiology, preferences, education, socioeconomic level, religion, customs, etc. All of these factors induce high variability and uncertainity on the disease transmission process. To confront the epidemic, a large number of modellers used variants of the family of so-called Kermack-McKendrick models. The Kermack-McKendrick models were first published in a series of papers in early decades of the XX century. These models are compartmental in nature and follow the fate of the individuals in the population where an infectious disease is present. One of the equations follows the prevalence of the disease, which, in the most classical SIR model, describes a bell-shaped curve with a unique maximum and where both initial growth and final decline are exponential in nature. This model originally was used to describe the bubonic plague epidemic [1]. Anderson G. McKendrick was a Scottish medical practitioner born at the end of the XIX century. He worked in Sudan and India where he learned mathematics by himself [2]. As a result from this experience, he published a first version of his now famous model [3], which later in his life was further developed with the help of W.O. Kermack in a series of landmark papers. In 1927, William O. Kermack and McKendrick started a series of papers entitled Contributions to the Mathematical Theory of Epidemics that together constitute the fundamental background of mathematical epidemiology [1, 4–7]. Infectious diseases are transmitted through contacts between susceptible and infectious individuals. The models that we will comment on in the following sections assume that all individuals are exactly equal and can be unequivocally classified into distinct classes that correspond to their physiological disease status: susceptible, exposed, infectious, recovered, quarantined, etc. During this long pandemic of SARS-CoV-2, many papers have been published where many more compartments are added to the basic transmission model (hospitalized, asymptomatically infected, presymptomatically infected, isolated individuals and so on). This increase in the number of compartments gives the illusion of realism but at the price of increasing the number of parameters -two per new compartment- thus requiring either estimating all parameters or assigning values to some of them for the purpose of inference, simulation, forecast and prediction. Modelling has to deal with two problems, one is lack of identifiability, the other, overfitting. Many of the parameter values are taken from the medical and epidemiological literature and assumed to be true. This form of "parameter reduction" does not necessarily diminish the sensitivity of the model solutions to variations in these parameter values. Mathematical models are tools to study natural phenomena. Models can certainly be used to predict, but they can also be used to explain and understand the mechanisms and causes of a given natural phenomenon. Kermack-McKendrick models are excellent strategical tools of this type. Their objective is then not so much to forecast incidence, or number of deaths and hospitalized individuals, for example, but to generate scenarios and explanatory hypotheses that may be of helpful for those engaged in model forecasting. In this pandemic, plenty of data has been made available to the general public since the initial stages. An epidemic is a biological and social process that first has to be understood in those terms. The analysis of this information for each national regional, local epidemic is essential to understand and correctly design mathematical models with technical power and biological feasibility and consistency that would make them useful tools to design and execute adequate public policies. Fitting curves and models to epidemics is only a part of it.

2 BASIC RESULTS OF THE KERMACK-MCKENDRICK MODEL

Mathematical models have been deployed during the present sanitary emergency in a variety of ways but mainly to forecast its course. The basic mathematical model that has been used for such an aim is the classical Kermack-McKendrick SIR mathematical model. The SIR model is a compartmental system of differential equations that models disease transmission of communicable diseases by subdividing the population into three classes: the susceptible class that contains individuals that are not immune to the disease and are at risk of contagion; infected individuals that can also transmit the disease, that is, they are also infectious, and the class of recovered or dead individuals. Recovered individuals are immune to the disease. The model stands as follows

$$\begin{aligned} S' &= -\beta S I \,, \\ I' &= \beta S I - \gamma I \,, \\ R' &= \gamma R \,, \end{aligned} \tag{4.1}$$

with initial conditions $S(0) = S_0$, $I(0) = I_0$ and $R(0) = R_0$ and where $\beta = \phi c$ is the effective contact rate with ϕ the probability of infection per contact, and c the number of contacts per capita per unit time of a typical individual in the population. Note that all individuals are exactly equal with respect to the disease. We will elaborate on this aspect of the model later in this text; γ is the recovery rate. Note that in the absence of new infections, $I(t)/I_0 = \exp(-\gamma t)$, where $I(0)$ is the initial number of infectious cases, and therefore

$$\frac{1}{\gamma} = \int_0^\infty e^{-\gamma t} dt$$

is the mean residence time in the infectious compartment. Summing the equations in (4.1) we see that $S(t) + I(t) + R(t) = N$ is constant for all t. It is more convenient to work with fractions instead of absolute densities. Therefore, in what follows, we take $N = 1$. From the first and the second equations, the solution curves can be found by solving

$$\frac{dI}{dS} = -1 + \frac{\gamma}{\beta S},$$

and thus $I = 1 - S + \gamma \log(S/S_0)/\beta$. We have the following Theorem [8]:

Theorem 2.1 *Let $S(t), I(t)$ be solutions of (4.1). Define $R_0 = \beta S_0/\gamma$. If $R_0 \leq 1$, then $I(t)$ decreases to zero as $t \to \infty$; if $R_0 > 1$, then $I(t)$ first increases up to a maximum value equal to $1 - \gamma/\beta - \gamma \log(R_0)/\beta$ and then decreases to zero as $t \to \infty$. The susceptible fraction $S(t)$ is a decreasing function, and the limiting value $S(\infty)$ is the unique root in $(0, \gamma/\beta)$ of the equation*

$$1 - S(\infty) + \log(S(\infty)/S_0)\frac{\gamma}{\beta} = 0.$$

The SIR equations (4.1) describe a single epidemic outbreak where demographic processes (births, death, immigration, and emigration) do not play a role and where immunity is complete. An implicit assumption is that the behavior of the individuals in the population is always constant and homogeneous. This means that the effective contact rate is the same for all, so that there are no groups of people with different contact rates and probability of infection. This is clearly an oversimplification but also something that a careful reading of the model equations leaves clear. When vital dynamics is introduced, the SIR model becomes

$$\begin{aligned} S' &= \mu - \beta S I - \mu S, \\ I' &= \beta S I - (\gamma + \mu) I, \\ R' &= \gamma I - \mu R, \end{aligned} \tag{4.2}$$

where μ is the birth and death rate. Since $R(t) = 1 - S(t) - I(t)$, this system has a biologically feasible interpretation in the triangle Δ bounded by the S and I axes and the line $S + I = 1$. Given the initial conditions $S(0) > 0$, $I(0) > 0$, $R(0) \geq 0$ with $S(0) + I(0) + R(0) = 1$, we can establish the following Theorem [8].

Theorem 2.2 *Let $S(t), I(t)$ be solutions of (4.2). Define $R_0 = \beta S_0/(\mu + \gamma)$. If $R_0 > 1$ then there exists a globally stable endemic equilibrium point in $\Delta - \{(S, 0) : 0 \leq S \leq 1\}$ given by $E_1 = (1/R_0, \mu(R_0 - 1)/\beta)$. If, on the contrary, $R_0 \leq 1$, the disease-free equilibrium is globally asymptotically stable in Δ.*

To appreciate the effect of temporary immunity on disease dynamics, let us suppose that the immunity conferred by the disease is short lived. Given the absence of vital dynamics, this model is only valid for short time scales (as the original SIR model (4.1) is). However, it serves our purpose of showing the characteristic oscillatory dynamics imposed by the reintroduction of recovered individuals into the susceptible class. The model is as follows:

$$\begin{aligned} S' &= -\beta SI + \omega R\,, \\ I' &= \beta SI - \gamma I\,, \\ R' &= \gamma I - \omega R\,, \end{aligned} \tag{4.3}$$

As mentioned above, the dynamics shares characteristics with model (4.1). If $R_0 = \beta S_0/\gamma > 1$ the number of infected individuals will increase, reach a maximum when $S = \gamma/\beta$ and then decrease. However, notice that S is no longer a nonincreasing function of time. The fact that immunity lasts only about $1/\omega$ units of time indicates that the susceptible pool is replenished as more people that where infected recover and then lose their immunity. This imposes a transient dynamic that consists of damped oscillations until the disease vanishes in the population (see Fig. 1).

To finish this preliminary introduction, we present another Kermack-McKendrick model that

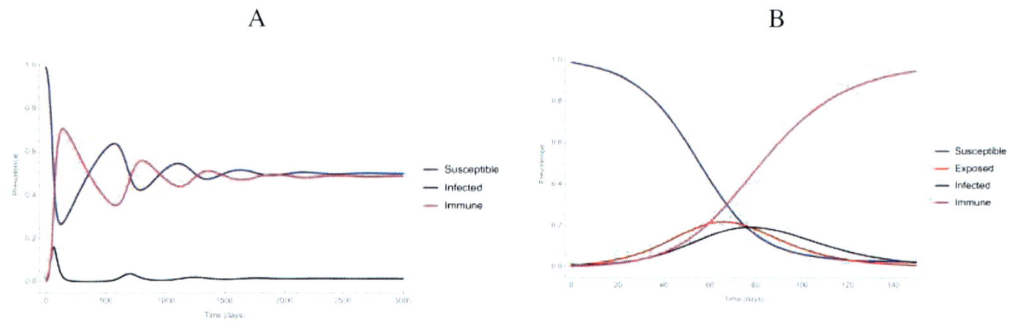

Figure 1: A) Dynamics of the model SIR with temporary immunity (4.3), B) Dynamics of the SEIR model (4.4)

has found multiple applications in the present pandemic. This is the SEIR model given by:

$$\begin{aligned} S' &= -\beta S I\,, \\ E' &= \beta S I - \eta E\,, \\ I' &= \eta E - \gamma I\,, \\ R' &= \gamma I\,, \end{aligned} \tag{4.4}$$

Here, the only new parameter is η, the incubation rate; as before, $1/\eta$ is the mean residence time that a person spends incubating the virus before becoming infectious. E is a compartment that contains the exposed individuals, defined as those that have been infected but are not yet infectious. It has similar properties to the SIR model but now presents two peaks: one corresponds to the prevalence of exposed and other to the prevalence of infectious individuals. Note that the typical form of an epidemic outbreak, common to all three models, is a bell-shaped epidemic curve that initially grows exponentially. For the SIR model (eq. 4.1) this can be easily illustrated. At the beginning of the epidemic, we can assume S is approximately constant and equal to S_0, thus, since $R_0 = \beta S_0/\gamma$,

$$I(t) = I(0)e^{\gamma(R_0-1)t}\,,$$

which allows us to define the population growth rate as $r = \gamma(R_0 - 1)$ which then implies that

$$R_0 = 1 + \frac{r}{\gamma} \approx 1 + \frac{T_R}{T_D},$$

where T_R is the recovery time and T_D is the doubling time of the epidemic, roughly equal to $1/r$. A similar expression can be found for the reproduction number of the SEIR model (eq.4.4). Linearizing the system around the disease-free equilibrium and finding the dominant eigenvalue, we obtain that

$$R_0 = \left(1 + \frac{r}{\gamma}\right)\left(1 + \frac{r}{\eta}\right).$$

A basic condition of the above two formulas strongly relies on the assumption that the probability distribution of the incubation and recovery periods is exponential

$$p_I(u) = e^{-\eta u}, \qquad p_R(u) = e^{-\gamma u}.$$

This is only an approximation. In reality, the distributions of these times are Gamma distributions, not exponential, a fact that is important for the correct estimation of the basic reproductive number and the initial epidemic growth rate.

3 MORE GENERAL MODELS

During the epidemic, many generalizations of the basic model SIR or SEIR were developed that included compartments for presymptomatic, symptomatic, asymptomatic, hospitalized, ICU, recovered and dead individuals respectively, just to list a few (see e.g.,[9–15]). Many of the residence times for these compartments, because of the nature of the differential equations of the Kermack-McKendrick models, are assumed to be exponential when in reality they are not. They are usually Beta or Gamma distributions that may also vary as the epidemic evolves [16].

In Fig. 2, we show the distributions of several important variables obtained from the Mexican Federal Government open data [17]. These four distribution functions determine in a significant way how individuals are allocated to different model compartments after the transmission event occurs. It is clear that none of them follows the hypothesis of exponentially distributed residence times assumed in Kermack-McKendrick models. Fig. 2A shows the empirical distribution and theoretical fit of a Gamma distribution for the time it takes a person to present a severe disease once he/she has shown symptoms. This distribution is fundamental to estimate hospitalization rates. Fig. 2B is the distribution of time from severe symptom onset to death as the epidemic develops, Fig. 2C records the probability of presenting severe symptoms if symptomatic. This probability distribution has been obtained for the whole population of Mexico. Clearly, it should be estimated by age and conditional on individuals presenting key comorbidities; finally, Fig. 2D presents the probability of dying once showing severe symptoms, which is necessary to estimate the expected IFR (infection fatality rate).

One other important distribution, perhaps the most important of them, is the one for the generation and serial interval of the infection. The generation interval is the time that passes between the infection of the infector and the infection of a secondary infectee. It is the fundamental basis for the estimation of the basic reproductive number [18–20]. The serial interval is an approximation to the generation interval and measures the time between symptom onset in the infector and symptom onset in the infectee. A recent study in China gives an estimate of the serial interval of 5.3 days with an interquartile range of 2.7 to 8.3 days, the generation interval has the same median but the interval of variation is a bit moved to the right, from 3.1 to 8.7 [21]. When mitigation measures are applied, however, the timing of their application becomes important. Still following Sun and coauthors [21], the median generation interval increases 4 days when cases are isolated 2 days after symptom onset, and increases to 7 days when the isolation occurs more than 6 days after symptom onset.

Given this variability, the great spread in the estimations of the basic reproduction number show is not surprising. For China, Hunan province outbreak [21] gives $R_0 = 2.19$ while [22] gives $R_0 = 5.7$. This fact highlights the importance of a clear understanding of the underlying hypothesis of the Kermack-McKendrick model, particularly on those that relate to the transmission process, namely, R_0. The SIR and SEIR models, described in the previous section, yield a basic

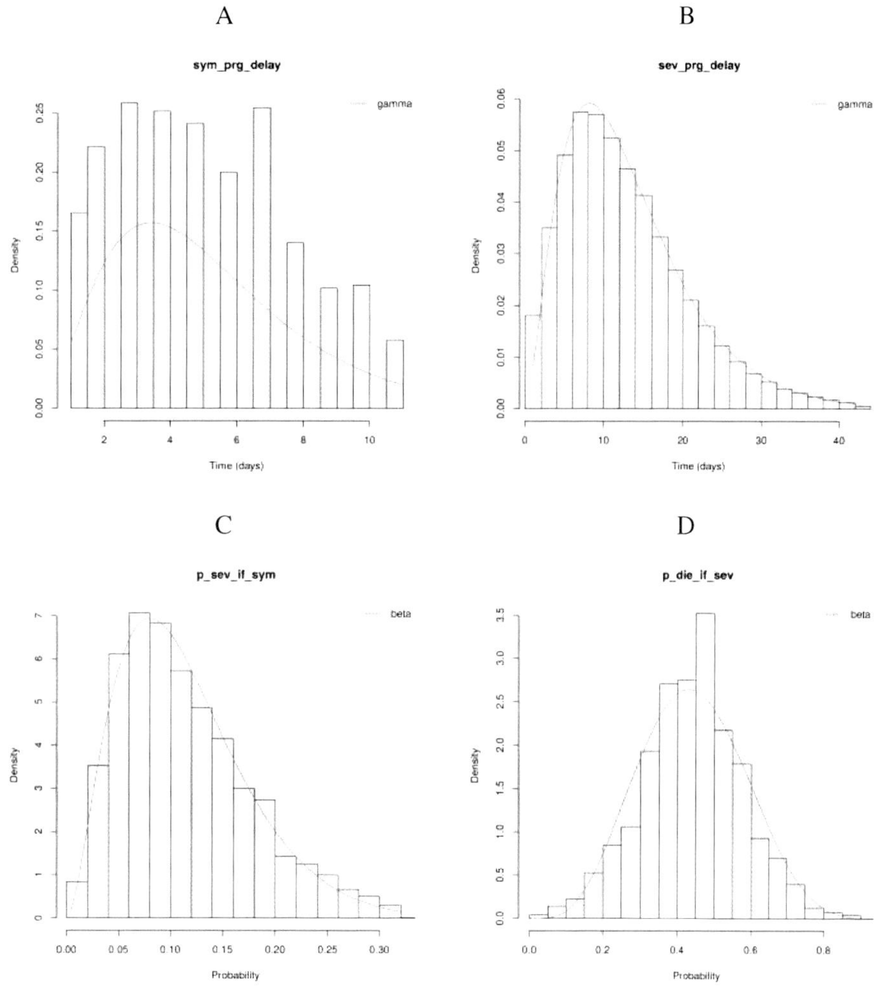

Figure 2: Data from the Mexican Federal Government open database consulted on February 24,2020. A) Fitted density function of the time from symptom onset to severe disease. B) Fitted density function of the time from severe symptom onset to death. C) Fitted density function of the probability of presenting severe symptoms if symptomatic. D) Fitted density function of the probability of dying if showing severe symptoms

reproductive number of the form $R_0 = \beta/\gamma$ which means that the serial or generation interval is approximated by the recovery time $T_R = 1/\gamma$. According to the CDC [23], the recovery period for COVID-19 in adults with mild disease is 10 days, and for those with severe disease is no longer than 20 days, numbers that are about two or three times larger than the serial interval, implying a possible overestimation of R_0 done directly from the Kermack-McKendrick model.

Moreover, in all of these generalized Kermack-McKendrick models, the core of the structure resides in the mixing function used. The mixing function represents the way in which individuals in the population come together and make contact with each other that results in a transmission event. The models in the previous section assume that the mixing is random and it is represented by the law of mass action $S \times I$, valid when the population is homogeneous and there are no differences due to age, gender, preferences or any other factor. Define c_{ij} as the proportion of contacts that group i has with group j. These contact rates must satisfy the following conditions [24, 25]:

1. $c_{ij} \geq 0$,
2. $\sum_{j=1}^{n} c_{ij} = 1$ for $j = 1, ..., n$,
3. $a_i N_i c_{ij} = a_j N_j c_{ji}$,

where N_i is the size of group i and a_i is the activity or risk level of group i. Proportional mixing between groups i and j can be obtained by assuming that $c_{ij} = c_i^a c_j^b$ and then axioms 2 and 3 above yield $c_{ij} = C c_j^b = \hat{c}_j$ with

$$\hat{c}_j = \frac{a_j N_j}{\sum_{i=1}^{n} a_i N_i} .$$

Preferential mixing assumes that the contacts of a given group i consists of reserving a fraction ϵ_i of contacts for within-group contacts (group i) and a fraction $1 - \epsilon_i$ which is distributed among all other groups according to

$$c_{ij} = \epsilon_i \delta_{ij} + (1 - \epsilon_i) \frac{(1 - \epsilon_j) a_j N_j}{\sum_{i=1}^{n} (1 - \epsilon_i) a_i N_i} , \tag{4.5}$$

with $\delta_{ij} = 0$ if $i = j$ and $\delta_{ij} = 1$ if $i = j$. Heterogeneity is a property of human populations. The mass action mixing function clearly oversimplifies the way groups of individuals interact. It is true that it can render reasonable approximations at a very general level, but one has to be cautious in this respect.

Many mathematical models for COVID-19 include several types of infectious individuals, including presymptomatic ones, that still follow the mass action law for their contacts, allowing only for a reduction or increase in the probability of infection. In Fig. 3, we show a typical contact matrix obtained from an extensive study on influenza-like illnesses [26]. The clear diagonally dominant pattern is shown.

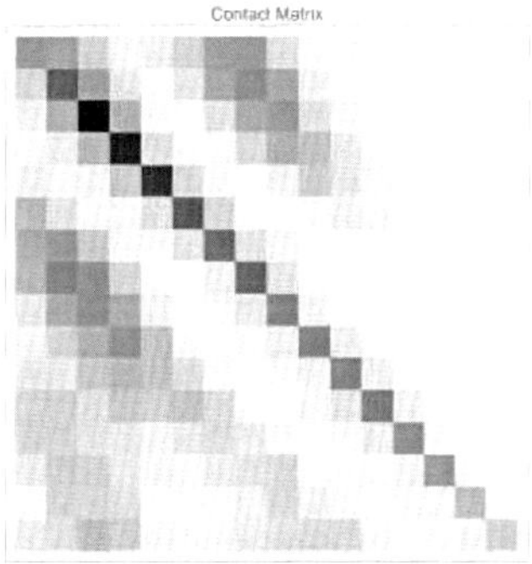

Figure 3: Contact matrix for a home environment modified from [26]. Each row is an age group of 5 years for a total of 16 age groups

The use of contact matrices is of fundamental importance when designing protocols for ending lockdowns or vaccination strategies. Age is a natural risk factor for this disease and that can be directly incorporated into the Kermack-McKendrick framework. As a representative example, we follow the model in another study [15]. This model was constructed to help in the design of a strategy to reopen the economy after the ending of strict lockdowns in many regions of the world. Risk of contagion has different characteristics depending on age. It is known, for example, that the IFR (infection fatality rate) is higher in older people (60 yrs old and older). Therefore, the release of restrictions in older adults at the same time than younger individuals may increase the IFR because of the higher transmission and mortality in the older adults age group [27]. To design a sound strategy, models have to include age as a new variable and, more importantly, consider that because of the mitigation measures, the structure of pre-pandemic contact patterns most likely has changed. The model [15] introduces seven compartments for each age class considered, which are S_i susceptible, E_i exposed, A_i asymptomatically infected, I_i symptomatically infected, H_i hospitalized, R_i recovered and M_i dead individuals where i refers to the age class. There are three age classes: 0-44 years old, 45-64 years old, and older than 65 years old. For each age class, the parameters are $1/k_i$ mean latent period, $1/\gamma_i$, $1/\gamma_{ia}$ mean infectious period for symptomatic and asymptomatic individuals respectivelly, η_i the average rate of transition form I_i to H_i, ϕ_i the rate at which individuals abandon the H_i compartment, where q_i is the proportion of these that die, p_i is the proportion of infections that develop symptoms, and θ_i and ξ_i denote the proportional reduction of infectivity, with respect to symptomatic cases, to asymptomatic and hospitalized individuals of age class i. The force of infection for each age class in this model incorporates the contact structure:

$$\lambda_i(t) = \sum_{j=1}^{3} a_i(t) c_{ij} \frac{I_j + \theta_j A_j + \xi_j H_j}{N_j}$$

where c_{ij} is defined as in (4.5). The equations are

$$\begin{aligned} S_i' &= -S_i \lambda_i(t)\,, & H_i' &= \eta_i I_i - \phi_i H_i\,, \\ E_i' &= S_i \lambda_i(t) - k_i E_i\,, & R_i' &= \gamma_{ia} A_i + \gamma_i I_i + (1 - q_i)\phi_i H_i\,, \\ A_i' &= (1 - p_i) k_i E_i - \gamma_{ia} A_i\,, & M_i' &= q_i \phi_i H_i + \delta_i I_i\,, \\ I_i' &= p_i k_i E_i - (\gamma_i + \eta_i + \delta_i) I_i\,, \end{aligned}$$

where $i = 1, 2, 3$ denote the age classes previously discussed. The main conclusion of this work is "...that the early release of low-risk young may protect older and more vulnerable individuals from severe health risks. As an added benefit, the staggered-release policy allows for more activity in the population at an earlier date than the delayed simultaneous release policy would. Thus staggered release policies can positively impact everyone involved by allowing people to return to their lives without putting them at risk" [15].

4 MODIFICATION OF THE BASIC MODELS

One of the important measures taken to control the spread of the epidemic was the application of mitigation measures expressed in total or partial lockdowns, social distancing, use of facemasks and frequent washing of hands among others. We will review here the model developed in Santana Cibrian et al [28] for a partial lockdown. The epidemiological model consists of the compartments of susceptible, exposed, asymptomatically infected, symptomatically infected, reported, recovered, and death individuals. It is assumed that the population is split into two different subpopulations, one that fully complies with social distancing, use of face masks, mobility restrictions, etc., and another group with lower compliance. These different levels of compliance affect the reduction of the effective contact rate under lockdown. We also consider that individuals under lockdown get tired of it and start to have high risk behaviours that equal their lower contact rates with those of the group with lower compliance. An important parameter in this model is $\omega(t)$, variable rate of mobility of the population in lockdown. We now present the model where the indices $i = 1, 2$ represent the two groups, $i = 1$ high compliance, $i = 2$ lower compliance:

$$\begin{aligned}
S_i' =& \ \mu_h (S_i + E_i + I_{ai} + I_{si}) + [(2-i)\,q + (i-1)(1-q)]\,\mu_h (I_r + R) \\
& -\beta_i(t)(I_{si} + I_{ai}) \tfrac{S_i}{N^*} + (-1)^i \omega(t) S_1 - \mu_h S_i + (1-i)^i \chi_r R\,, \\
E_i' =& \ \beta_i(t)(I_{si} + I_{ai}) \tfrac{S_i}{N^*} - \gamma E_i + (-1)^i \omega(t) E_1 - \mu_h E_i\,, \\
I_{ai}' =& \ \rho\gamma E_i - \eta_a I_{ai} + (-1)^i \omega(t) I_{a1} - \mu_h I_{ai}\,, \qquad\qquad (4.6)\\
I_{si}' =& \ (1-\rho)\gamma E_i - (\eta_s + \delta_s) I_{si} + (-1)^i \omega(t) I_{s1} - \mu_h I_{si}\,, \\
I_r' =& \ \delta_s (I_{s1} + I_{s2}) - \delta_r I_r - \mu_h I_r\,, \qquad D' = \mu\delta_r I_r\,, \\
R' =& \ \eta_a (I_{a1} + I_{a2}) + \eta_s (I_{s1} + I_{s2}) + (1-\mu)\,\delta_r I_r - \mu_h R - \chi_r R\,,
\end{aligned}$$

where $N^* = \sum_{i=1}^{2} (S_i + E_i + I_{ai} + I_{si}) + R$, $i = 1, 2$; μ_h, is the birth rate and natural death rate of the population, and χ_r^{-1}, the average time of temporal immunity. Individuals can abandon the group with higher compliance at a rate ω, γ^{-1} is the incubation period , ρ is the proportion of individuals that become asymptomatically infected, η_a^{-1} is the average recovery time for asymptomatic individuals, η_s^{-1} is the average recovery time for symptomatic individuals, $\delta_s^{-1}$is the average time that takes one individual to seek medical attention, δ_r^{-1} is the average time until recovery and μ is the proportion of individuals that die.

The effective contact rate for each group, $\beta_i(t)$, decreases after the implementation of the lockdown but is not the same for each subpopulation. There are many alternatives to model this behavior. One way is to define the following:

$$\beta_i(t) = \begin{cases} bq_1, & \text{if } t < T, \\ bq_2, & \text{if } t \geq T, \end{cases}$$

where $q_1, q_2 \in [0, 1]$ and $(1 - q_i) \times 100$ are the percentage reduction of the original (pre-lockdown) contact rate, and b is a step function.

This model allows us to explore the changes in the epidemic curve when the effective contact rate has a sudden increase because of, for example, short bursts of heightened mobility. Increases in the effective contact rate are related to human behavior. The reasons behind violating the rules of lockdowns are very varied and very rarely predictable, except perhaps, when holidays, vacations of other festivities that have a social component of family, religious, or political nature occur. These atypical events during the epidemic can be characterized as superspreading events (events with increased transmission in the large scale) that, in the context of the model in this section, we associate with the rate ω that represents the loosening of compliance because individuals in lockdown move out of it and become, de facto, members of the low compliance group.

An atypical increase in mobility is modeled as follows [29]: First, the increase in mobility lasts only for a period of τ days; second, the change in mobility is reflected on ω_0 by a factor k, i.e., for the superspreading period, the new compliance failure rate is $k\omega_0$ baseline mobility rate; third, the behavioral change is not instantaneous but modelled as

$$\beta_i(t) = \begin{cases} b - \frac{(1-q_i)}{\theta} b\,(t - T), & \text{if } T \leq t < T + \theta, \\ q_i b, & \text{if } t \geq T + \theta, \end{cases}$$

where θ is the period where the contact rate declines, and q_i is the proportion of reduction of the baseline effective contact rate for each subpopulation.

As an example of the results, we assume that no reinfections occur ($\chi_r = 0$) and simulate one atypical event where mobility increases for three days by a factor of $k = 10$ times the baseline failure rate, i.e. $\omega = 10\omega_0$, with $\omega_0 = 0.005$). We simulate several events before or after the baseline incidence peak.

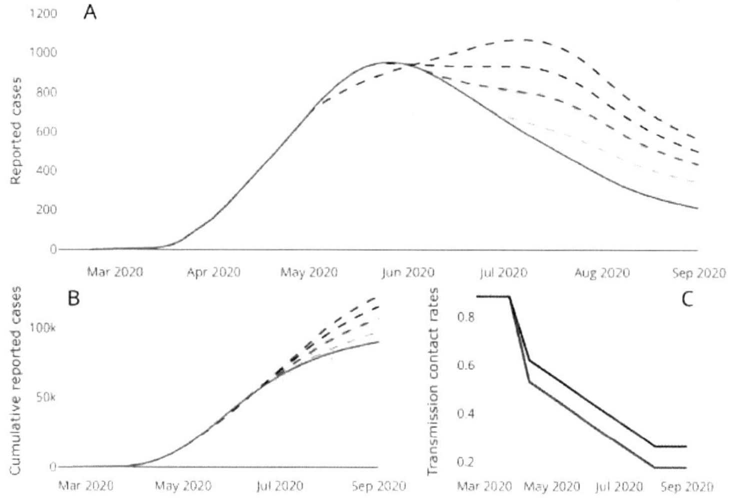

Figure 4: Impact of different times of mobility increase on the epidemic curve. Mobility increase is given by $10\omega_0$ ($\omega_0 = 0.005$). A) The green line is the baseline epidemic curve. Blue, black, red, and yellow discontinuous lines illustrate the scenarios when the mobility event starts, four weeks before, a week before, a week after, and four weeks after the peak incidence, respectively. B) Cummulative incidence, C) effective contact rate

In Fig. 4, the green solid line is the baseline epidemic curve, normal Kermack-McKendrick dynamics. Note that the worst-case scenario (blue dashed line) occurs when the atypical event is located on the exponential growth phase of the curve and relatively far from the maximum incidence. The most benign scenario occurs when the superspreading event happens after the incidence peak (dashed yellow line). When the superspreading event occurs just before (black dashed line) or just after (red dashed line) the peak of the curve, a plateau that lasts several weeks is formed. Fig. 4B shows the cumulative incidence for each case and shows that, regardless of the timing of increased mobility, there is a similar increment in cases. Fig. 4C illustrates the shape of the effective contact rates. Further details can be found in Santana Cibrian et al [29].

This model was applied to the epidemic in Mexico City. One of the important conclusions was the accurate prediction of the time when the maximum incidence would be reached that was located towards the end of May. With this model, the entrance of the epidemic to a long plateau was also correctly predicted.

5 EPIDEMIC CURVES

Kermack-McKendrick models have, all of them, an initial exponential growth and then, after reaching a maximum, the epidemic curve decreases also exponentially. In Fig. 5, the epidemic curves of Spain and Mexico, from the initial case up to March 9, are plotted.

The differences of both curves are striking. Spain reached the epidemic peak very fast (around day 50), reaching almost 10 000 cases per day at the acme, and then, because of the strongly enforced lockdown measures, the first epidemic outbreak practically died out (Fig. 5A and C); in contrast, the epidemic in Mexico grew very slowly likewise reaching almost 10 000 cases per day but until the 100th day of the epidemic; then because of the very weak mitigation measures, the epidemic reached a plateau and stayed there for several months until mid September where the second major outbreak started (Fig. 5B and D). The initial growth of the Spanish curve is compatible with exponential growth, while the Mexican curve grows practically in a linear way. This peculiar behavior is observed in many epidemic growth curves around the world, which has been explored in Thurner et al [30], who have provided an explanation for this linear growth that involves the structure of the underlying contact network of individuals and the maintenance of the effective reproduction number around $R_t \approx 1$ for sustained periods of time. This phenomenon can be better appreciated in the epidemic of Mexico City (Fig. 6).

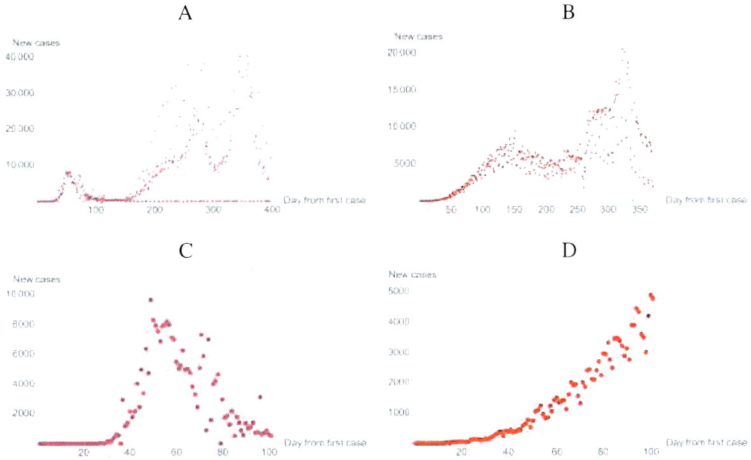

Figure 5: Comparative plots of the epidemic curves for Mexico and Spain. A) and B) Epidemic curve of Spain and Mexico, respectively, from the first case to early March 2021; C) and D) initial epidemic growth of Spain and Mexico, respectively, up to day 100 of their respective epidemics. Data from Our World in Data web page

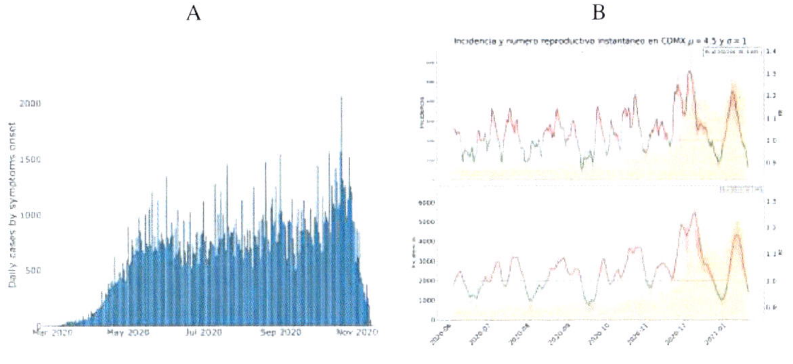

Figure 6: A) Epidemic curve for Mexico City. The initial linear growth and the plateau reached after May 30th can be identified until about mid-September, B) Evolution of the instantaneous reproductive number R_t for México City from June 1 2020 to the end of February 2021. The erratic oscillations around $R_t = 1$ are clear. Lower panel in B shows an smoothed version of R_t

From the results of model (4.6) and the mitigation measures applied in the Mexico City epidemic, we can deduce that the initial slow growth was the product of an early application of the weak mitigation measures. Indeed, the first case in Mexico occurred by the end of February 2020 and the first mitigation measures where applied on March 23th, about 25 days after the initial case. From [9, 28] and the results of model (4.6) discussed in the previous section, we can conclude that there were superdispersion events in Mexico City in early May (particularly April 30th to May 10th) that shifted the expected day of maximum incidence towards the end of the month and also sent the epidemic into a quasi-stationary state characterized by values of $R_t \approx 1$. In contrast, in Spain the first case was recorded by the end of January and the lockdown was imposed on March 14, more than 40 days after the initial case. Given the stricter nature of the lockdown, the initial outbreak was controlled and resolved by the 100th day of the epidemic.

6 EPIDEMIC INTERACTIONS

Vaccine application to protect against severe acute respiratory infections is a priority around the globe as new waves of COVID-19 occur in many countries and there is increasing pressure on health care systems to accommodate the growing numbers of severe cases. In addition to this, acute respiratory infections occur as annual or biannual epidemics as is the case for influenza.

With the presence of SARS-CoV-2 we will have to deal with an scenario where this virus will cocirculate with the influenza virus the whole year but particularly in the fall and winter seasons in each hemisphere. Fortunately, there are vaccines for influenza and therefore, influenza vaccination can potentially reduce its prevalence and reduce symptoms that might be confused with those of COVID-19 [31].

In Acuña-Zegarra et al [32], a mathematical model is presented for the cocirculation of SARS-CoV-2, and influenza under the assumption that a vaccine exists for both viruses. The model explores the effects of coverage, efficacy, induced temporal immunity on the dynamics of this coupled system.

$$
\begin{aligned}
s' &= \mu - \left(\beta_i(t)(i + i_{r_y}) + \beta_y(t)(y + y_{r_i})\right) s + \theta_i r_i + \theta_y r_y + \theta r - (\mu + \phi_i + \phi_y)s\,,\\
i' &= \beta_i(t)(i + i_{r_y})s - \alpha\beta_y(t)iy - (\eta_i + \mu)i\,,\\
y' &= \beta_y(t)(y + y_{r_i})s + \alpha\beta_y(t)iy - (\eta_y + \mu)y\,,\\
r_i' &= \phi_i s + \eta_i i - (1 - p_i)\beta_y(t)r_i(y + y_{ri}) - (\phi_y + \theta_i + \mu)r_i\,,\\
r_y' &= \phi_y s + \eta_y y - \beta_i(t)r_y(i + i_{ry}) - (\phi_i + \theta_y + \mu)r_y\,,\\
y_{r_i}' &= (1 - p_i)\beta_y(t)r_i(y + y_{ri}) - (\omega_y + \mu)y_{r_i}\,,\\
i_{r_y}' &= \beta_i(t)r_y(i + i_{ry}) - (\omega_i + \mu)i_{r_y}\,,\\
r' &= \omega_y y_{r_i} + \omega_i i_{r_y} + \phi_y r_i + \phi_i r_y - (\theta + \mu)r\,,
\end{aligned}
$$

where s, i, y, r_i, r_y, y_{ri}, i_{ry}, r represent, respectively, the individuals that are susceptible, infected by influenza, infected by coronavirus, immune against influenza, immune against coronavirus, infected by coronavirus while immune to influenza, infected by influenza while immune to coronavirus and immune to both diseases. The model couples two SIR models where vaccinated and naturally immune individuals for a given disease (i.e., individuals that are immune after recovering from an infection) are pooled together in the same compartment); η_k, ω_k, θ_k, θ, ϕ_k are the recovery from a primary infection, recovery from a secondary infection, waning from a primary infection/vaccination, waning from a secondary infection/vaccination, and vaccination rates for influenza ($k = i$) or coronavirus ($k = y$), respectively. Finally, $\beta_k(t)$ are the time-dependent effective contact rates and α is a coefficient that introduces the hypothesis that a host already infected by the influenza virus can be infected by the coronavirus, resulting in the effective displacement of influenza from that host.

As mentioned earlier, the flu season of 2019-2020 has been atypical. There has been a significant decrease of influenza cases in the season that, at the time of writing, is about to end, and SARS-CoV-2 has been the dominant respiratory disease from the beginning of 2020 [33]. There are several issues dealt with in the paper where this model was presented [32] that have to do with the indirect protective effect of the influenza vaccine against coronavirus infection, and the consequences of deficiencies in coverage and vaccine efficacy on the persistence of one or both diseases. We concentrate here in a particular phenomenon of the epidemic.

At the time of writing, the world was in the midst of a vaccination campaign that aimed at controling epidemic growth by decreasing the risk of infection, which would allow everybody to return to a new normality. The question, however, is whether the coronavirus will really go away. The basic SIR and SEIR models presented in the first section of this chapter can provide plausible scenarios and clues to consider and evaluate. To study the long-term behavior of both epidemics, we need to assume that the effective contact rates are time dependent. Take $\beta_k(t) = a_k(1+\cos(2\pi t/365))$ which is a periodic function with a period equal to 365 days, then the question is if the coronavirus persists as an endemic disease, what kind of dynamics will it have? Will it become similar to influenza with annual or biannual epidemic peaks? Will influenza maintain the same trend as the one observed until 2019?

The results of some of the simulations are shown in Fig. 7. It can be seen that influenza and coronavirus can present epidemic episodes with alternating dominance by one or the other. Note also that when one virus dominates, the other one still presents cases but at a much lower level. The possibility of having simultaneous epidemic episodes is also explored in Acuña-Zegarra et al [32].

Influenza and influenza-like illnesses cocirculating with the coronavirus constitute a single group of infectious agents that interact with SARS-CoV-2. The large disruptions that lockdowns and other mitigation measures caused in the world, impacted control programs for many other diseases. Vaccination campaigns were disrupted for measles, nebulization and mosquito control programs against Dengue. Zika, Chikungunya, Malaria also were severely disrupted. Models are needed to evaluate the current condition of these diseases and to design adequate ways to reduce the morbidity that the post-coronavirus emergency will bring.

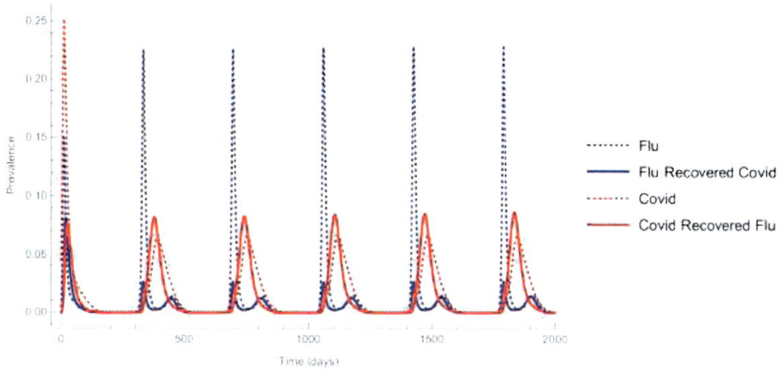

Figure 7: Outbreaks of coronavirus and influenza undergo alternate occurrences both for primary and secondary infections. Shown are primary coronavirus cases (dashed red), secondary coronavirus cases (solid red), primary influenza cases (dashed blue lines), and secondary influenza cases (solid blue)

7 CONCLUDING REMARKS

The mathematical modelling of infectious diseases took the center stage during the past year. Many of the models that are being used to inform public health policy are of the Kermack-McKendrick type constructed by multidisciplinary teams of many types of professionals but where epidemiologists and medical practitioners play an important role as experts in the field. In one of the latest and interesting (and useful) applications, we find two works [27, 34]. In a study [27], several mathematical models are used to explore strategies that might be optimal for vaccine application, now that vaccines are scarce in many regions of the world. The conclusions are that prioritizing age groups between 20 and 49 years old minimizes cumulative incidence, but targeting age classes 60 years and older, mortality and years of life lost are minimized. The authors conclude their work pointing out the multifacetic problem of deciding which group should be first in receiving the vaccine. Like in other pandemics, the burden associated with COVID-19 has been particularly high for certain economically deprived population groups. The assignment of priorities derived from the analysis of these models where the main risk factor is age, has to be complemented with other measures of risk. Mathematical models are essential tools supported by the hypothesis that researchers introduce to construct them. Age is not the only risk variable that can be considered. In Latin American countries, comorbidities (diabetes, hypertension, obesity) have an increased fatality rate in younger people and socioeconomic inequalities threaten the timely access to vaccines. These factors need to be integrated at regional and local levels to evaluate in a more comprehensive way the optimal priorities in the application of vaccines.

According to Subramanian et al [34], the problem of the impact on the transmission of a large pool of asymptomatically infected individuals, characteristic of SARS-CoV-2, is addressed. In these sets of models, another important compartment is introduced, that of pre-symptomatic individuals, and a basic public health tool, unfortunately scarce in many Latin American countries: testing capacity and strategies.

Several issues have not been addressed in this chapter, which represent opportunities for research in areas related to quantitative epidemiology: the role of heterogeneity in the transmission of SARS-CoV-2 [21], the need to perform prevalence estimation to monitor the true behaviour of the epidemic [35], the role of testing as a way to successful screening of populations [36] and the dynamics of whithin-host viral interactions [37].

Finally, a few comments on the use of models in this pandemic. Public opinion on the usefulness and value of models has shifted during this pandemic (e.g, [38]), going from a very positive perspective in the initial months, to an esceptical and sometimes disqualifying attitude in recent times. Many Kermack-McKendrick variants were used in the early times of the emergency to forecast its development and many of them failed when the biological, social, and behavioral evolving nature of the epidemic started to act. Experts were not surprised by this development, but many researchers and politicians were indeed. Epidemiological models in pandemic times are immensely valuable tools that, as any other tool, require careful design and application by multidisciplinary teams and interdisciplinary approaches to be effective. They also require adequate public communication and dissemination of results. The mathematical models included in this paper are meant to illustrate their use for so-called strategic objectives. In these models, the aim is not to fit curves with 95% confidence intervals and then extrapolate the incidence to see when the epidemic will end, but to understand the basic mechanisms of the problem and provide scenarios supported by current epidemiological and medical knowledge on the pandemic. The examples have been chosen subjectively, on the ground that they are interesting and informative. I hope to have transmitted to the reader that strategic mathematical models are powerful conceptual tools that can inform in a very effective way public health decisions. Model fitting is but one component of mathematical modelling whose usefulness is conditioned by a conceptually sound and well-thought mathematical model.

8 CONSENT FOR PUBLICATION

Not applicable.

9 CONFLICT OF INTEREST

The authors declare no conflict of interest, financial or otherwise.

10 ACKNOWLEDGEMENTS

I am very grateful to the enjoyable and fruitful collaborations that started early last year and have continued into the present time, with my colleagues Adrián Acuña Zegarra, Mario Santana Cibrián, Mayra Núñez López, Fernando Saldaña García and Ruth Corona-Moreno. I acknowledge support from DGAPA-PAPIIT-UNAM grant IV100220 (convocatoria especial COVID-19) and DGAPA-PAPIIT-UNAM grant IN115720.

References

[1] Kermack WO, McKendrick A. A contribution to the mathematical theory of epidemics. Proceedings of the Royal Society of London. Series A, Containing Papers of a Mathematical and Physical Character [Internet]. 1927 Aug [cited 2021 Oct 1];115(772):700–21. Available from: https://doi.org/10.1098/rspa.1927.0118

[2] Bacaer N. A short history of mathematical population dynamics. Choice Reviews Online [Internet]. 2011 May 1 [cited 2021 Oct 1];48(09):48–5141. Available from: https://doi.org/10.5860/choice.48-5141

[3] Kermack W, Mckendrick A. Contributions to the mathematical theory of epidemics–I. Bulletin of Mathematical Biology [Internet]. 1991 [cited 2021 Oct 1];53(1-2):33–55. Available from: https://doi.org/10.1016/s0092-8240(05)80040-0

[4] Kermack W, Mckendrick A. Contributions to the mathematical theory of epidemics–II. the problem of endemicity. Proceedings of the Royal Society of London. Series A, Containing Papers of a Mathematical and Physical Character [Internet]. Oct 1932 [cited Oct 2, 2021];138(834):55–83. Available from: https://doi.org/10.1098/rspa.1932.0171. Also in: Bulletin of Mathematical Biology [Internet]. 1991 [cited Oct 2, 2021];53(1-2):57–87. Available from: https://doi.org/10.1016/s0092-8240(05)80041-2

[5] Kermack W, McKendrick A. Contributions to the mathematical theory of epidemics. III.–Further studies of the problem of endemicity. Proceedings of the Royal Society of London. Series A, Containing Papers of a Mathematical and Physical Character [Internet]. Jul 3, 1933 [cited Oct 2, 2021];141(843):94–122. Available from: `https://doi.org/10.1098/rspa.1933.0106`. Also in: Bulletin of Mathematical Biology [Internet]. 1991 [cited Oct 2, 2021];53(1-2):89–118. Available from: `https://doi.org/10.1016/s0092-8240(05)80042-4`

[6] Kermack WO, McKendrick AG. Contributions to the mathematical theory of epidemics: V. Analysis of experimental epidemics of mouse-typhoid; a bacterial disease conferring incomplete immunity. Journal of Hygiene [Internet]. May 1939 [cited Oct 2, 2021];39(3):271–88. Available from: `https://doi.org/10.1017/s0022172400011918`

[7] Kermack WO, McKendrick AG. Contributions to the mathematical theory of epidemics IV. Analysis of experimental epidemics of the virus disease mouse ectromelia. Journal of Hygiene [Internet]. 1937 Apr [cited 2021 Oct 1];37(2):172–87. Available from: `https://doi.org/10.1017/s0022172400034902`

[8] Hethcote HW. Qualitative analyses of communicable disease models. Mathematical Biosciences [Internet]. 1976 Jan [cited 2021 Oct 1];28(3-4):335–56. Available from: `https://doi.org/10.1016/0025-5564(76)90132-2`

[9] Acuña-Zegarra MA, Santana-Cibrian M, Velasco-Hernandez JX. Modeling behavioral change and COVID-19 containment in Mexico: A trade-off between lockdown and compliance. Mathematical Biosciences [Internet]. 2020 Jul [cited 2021 Oct 1];325:108370. Available from: `https://doi.org/10.1016/j.mbs.2020.108370`

[10] Li Q, Tang B, Bragazzi NL, Xiao Y, Wu J. Modeling the impact of mass influenza vaccination and public health interventions on COVID-19 epidemics with limited detection capability.

Mathematical Biosciences [Internet]. 2020 Jul [cited 2021 Oct 1];325:108378. Available from: https://doi.org/10.1016/j.mbs.2020.108378

[11] Magal P, Webb G. The parameter identification problem for SIR epidemic models: identifying unreported cases. Journal of Mathematical Biology [Internet]. 2018 Jan 13 [cited 2021 Oct 1];77(6-7):1629–48. Available from: https://doi.org/10.1007/s00285-017-1203-9

[12] Mena RH, Velasco-Hernandez JX, Mantilla-Beniers NB, Carranco-Sapiéns GA, Benet L, Boyer D, Castillo IP. Using posterior predictive distributions to analyse epidemic models: COVID-19 in Mexico City. Physical Biology [Internet]. 2020 Sep 22 [cited 2021 Oct 1];17(6):065001. Available from: https://doi.org/10.1088/1478-3975/abb115

[13] Mukandavire Z, Malunguza NJ, Cuadros DF, Shiri T, Musuka G, Nyabadza F. Quantifying Early COVID-19 Outbreak Transmission in South Africa and Exploring Vaccine Efficacy Scenarios. SSRN Electronic Journal [Internet]. 2020 [cited 2021 Oct 1]. Available from: https://doi.org/10.2139/ssrn.3576901

[14] Wu JT, Leung K, Leung GM. Nowcasting and forecasting the potential domestic and international spread of the 2019-nCoV outbreak originating in Wuhan, China: a modelling study. The Lancet [Internet]. 2020 Feb [cited 2021 Oct 1];395(10225):689–97. Available from: https://doi.org/10.1016/s0140-6736(20)30260-9

[15] Zhao H, Feng Z. Staggered release policies for COVID-19 control: Costs and benefits of relaxing restrictions by age and risk. Mathematical Biosciences [Internet]. 2020 Aug [cited 2021 Oct 1];326:108405. Available from: https://doi.org/10.1016/j.mbs.2020.108405

[16] Ali ST, Wang L, Lau EH, Xu XK, Du Z, Wu Y, Leung GM, Cowling BJ. Serial interval of SARS-CoV-2 was shortened over time by nonpharmaceutical interventions. Science

[Internet]. 2020 Jul 21 [cited 2021 Oct 1];369(6507):1106–9. Available from: https://doi.org/10.1126/science.abc9004

[17] SSA. Gobierno de México: Información referente a casos COVID 19 en México. Technical report, Secretaría de Salud, 2021.

[18] Champredon D, Dushoff J. Intrinsic and realized generation intervals in infectious-disease transmission. Proceedings of the Royal Society B: Biological Sciences [Internet]. 2015 Dec 22 [cited 2021 Oct 1];282(1821):20152026. Available from: https://doi.org/10.1098/rspb.2015.2026

[19] Park SW, Champredon D, Dushoff J. Inferring generation-interval distributions from contact-tracing data. Journal of The Royal Society Interface [Internet]. 2020 Jun [cited 2021 Oct 1];17(167):20190719. Available from: https://doi.org/10.1098/rsif.2019.0719

[20] Wallinga J, Lipsitch M. How generation intervals shape the relationship between growth rates and reproductive numbers. Proceedings of the Royal Society B: Biological Sciences [Internet]. 2006 Nov 28 [cited 2021 Oct 1];274(1609):599–604. Available from: https://doi.org/10.1098/rspb.2006.3754

[21] Sun K, Wang W, Gao L, Wang Y, Luo K, Ren L, Zhan Z, Chen X, Zhao S, Huang Y, Sun Q, Liu Z, Litvinova M, Vespignani A, Ajelli M, Viboud C, Yu H. Transmission heterogeneities, kinetics, and controllability of SARS-CoV-2. Science [Internet]. 2020 Nov 24 [cited 2021 Oct 1]:eabe2424. Available from: https://doi.org/10.1126/science.abe2424

[22] Sanche S, Lin YT, Xu C, Romero-Severson E, Hengartner N, Ke R. High Contagiousness and Rapid Spread of Severe Acute Respiratory Syndrome Coronavirus 2. Emerging Infectious Diseases [Internet]. 2020 Jul [cited 2021 Oct 1];26(7):1470–7. Available from: https://doi.org/10.3201/eid2607.200282

[23] CDC. Interim Guidance on Duration of Isolation and Precautions for Adults with COVID-19. Technical report, Centers for Disease Control, 2021.

[24] Busenberg S, Castillo-Chávez C. A general solution of the problem of mixing of subpopulations and its application to risk- and age-structured epidemic models for the spread of AIDS. Mathematical Medicine and Biology [Internet]. 1991 [cited 2021 Oct 1];8(1):1–29. Available from: `https://doi.org/10.1093/imammb/8.1.`

[25] Glasser J, Feng Z, Moylan A, Del Valle S, Castillo-Chávez C. Mixing in age-structured population models of infectious diseases. Mathematical Biosciences [Internet]. 2012 Jan [cited 2021 Oct 1];235(1):1–7. Available from: `https://doi.org/10.1016/j.mbs.2011.10.001`

[26] Prem K, Cook AR, Jit M. Projecting social contact matrices in 152 countries using contact surveys and demographic data. PLOS Computational Biology [Internet]. 2017 Sep 12 [cited 2021 Oct 1];13(9):e1005697. Available from: `https://doi.org/10.1371/journal.pcbi.1005697`

[27] Bubar KM, Reinholt K, Kissler SM, Lipsitch M, Cobey S, Grad YH, Larremore DB. Model-informed COVID-19 vaccine prioritization strategies by age and serostatus. Science [Internet]. 2021 Feb 26 [cited 2021 Oct 1];371(6532):916–21. Available from: `https://doi.org/10.1126/science.abe6959`

[28] Santana-Cibrian M, A Acuña-Zegarra M, X Velasco-Hernández J. Lifting mobility restrictions and the effect of superspreading events on the short-term dynamics of COVID-19. Mathematical Biosciences and Engineering [Internet]. 2020 [cited 2021 Oct 1];17(5):6240–58. Available from: `https://doi.org/10.3934/mbe.2020330`

[29] Santana-Cibrian M, Acuña-Zegarra MA, Angulo MT, Hernández-Vargas EA, Velasco-Hernández JX. Modeling SARS-CoV-2: mitigation interventions and increased

mobility events. In T. Azar and A. Hassanien, editors, Modeling, Control and Drug Development for COVID-19 Outbreak Prevention, chapter 16, page 690. Springer International Publishing, Switzerland, 2021.

[30] Thurner S, Klimek P, Hanel R. A network-based explanation of why most COVID-19 infection curves are linear. Proceedings of the National Academy of Sciences [Internet]. 2020 Aug 24 [cited 2021 Oct 1];117(37):22684–9. Available from: https://doi.org/10.1073/pnas.2010398117

[31] Sultana J, Mazzaglia G, Luxi N, Cancellieri A, Capuano A, Ferrajolo C, de Waure C, Ferlazzo G, Trifirò G. Potential effects of vaccinations on the prevention of COVID-19: rationale, clinical evidence, risks, and public health considerations. Expert Review of Vaccines [Internet]. 2020 Oct 2 [cited 2021 Oct 1];19(10):919–36. Available from: https://doi.org/10.1080/14760584.2020.1825951

[32] Acuña-Zegarra MA, Núñez-López M, Comas-García A, Santana-Cibrian M, Velasco-Hernández JX, Co-circulation of SARS-CoV-2 and Influenza under vaccination scenarios, 2021, medRxiv, Available from: http://medrxiv.org/content/early/2021/01/04/2020.12.29.20248953.abstract

[33] World Health Organization. Influenza Update 380. Technical Report November, World Health Organization, 2020

[34] Subramanian R, He Q, Pascual M. Quantifying asymptomatic infection and transmission of COVID-19 in New York City using observed cases, serology, and testing capacity. Proceedings of the National Academy of Sciences [Internet]. 2021 Feb 10 [cited 2021 Oct 1];118(9):e2019716118. Available from: https://doi.org/10.1073/pnas.2019716118

[35] Clark SJ, Turner AN. Monitoring epidemics: Lessons from measuring population prevalence

of the coronavirus. Proceedings of the National Academy of Sciences [Internet]. 2021 Feb 24 [cited 2021 Oct 1];118(9):e2026412118. Available from: https://doi.org/10.1073/pnas.2026412118

[36] Larremore DB, Wilder B, Lester E, Shehata S, Burke JM, Hay JA, Tambe M, Mina MJ, Parker R. Test sensitivity is secondary to frequency and turnaround time for COVID-19 screening. Science Advances [Internet]. 2020 Nov 20 [cited 2021 Oct 1];7(1):eabd5393. Available from: https://doi.org/10.1126/sciadv.abd5393

[37] Hernández-Vargas EA, Velasco-Hernández JX. In-host Mathematical Modelling of COVID-19 in Humans. Annual Reviews in Control [Internet]. 2020 [cited 2021 Oct 1];50:448–56. Available from: https://doi.org/10.1016/j.arcontrol.2020.09.006

[38] Kreps SE, Kriner DL. Model uncertainty, political contestation, and public trust in science: Evidence from the COVID-19 pandemic. Science Advances [Internet]. 2020 Sep 25 [cited 2021 Oct 1];6(43):eabd4563. Available from: https://doi.org/10.1126/sciadv.abd4563

CHAPTER 5

Data Science: A Useful Tool for Understanding SARS-CoV-2 Information Facts

Nicandro Cruz-Ramírez[1], Guillermo-de-Jesús Hoyos-Rivera*[1]
Sonia-Lilia Mestizo-Gutiérrez[2] and Horacio Tapia-McClung[1]

* **Corresponding author:** ghoyos@uv.mx, Phone: +52 2288 421700 ext. 10211
[1] Artificial Intelligence Research Institute, Universidad Veracruzana, Xalapa, Veracruz, Mexico
[2] Faculty of Chemical Sciences, Universidad Veracruzana, Xalapa, Veracruz, Mexico

Abstract. By the end of 2019, a local pneumonia outbreak in Wuhan, China, was determined to be caused by a novel form of coronavirus named Severe Acute Respiratory Syndrome Coronavirus 2 (SARS-CoV-2), which, since then, has spread worldwide thus becoming the most important public health issue of the beginning of the 21st century. As a response, governments and health organizations started collecting data about this disease for analyzing it, trying to draw conclusions that could lead to a better understanding of it, and eventually to alleviate its effects. Through the analysis of the available data, our area of interest has to do with finding possible correlations among the variables related to COVID-19 cases which could give some insights. For example, which factors make a given patient to present an aggravated form of this illness, or even a higher risk of dying? Does the level of poverty make some people prone to get ill? What about the place where people live in? These and other questions can be answered based on the analysis of the available data. In this chapter, we give a brief introduction to Data Science (DS), a field of Artificial Intelligence (AI), and present some data analysis using publicly available COVID-19 data sets provided by the Mexican government. This allows us to show how AI tools and techniques can help us to better understand some aspects of this kind of situation, and in this way, hopefully helping health officials and providers to create better health policies and services and succeeding in their goal: saving lives.

Key words: Artificial Intelligence, Bayesian Network, COVID-19, Database, Data Science, Decision Tree, Entropy, Epidemiology, Health, Information, Knowledge, Pandemic, SARS-CoV-2, Workflow

1 INTRODUCTION

1.1 Importance

This chapter highlights the potential impact of Data Science, as a branch of Artificial Intelligence, in unveiling relevant associations related to COVID-19. Data Science provides tools to find meaningful associations from large databases, which can later be tested with more specific analytical techniques. A better understanding of the causation web around this disease is a key factor to design and implement strategies to cope with the pandemic.

1.2 Preliminaries

Ipsa scientia potestas est. This phrase means "knowledge itself is power". It appears in Meditationes Sacræ[1], which was written by Sir Francis Bacon (1561-1626), and is of an astonishing relevance at the present time. In fact, this was not the first time humankind realized that knowledge is worth, frequently even more than wealth. Other ancient references exist in this same sense, which confer great importance to knowledge.

But, what is knowledge, and is it really as important as we think? How is knowledge related to information and data? There is not a unified consensus on how these concepts are related, since each source assumes slightly different points of view, and even their definitions are constructed cross-reference to the other ones. For example, as stated in the Merriam-Webster dictionary [2], knowledge, information, and data are defined as:

Knowledge:

1. The fact or condition of knowing something with familiarity gained through experience or association.
2. The range of one's information or understanding.
3. The fact or condition of having information or of being learned.

Information:

1. Knowledge obtained from investigation, study, or instruction.
2. A signal or character (as in a communication system or computer) representing data.
3. Something (such as a message, experimental data, or a picture) which justifies change in a construct (such as a plan or theory) that represents physical or mental experience or another construct.

Data

1. Factual information (such as measurements or statistics) used as a basis for reasoning, discussion, or calculation.
2. Information in digital form that can be transmitted or processed.

3. Information output by a sensing device or organ that includes both useful and irrelevant or redundant information and must be processed to be meaningful.

As we can easily see from these three definitions, it may be not completely clear how they relate to each other, and cross references among them are not helpful. Somehow, we can see that all of them are related to a type of of nontangible "artifact" that resides in our state of mind, or that can modify it.

One way of easily stating the relation among these terms is to assume a pyramidal representation, considering knowledge, the most elaborated concept, as a state of mind; information, an intermediary one, as something capable of modifying one's state of mind, and finally data, the simplest of the three, the minimal piece of information, which is nonsense unless it is placed into a context. A simple fact. This idea is shown in Fig. 1.

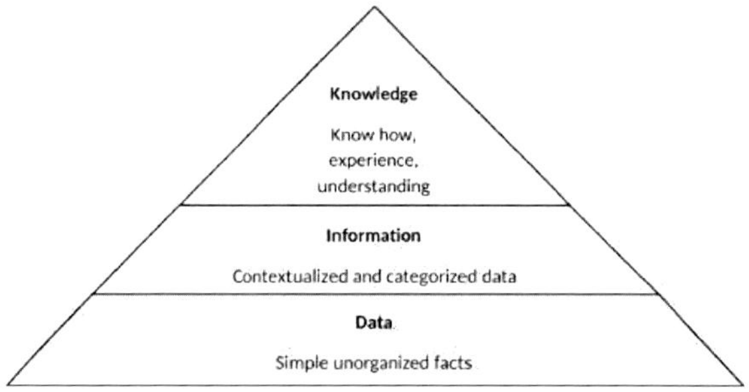

Figure 1: Pyramidal approach of Data, Information and Knowledge relations

In this way, if the number 54 is presented to us, we can only consider it a datum, since no context, or multiple contexts can be associated with it. In other words, the number 54 can be anything that can be numerable: age, size, weight, etc. On the other hand, if we see this same number accompanied by the word "years", it becomes information, since now we know that this number refers to a time span, maybe, an age, and that is completely different if we say, for example, 54 pounds. If it means the age of a living being, it will tell us whether that living being is old or not, depending on the species. Finally, when I know that my new teammate is 54 years old, I acquire knowledge, which allows me to make decisions according to what can I expect from him/her, and how we will possibly relate to each other; for example, if I should talk to him/her respectfully or not, depending on my own age, and our respective positions in the organization.

Battles have been won or lost because of the availability of quality information. Fortunes have been raised or completely lost because of decisions made based on good or wrong market information. Our own lives are the way they are because of the good and bad decisions we have made during our lifetime, and the quality of the information available when making these decisions.

Data is everywhere and is up to us to decide what to do with it. Sometimes it is easily available, but some other times it is hidden somehow, and we must make some effort to get it. It is true that in past times data were scarce or difficult to access, and that interested people, such as statisticians, had to work hard to get it. At present, however, with the exponential growth of the availability of computers, the rise of Internet-based communications, the creation of the so-called Social Networks[1], the increase of the Internet of Things (IoT) devices available almost everywhere, the amount of data available has increased in such an impressing way, that sometimes we start having difficulties in processing it.

One of the most important fields where good quality information is of crucial importance is people's health. Human body is a highly complex system, and it is often hard to understand all small intricate mechanisms that make it keep going. Several facts are still beyond our understanding about how cells work, how they interact, and how different substances or microorganisms that enter into the human body, such as viruses and bacteria, can affect it. Sometimes we know the effects but not the causes. Viruses are of special interest in this study, particularly since the beginning of the COVID-19 pandemic, by the end of 2019.

Several months have passed since the first COVID-19 case appeared in Wuhan city, in the People's Republic of China, and we are witnessing everyday numerous scientific teams hardly

[1]The Social Network concept is defined in [3] as "a network of individuals (such as friends, acquaintances, and coworkers) connected by interpersonal relationships)", and originally had nothing to do with computers and the Internet-based Social Networks, which is a rather new concept.

working, without being able to completely understand its behavior, nor even control it. Medical teams have proposed several treatment options, none of them a real complete solution to the problem. There are some medical teams which affirm that SARS-CoV-2 affects mainly the respiratory system, particularly the lungs and bronchi, and others say that it concerns mainly the circulatory system, producing micro-hemorrhages that cause the sensation of suffocation. Even more, there are supposed collateral effects, such as hearing or vision problems, which seem to appear after the end of the infection. In fact, we have not even understood how the infection is propagated, because there are literally millions of asymptomatic cases, which hinder the tracking of the contagion chain [3, 4].

In such a complex environment and having literally thousands of researchers around the world intensively working on finding a solution to this problem from different approaches, several terabytes of data are being generated worldwide every single day and analyzing all that data is not a simple task. This is mainly because, in the presence of the big quantity of available variables, which may be very diverse, a big number of examples, and the diversity of them depending on the principles guiding their collection, it is not easy to draw conclusions about the implications of the collected facts.

Causality is the holy grail of data analysis and the repository of possible correlations hidden in data. This is the problem that DS pretends to tackle. It is not an absolutely easy-to-achieve goal, and requires a careful analysis of the data, trying to understand which facts offer more information than the other, and then feeding classification algorithms with it, with the hope that we will find some relevant information in it, leading, in this way, to a better understanding of the pandemic, and how to act to minimize its effects.

In this chapter, we focus on the COVID-19 data generated by the Mexican government and use them as the input to classification algorithms leading to some interesting conclusions. The results of these algorithms allow to confirm, through hard data, that the initial assumptions, generally obtained in an intuitive way, are as we thought they were.

2 ARTIFICIAL INTELLIGENCE: THE NEW BOOM

Much has been said about AI. The name itself sounds sophisticated, modern, with a very high-tech style, leaving a lot to the imagination. However, this is not a new idea just recently coined as it dates back a long time ago.

In the Greek mythology we can find one of the oldest references to this subject: a humanoid bronze giant automaton, called Talos, created by the god Hephæstus, whose purpose was to guard the island of Crete, where Europa lived, and protect her from pirates and invaders. Since then, the human being has fancied with the possibility of artificially creating a type of intelligent being, or at least simulating intelligent behavior.

It is not until the twentieth century, with the invention of computers, and their increasing computing power, that the dream was retaken, then with another approach: looking for the creation of artificial artifacts, either anthropomorphic or not, which, having a computer as "brain", could behave as humans do.

AI has experienced periods of good and bad reputation, alternating booms with periods in which the originally set goals were far from being achieved. These were dubbed the winters of AI.

The first boom of AI happened by the end of the sixties of the twentieth century when, after World War 2, the countries' economies were recovering, and the development of computers was increasing its pace. At that time, researchers like Allen Newell, Herbert Simon, John McCarthy, and Marvin Minsky made very interesting proposals in both the philosophical and the technical field. By then, proposals such as the one called General Problem Solver [5], which pretended to be an automatic theorem prover, created great expectations: the possibility of building, in the short time, intelligent devices. However, that was not the case, and disappointment replaced all previous enthusiasm. This was called the first winter of the AI.

The second boom came about twenty years later, by the end of the eighties. Two of its main actors were Edward Feigenbaum and Rodney Brooks. Proposals such as DENDRAL, MYCIN, and new programming languages such as Prolog and Lisp, gave rise to a new wave where imagination created a future where expert systems would replace human's expertise, and medical diagnoses could then be made by consulting a machine, instead of a physician. Concerning the programming language, experts thought that it would be possible to create self-improving programs, which, through the modification of its own code, would be able to evolve and improve every day. However, this did not happen either, and AI fell into a second winter of disappointment.

Finally, a third boom of AI is now under way, and again great expectations exist around its magnitude and future development. The history is being written day after day. Eloquent examples are autonomous vehicles, computer programs that can beat Go and chess world champions, win the Jeopardy contest, do social manipulation and create intelligent weapons.

One of the main reasons for this third AI boom is the increasing availability of amazing amounts of computing power, previously unavailable, which has allowed to retake ancient AI techniques that had been relegated due to the impossibility of implementing operational computer programs to solve problems using them was literally impossible. One clear example is Artificial Neural Networks (ANN) [6], originally proposed by Warren McCulloch and Walter Pitts in 1943. Even if the idea was of astonishing originality, inspired by the way the human brain works, it was unfeasible to solve real problems with the computing power available at that time.

There are good and bad applications of modern AI techniques, not attributed to the tool itself, but to its practical use, which support both hope and fear about the future of AI, and whether it may evolve and represent a threat to humankind, such as depicted in several science fiction films, such as 2001: A Space Odyssey by Stanley Kubrick, Terminator by James Cameron, or the Matrix trilogy by Lana and Lilly Wachowski (as the Wachowski Brothers).

It is not sure that this kind of event could happen. Getting AI to reach the so-called singularity, the moment when it becomes autonomous from human beings and uncontrollable, is not something what we should worry about soon, and perhaps it will never happen. However, despite the bad use of AI, there is a light of hope, talking about applications that could lead to a better understanding of nature evolution, healthcare, and in this way, lead us to a higher standard of living.

This may be the case with the COVID-19 pandemic. We have largely seen how explosive was its evolution since it started, and how little we know about it, leading to literal thousands of deaths in only a few months. Despite the enormous efforts devoted by high-level scientists and physicians worldwide, there remain many unkowns about it both from the clinical and epidemiological point of view.

There is no consensus on how SARS-CoV-2 is transmitted, why there are asymptomatic patients, and others with mild, moderate, or even severe symptoms, and others with many complications leading to death. In some cases, symptoms and complications are fulminant, and in others they imply many days in ICU until the death of the patient. Moreover, for those who survive, particularly if they present moderate or severe symptoms, recovery may be slow, with sequels that can deeply affect their quality of life. The main sequel, although not the only one, seems to be lung fibrosis [7, 8].

Data collection in Mexico started since April 12th, 2020 [9], very early with respect to the beginning of the COVID-19 pandemic (February 26th was the first date with three confirmed cases in the country), and a new incremental database is generated daily with additional information. In these databases, each example corresponds to a single case of a person suspected of being infected by SARS-CoV-2, and more than 35 attributes[2] are collected for each one of them, such as age, date of first symptoms, date of hospitalization, date of death, if ever, whether the patient presents comorbidities, etc. By March 6th, 2021, there were 5,608,962 single registered cases, producing a single CSV file of 867 Mb containing all data.

Many inferences can be drawn from these data. For example, that there is a positive correlation between the age of the patient and the risk of dying, that diabetic patients have a higher risk of dying, or that patients without specific comorbidities have greater chances of survival and recovery. These, however, are simple associations with many exceptions in practice: diabetic patients who recover completely after getting infected, older people with mild symptoms, or asymptomatic at all, and young and healthy people who die.

[2]The number of attributes registered in this database raised from 35 to 38 since October 7, 2020; the data analysis presented in this chapter corresponds to the first version of the database.

What is it happening in these cases? What do we ignore about each atypical case? Which variables are correlated with others, and which represent causal associations? AI, through DS, offers tools that provide some clues to answer these and other questions. Efforts in other fields of AI are also under development; for example, the use of AI image classification methods to try to detect as early as possible pneumonia cases that could get worse in the following hours and that require quick medical attention [10]. Another possibility is trying to find in DNA whether there exist some traits that characterize patients who recover, and patients whose situation gets aggravated.

Sine-qua-non conditio using AI techniques to improve our knowledge of COVID-19 is quality data. If we have quality data as input, the use of these techniques may plausibly allow us to get interesting results. However, if the data do not have a minimal level of quality, or if there are too many missing values, or even if some specific data are not available at all, we could get not very trustworthy results.

Therefore, as we have more data, we can potentially carry out more accurate analyses. Unfortunately, specific data are not always available when we need them, and as a consequence, our analyses may have limitations.

3 GENERAL FRAMEWORK OF DATA SCIENCE PROJECTS

We live in a continuously connected world. Digital Social Media, services request, purchases, activity tracking, reading, etc., and most of our daily activities generate data, and aggregated data from everybody poses both technical and analytical challenges. This is the origin of DS, a set of tools developed and designed to extract the knowledge and value of all available data on a particular subject or event. Due to the recent COVID-19 outbreak, several open-source data sets are available for most countries, and Mexico is no exception. It is possible to combine these datasets with others containing socio-economic information that make them suitable for use in mathematical models and AI. Before merging different datasets that serve this purpose, it is necessary to prepare and possibly clean them. In this section of the chapter, we describe the general process of a traditional DS workflow.

DS is a recently coined name for the application of combined knowledge and skills from different disciplines to study problems based on data and its analysis. DS uses techniques from Computer Science, Statistical Analysis, mathematics, physics, engineering, and specific domain knowledge, to leverage the use of data as a powerful tool to tackle, understand, and solve problems, but particularly to take advantage of the knowledge generated from the analysis of the available data of the phenomenon under study.

In this text we look at some aspects of the COVID-19 pandemic from the DS perspective. This type of analysis is of the highest importance before attempting to construct mathematical models that account for more realistic results. Models do not only help to understand disease-related issues such as infection spread or containment, patient recovery, etc., but also enhance our understanding of infectious disease dynamics. Therefore, we must be sure that we understand the data, its contents, how it is collected, etc., to assure that any model built using it will be accurate and possibly generalizable.

Every DS project/workflow begins with questions about the process or the problem we are interested in. The origin of this question can come from the available data or likewise the data can be acquired/generated to answer a specific question. In the case of the COVID-19 pandemic, there are many questions; we know it is caused by a previously unknown virus, a member of a family of widely known viruses, and we know that it is highly contagious. Unfortunately, there is more about the virus that we do not know. What we want to do is to use the tools developed for DS workflow to understand the data that has been generated based on information gathered related to the epidemic in Mexico.

In general, data comes from a variety of sources and in a variety of forms: numbers, text, images, audio, video, and any kind of signal we can digitally acquire, collect, keep, and process using DS techniques. Unfortunately, we cannot use many of the most "powerful" techniques and results, like AI, right away when we are conceiving a DS project. Once we have access to the right data, it must be prepared for its use. Data seldom comes ready to use in models and for prediction.

3.1 The Data Science Workflow

Although a typical implementation of a DS workflow is, like any scientific endeavor, an iterative task, it is possible to encapsulate it as a process with at least the following steps:

1. Definition of the problem.
2. Acquisition of a labelled dataset.
3. Exploration of the data and model definition.
4. Building of an initial version of the model.
5. Testing of the model and iteration to improve it.
6. Repetition of steps 3-5 until appropriate performance is achieved.
7. Deployment and user monitoring and interaction.

When we systematically apply steps 3 through 6, we are effectively doing what in the media and literature is referred to as DS: a systematic problem solution strategy based on a scientific approach to the study of the available data and its analysis.

In the remaining of this section, we describe in more detail step 3 of the above list, which is fundamental to make sure that the data has the required quality. But first a couple of words on steps 1 and 2 about the problem we are tackling. As previously stated, we will present the general DS workflow using as example the case of COVID-19 in Mexico between March and October 2020. For that, we use the publicly available data from the Mexican *Dirección General de Epidemiología*, which is published every day [11].

The data contains information of the registered cases of patients presenting COVID-19 symptoms in Mexico and is presented as a structured table. Each row contains the information of a case registered in the dataset, i.e., a patient registered as being possibly affected by COVID-19. The information associated to each case is displayed in columns, called attributes. These attributes are, in general, self-explanatory as given by the column names. In summary, for the database of October 1st, 2020, which is the one that we took for our experiments, the data contains 1,721,871 rows and 35 columns which amount to 60,265,485 entries of many different formats. Precise description of the data as provided by the DGE is found in the associated data dictionary, also available as open data [12].

3.2 Exploratory Data Analysis and Preprocessing

Pre-processing entails performing certain explorations and eventually some transformations to detect missing or erroneous data, since wrong values that could have been corrupted during data generation or capture can potentially cause problems in the results and their interpretation.

There are many reasons why we must devote all the necessary time to explore the available data. It is always possible that in such relatively big data sets, such as the one we are exploring, errors occur which are very hard to detect without deep exploration. For example, imagine a record corresponding to an instance of a male subject that has the "pregnant" field marked as Yes. This is clearly a mistake that could happen, so it is a good practice to check for this implausible kind of error to appear in a dataset prior to its further use and analysis.

Fortunately, the data from DGE has been carefully revised when produced, so that the results arising from the analysis are supported by sound data, and errors are infrequent. In most cases, having the right data is more important than anything else.

The type of exploration that is performed to check the existence of these and similar errors, without trying to determine the source that originated them, which can be an impossible task, is part of the data pre-processing. There are many ways to explore the available data, and a whole line of research is being developed to provide better ways to present information in such a way that it provides useful insights to the Data Scientist. When a dataset is arranged in big-sized structured tables, it cannot be analyzed by simple visual inspection of the raw data and often requires intensive computer processing to get some understandable representation. Some of these analyses consist only of general explorations of how values are distributed. Next, we present three cases of this kind of visual analysis.

In Fig. 2, we observe the age distribution of records in the data grouped by sex (female/male), which allow us to have an idea of how are distributed by sex, the ages of the people who have been suspicious of having been infected by COVID-19.

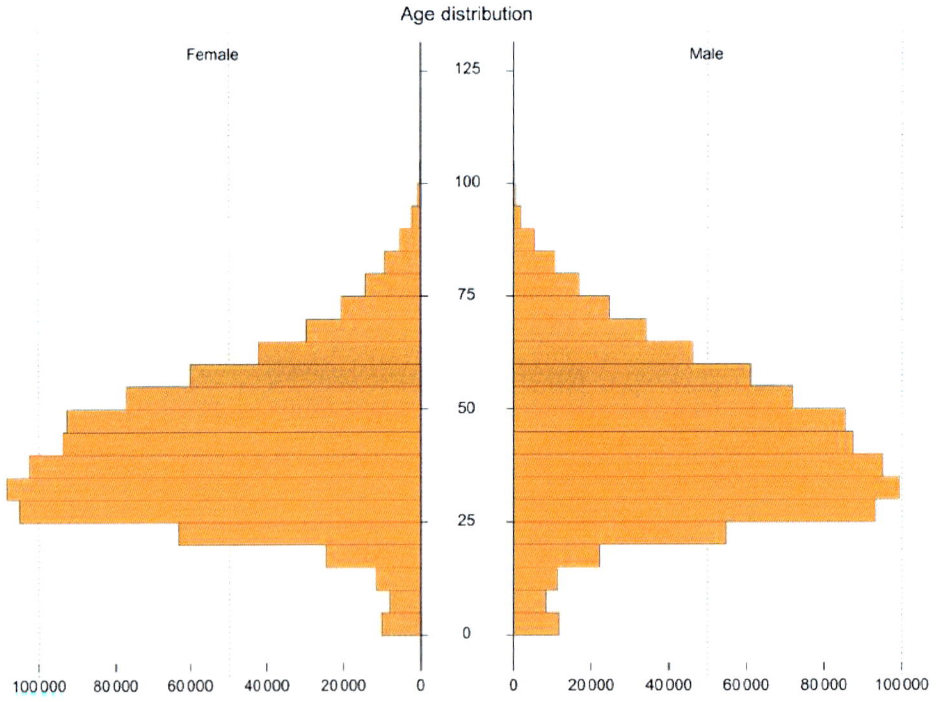

Figure 2: Age distribution grouped by sex from epidemiological data for Mexico up to October 1st, 2020

In Fig. 3, we can observe the distribution of the pandemic among Mexico States, which gives us an idea of how COVID-19 is affecting the population in different areas. This geographic distribution is essential to establish priorities and to design more in-depth analysis.

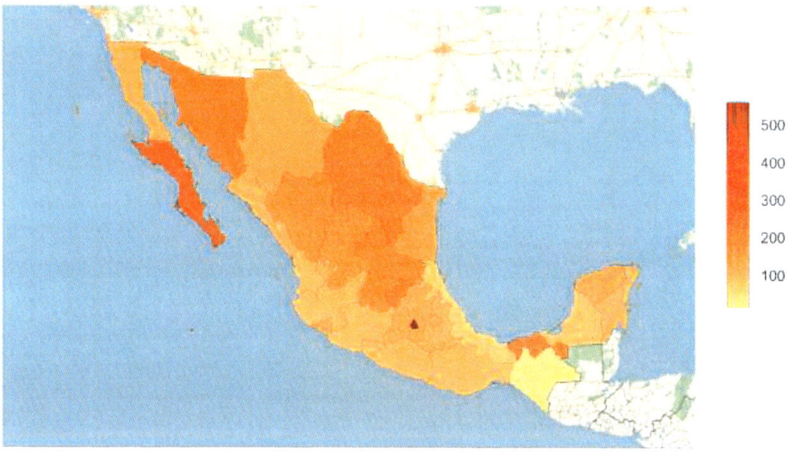

Figure 3: COVID-19 confirmed cases per 10,000 inhabitants in Mexico by entity as of October 21st, 2020; dark tones (red/orange) indicate a higher number of cases, while lighter (yellow) tones lower number

The next step is to transform and change the data to prepare it towards the model of interest. Care must be taken to avoid errors that can result from simple arithmetic operations, like dividing by zero. The use of statistics to inspect distributions among the values in the structured data and determine if any variable is skewed or normally centered around a mean value as well as exploring other properties of the data as a collection is the next step, allowing a more detailed or tailored exploration of the data.

Before modeling, an extra step is usually taken, which depends on the purpose of the study and consists of data transformation. This is the last step prior to feeding data to the model, usually known as feature engineering. This aspect is what will be explained in the next section.

4 CASE STUDY: THE MEXICAN COVID-19 DATA

In this section we present the analysis we performed on the previously mentioned data, provided by the Mexican government. All results correspond to the database of October 1st 2020, but the analysis can be applied to any other date.

4.1 The Database

Mexican COVID-19 database consists of a CSV file produced and published every single day since April 12th, 2020, which collects epidemiological data for each patient suspected to have been infected by SARS-CoV-2. The attributes collected and reported in this database are shown in Table 1 [3].

By simple scrutiny, several fields are clearly useless and can be discarded, such as "FECHA_ACTUALIZACION" which is fixed and previously established for each published database, and "PAIS_NACIONALIDAD" since most of the records correspond to Mexican citizens.

In addition to eliminating useless attributes, we changed the representation of some of them to make them easier to manipulate and understand, and added new attributes, some of them derived from those already in the data base, which could plausibly help us to get better classification results.

We decided to eliminate the attributes FECHA_ACTUALIZACION, ID_REGISTRO, ORIGEN, SECTOR, ENTIDAD_NAC, FECHA_INGRESO, FECHA_SINTOMAS, FECHA_DEF, NACIONALIDAD, HABLA_LENGUA_INDIG, MIGRANTE, PAIS_NACIONALIDAD and PAIS_ORIGEN since we consider they do not provide useful information for our classification. FECHA_ACTUALIZACION, as previously said, is eliminated because it contains the date of creation of the CSV file, which is the same value for all records, and only provides the date of the current dataset; ID_REGISTRO is an identifier that associates each case of the anonymized database with a case; ORIGEN and SECTOR, as well as all the data related to the nationality,

[3] Attributes names have been kept in Spanish to ease their identification in case the reader could be interested in downloading and processing the Mexican database.

Attribute Name	Attribute Meaning
FECHA_ACTUALIZACION	Data base update date
ID_REGISTRO	Anonymized patiens's register id
ORIGEN	The case comes from a respiratory diseases facility
SECTOR	Medical facility where the case was registered
ENTIDAD_UM	State where the medical facility is
SEXO	Patient sex
ENTIDAD_NAC	Patient's state of birth
ENTIDAD_RES	Patient's state of residence
MUNICIPIO_RES	Patient's municipality of residence
TIPO_PACIENTE	Patient type ([Am]bulatory or [Hos]pitalized)
FECHA_INGRESO	Date of admission in the medical facility
FECHA_SINTOMAS	Date when first symtomps appeared
FECHA_DEF	Date of decease (if ever)
INTUBADO	Need to intubate
NEUMONIA	The patient has pneumonia
EDAD	Patient's age
NACIONALIDAD	Patient's nationality
EMBARAZO	The patient was pregnant
HABLA_LENGUA_INDIG	Whether the patient speaks a native language
DIABETES	The patient is diabetic
EPOC	The patient has COPD
ASMA	The patient was asthmatic
INMUSUPR	The patient has immunosuppression
HIPERTENSION	The patient is hypertensive
OTRA_COM	The patient has another comorbidity
CARDIOVASCULAR	The patient has a cardiovascular disease
OBESIDAD	The patient has obesity
RENAL_CRONICA	The patient has a chronic renal disease
TABAQUISMO	The patient smokes
OTRO_CASO	Contact with another COVID-19 case
RESULTADO	Results of the SARS-CoV-2 test (+/-/pending)
MIGRANTE	The patient is migrant
PAIS_NACIONALIDAD	Patient nationality
PAIS_ORIGEN	Country of origin of the patient
UCI	Whether the patient was in ICU

Table 1: Attributes provided by the Mexican government

origin, citizenship, and whether the recorded case speaks a native language, do not offer any relevant information to our study and finally, the attributes containing the string FECHA_* were used to derive other attributes from the data, that for the purpose of our analysis, are better suited than in the way they are present in the original dataset.

Once eliminated the previously named attributes, we added the derived attributes RANGO_EDAD_10, RANGO_EDAD_20, and RANGO_EDAD_25, separating the age cases in groups of 10, 20, and 25 respectively, to ease some analysis towards the models we propose to apply. The variable DIAS_SINTOMAS_HOSPITAL was calculated as the difference between the date when a given patient was admitted into the hospital to be treated due to COVID-19-related causes, and the date symptoms started. We also defined and added the variable FALLECIDO, which indicates whether the patient died or not; this is calculated from the decease date in the original database, which contains a valid date if the patient died, and an invalid date (9999-99-99) otherwise. In fact, this last attribute was the one used as the predicting class attribute for the models presented in this text.

The attribute RESULTADO, which stores the result of the COVID-19 test as positive/negative/pending is also used. For consistency, we decided to eliminate all patients with the value "pending" on this variable and work only with confirmed cases either positive or negative. In this way, we can explore the effect on the model of appearing as a positive diagnosis with a probability of decease according to the data. A limitation of this database is that it does not specify which test was used to determine positive cases of SARS-CoV-2. Values for most of the fields are "Si" or "No".

Finally, we incorporated new attributes using an additional database obtained from the *Sistema Nacional de Información Municipal* (SNIM) [13], which contains relevant demographic data that complements our analysis. This information is integrated associating it with the ENTIDAD_RES and MUNICIPIO_RES attributes of each entry. This dataset dates back to the year 2015, since the last available information corresponding to the 2020 National Census was not yet published on the day of this analysis. As a result of all this processing a new database was obtained with attributes

Attribute Name	Attribute Meaning
ENTIDAD_UM	State where the medical facility is
SEXO	Patient's sex
ENTIDAD_RES	Patient's State of residence
MUNICIPIO_RES	Patient's Municipality of residence
TIPO_PACIENTE	Patient type ([Am]bulatory or [Hos]pitalized)
INTUBADO	Need to intubate
NEUMONIA	The patient has pneumonia
EDAD	Patient's age
RANGO_EDAD_10	Group by age of the patients in tens
RANGO_EDAD_20	Group by age of the patients in twenties
RANGO_EDAD_25	Group by age of the patients in twenty five
EMBARAZO	The patient was pregnant
DIABETES	The patient is diabetic
EPOC	The patient has COPD
ASMA	The patient is asthmatic
INMUSUPR	The patient has immunossupression disease
HIPERTENSION	The patient is hypertensive
OTRA_COM	The patient has another comorbidity
CARDIOVASCULAR	The patient has a cardiovascular disease
OBESIDAD	The patient has obesity
RENAL_CRONICA	The patient has chronic renal disease
TABAQUISMO	The patient smokes
OTRO_CASO	Contact with another COVID-19 case
RESULTADO	Results of the SARS-Cov-2 test (+/-/pending)
UCI	Whether the patient was in UCI
DIAS_SINTOMAS_HOSPITAL	Days passed since symptoms to admission
POBLACION_HOMBRES	Municipality's male population
POBLACION_MUJERES	Municipality's female population
POBLACION_TOTAL	Municipality's total population
INDICE_DESARROLLO_HUMANO	Municipality's human development index
GRADO_DESARROLLO_HUMANO	Municipality's human development degree
INDICE_SALUD	Municipality's health index
INDICE_EDUCACION	Municipality's education index
INDICE_INGRESO	Municipality's income index
INDICE_MARGINACION	Municipality's margination index
GRADO_MARGINACION	Municipality's margination degree
FALLECIDO	Whether the patient died or survived

Table 2: Attributes on which the data analysis process has been applied

shown in Table 2, where the newly added attributes are indicated using italic-bold font. All further analyses were performed on this dataset.

Two important remarks concerning this dataset are:

i) All municipality information is linked to the municipality of residence associated with each patient, so that patients can eventually be grouped by this criterion, and

ii) The FALLECIDO attribute values are "Si", for the case where patient died because of SARS-CoV-2, and "No" otherwise.

In fact, as mentioned earlier, FALLECIDO is the response or outcome variable and the one we use to train the model and to identify the most relevant variables in terms of predictive capacity. For this, two DS tools are useful: Bayesian Networks (BN) and Decision Trees (DT). Before presenting the models and the results obtained from them in the next sections, we comment on the performance of these classifiers, which have been evaluated according to the following criteria:

a) *Accuracy*: number of correct classifications divided by the size of the test set.

b) *Sensitivity*: proportion of real positive cases correctly classified as positive.

c) *Specificity*: proportion of real negative cases correctly classified as negative.

4.2 Bayesian Networks

A Bayesian Network (BN) is a graphical model that encodes probabilistic relationships among variables of interest in a specific problem [14]. It allows us, on the one hand, to visually represent those relationships and, on the other hand, to quantify their strength by means of local probability distributions. This concept is illustrated in Fig. 4.

Together, these two components permit us to recover a joint probability distribution from the local ones as shown in Eq. (5.1) this is the core of such a model. The central idea is then that of

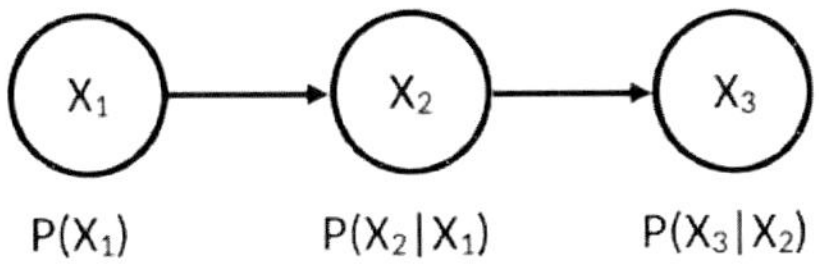

Figure 4: An example of a Bayesian Network

independence: "any node is conditionally independent of its nondescendants, given its parents", the so-called Markov condition [15]. Thus, X_3 is conditionally independent of X_1 given X_2

$$P(X_1, X_2, \ldots, X_n) = \Pi_{i=1}^{n} P(X_i | P_a(X_i)), \tag{5.1}$$

where $P(X_i)$ represents the parents of X_i. Here X_2's parent is X_1 and X_3's parent is X_2. Hence, the joint probability of X_1, X_2, and X_3 can be recovered from the product of their local distributions:

$$P(X_1, X_2, X_3) = P(X_1) \bullet P(X_2) \bullet P(X_3).$$

A BN can be constructed either manually, from prior knowledge, or automatically, from a dataset. We follow the latter since we want to take advantage of the previously COVID-19 dataset. Thus, in the context of our case study, we automatically build BNs because of two reasons:

1. To discover, from our data, the main relationships among the variables potentially related to COVID-19.
2. To assess the predictive power of such a model.

4.2.1 Learning Bayesian Networks Structures from Data

Various algorithms that automatically construct BNs from data have been proposed [15–19]. There are basically two approaches for doing this:

a. constraint-based methods and,

b. search and scoring procedures.

Constraint-based methods try to discover the dependence/independence relationships hidden in the data while search and scoring procedures look for a structure that maximizes/minimizes a specific metric. For the sake of brevity and clarity, we do not delve into the details here. Rather, we direct the reader to the corresponding references presented above. However, it is important to stress that both methods have parsimony as a main goal: models with a good balance between their goodness of fit and their complexity. We ran tests using two procedures: MOPSO-BN, which is a modification of the one proposed in [20], and Hill-Climbing, respectively [21]. Both were designed having parsimony in mind. Once the BN structures are built, they can be used to carry out different types of inferences. To that end, we used the Waikato Environment for Knowledge Analysis (Weka) [22] and the SamIam [23] software package. The results of these procedures are presented below.

4.2.2 Pre-Processing of Data

Before running the algorithm, we preprocessed the original dataset following the principles explained in the previous sections and decided to select 10% of those data and balance the class, i.e., to choose the same number of people who died and who survived. We did this using the "Resample" method included in Weka with default parameters, except for "biasToUniformClass", which we set to 1 to ensure a balanced class. Then, we carried out a feature selection procedure called "GainRatioAttributeEval" combined with a search method called "Ranker" with default parameters, both included in Weka as well. We selected the first seven attributes according to this metric.

4.2.3 Results

Fig. 5 shows the structures of the procedures MOPSO-BN and Hill-Climbing, respectively. Table 3 shows the predictive accuracy for the class variable FALLECIDO (Si/No) given by the two procedures. It also presents the sensitivity, specificity, PV+, PV- and the Kappa statistic of such BNs.

4.2.4 Discussion

Procedure MOPSO-BN builds models with a good trade-off between classification accuracy and MDL[4]. In other words, it searches for models that are well balanced regarding these two metrics since they are in conflict. It is this trade-off that achieves a more parsimonious model (compared to that of the other algorithms) at the expense of a slight reduction in accuracy. Although the BN structure yielded by Hill-Climbing is more complex (i.e., it contains more arcs) even when MDL is used as an objective too, it is more accurate than MOPSO-BN and the difference is statistically significant. However, the ultimate validation of such structures is that of the medical expert, who must decide, in the end, which one is more useful for a clearer understanding of the phenomenon under study. The number of possible BN structures is superexponential in the number of variables n, as Eq. (5.2) indicates:

$$f(n) = \sum_{i=1}^{n}(-1)^{i+1}\begin{pmatrix} n \\ i \end{pmatrix} 2^{i(n-i)} f(n-i), \tag{5.2}$$

If $n = 8$ (as in our case), the number of possible structures is 7.8×10^{11}; this is clearly a huge number and it is practically impossible to exhaustively test both quantitively and qualitatively, every one of them. Therefore, we need to resort to heuristic methods such as those used in our experiments. Prior knowledge can be inserted into the algorithm in the form of probability functions to guide the search. We do not do this here though. Our main goal is to present some examples of the potential these methods have to numerically determine the class to which a case belongs to as described above using the available information.

[4]Minimum Description Length is a metric which basically balances the goodness of fit and the complexity of a model; in other words, a model with a good MDL value (the lower the better) represents, in a compact way, the original data.

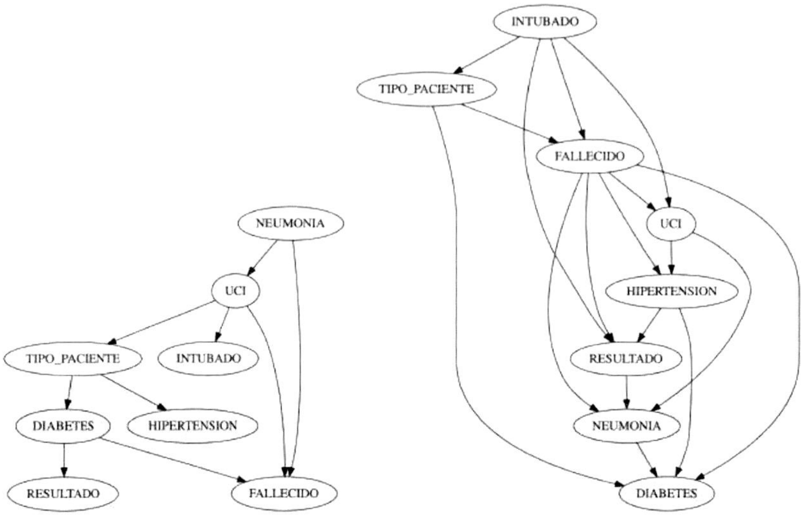

(a) (b)

Figure 5: (A) MOPSO_BN procedure, (B) Hill-Climbing procedure

Tests	Algorithms	
	MOPSO	**Hill Climbing**
Accuracy	90.52% (0.21)	90.76% (0.21) *
Sensitivity	95% (95-95)	95% (94-95)
Specificity	86% (86-86)	87% (87-87)
PV+	87% (87-88)	88% (88-88)
PV-	94% (94-95)	94% (94-94)
Kappa statistic	81% (81-81)	82% (81-82)

Table 3: Accuracy, sensitivity, specificity, PV+, PV- and Kappa statistics are given for the 2 procedures. For accuracy, the standard deviation is shown in parentheses. For the rest of the tests, 95% confidence intervals are shown in parentheses. An "∗" next to the accuracy of the procedure means that the result is statistically better (using a paired t-test with significance level = 0.05)

The BN of Fig. 5(A) identifies only 3 variables out of 7, as relevant in association with the patient's outcome and his/her death (DIABETES, UCI and NEUMONIA), while the BN of Fig. 5(B) identifies all variables as relevant. The structure of a BN is also useful for showing the relationships among attributes, which allows us to give possible explanations of the phenomenon under investigation.

With these models, and based on the available data, we can answer questions like these:

- What is the probability of dying if the patient was intubated?
- What is the probability of dying if the patient was diabetic and has hypertension?
- How much does pneumonia increase the probability of dying given that a patient tests positive for SARS-CoV-2?
- What are the most probable values for TIPO_PACIENTE, and DIABETES given that the patient has died?
- Are the result of the test and being dead conditionally independent given the presence of diabetes?

Notice that some of these queries may be ill-posed and only arise because of the probabilistic relations found by the models from the data that were available. The results do not imply that a patient will have a probability of dying by COVID-19 or not, only that given the available information, the models separate cases based on frequent conditions.

This kind of query can promptly be answered with such a model. To that end, we use the SamIam software (for the sake of brevity, we do not go into details here about how to use it). To answer the first 4 queries, which are of probabilistic nature, we need both the qualitative (structure) and the quantitative (local probability distribution) parts. The answers for those queries are, respectively, 0.88, 0.85, 0.38 (from 0.51 to 0.89) and TIPO_PACIENTE = "No" and DIABETES = "No" for the BN of Fig. 5(A). In the case of the BN of Fig. 5(B), the corresponding values are 0.98, 0.82, 0.28 (from 0.64 to 0.92) and TIPO_PACIENTE = "Am" and DIABETES = "No".

Now, to answer the last query, we only need the structure of the BNs. For the one of Fig. 5(A), the answer is "Si" (i.e., the result of the test and dying are conditionally independent given that the patient is diabetic) and for the BN of Fig. 5(B), the answer is "No" (the result of the test and dying are not conditionally independent given that the patient is diabetic). This is a qualitative inference and can be effectively carried out using a criterion called d-separation of the Markov condition mentioned above. All these queries are just some examples of what we can do with BN. For our problem, it is important to recall that, in these experiments, we selected only a subset of the attributes. If needed, we can include more variables and run similar queries. Since a BN represents a joint probability distribution, we can practically answer any query, as shown above. In fact, we ran tests including 22 variables and the results of accuracy and related measures are not so different to those presented here (91.52% for the 22-variable case). However, the structure is much more complex than that of Fig. 5 (for space reasons, we do not present it here). That is why we decided to carry out a feature selection procedure. The modeler can give different alternatives to the domain experts so that a thorough analysis of the problem can be performed.

Regarding the accuracy and related metrics, as we can see from Table 3, the performances of the two procedures are quite similar except for the accuracy, which is statistically better for Hill-Climbers than MOPSO-BN. Something important to note is that, for both models, we get better results for sensitivity than specificity. In other words, our models make fewer mistakes predicting cases where FALLECIDO has a value of "Si" than otherwise. The model including 22 attributes has the following values for sensitivity and specificity, respectively: 95% (94-95) and 88% (88-89). We can argue that, even when we consider more variables, the specificity result is nearly the same. This may be a certain indication that we could need to measure other variables so that we can improve specificity. The numbers suggest that the value of this test is the best we can get with this set of variables.

With all these results, those models can be considered powerful tools not only for classification accuracy but also for unveiling the phenomenon under investigation.

4.3 Decision Trees

Decision Trees (DT) are a widely used supervised learning technique for the classification of data. They combine interpretability and efficiency and offer excellent accuracy [24].

DTs represent decisions that serve to classify the data. A DT obtains rules that enable the classification of data and are formed by a group of nodes, leaves, and branches. The classification process begins with the so-called root node, with the lower-level nodes corresponding to each of the questions that relate to each one of the attributes of the problem. A child node corresponds to a possible response to the question. The branches that emerge from each node are labeled with the possible values of the attribute. The final nodes, or leaf nodes, correspond to a final determination, which coincides with one of the class variables of the problem to be solved.

The algorithm that generates DTs comprises two stages: the induction of the tree and the classification of data. In the first stage, the DT is constructed from the training set. In the second stage, each new case is classified using the created DT.

Some of the most widely used classification algorithms are ID3 and C4.5. ID3 uses the best attribute by means of the heuristic known as Information Gain. The most informative attribute is that with the least entropy or the maximum information gain [25]. The entropy is a measure of average uncertainty. It is calculated from the probability of occurrence of each event. If the target attribute takes different values for c, then S is the entropy for each value of c is defined as:

$$Entropy(S) = -\sum_{i=1}^{c} p_i \log_2 p_i,$$

where p_i is the probability of class i, divided by the probability that S belongs to class i. The information gain is the complement of entropy. A higher entropy means less information. Given a set of samples S with respect to an attribute A, the information gain is defined as:

$$Informationgain(S, A) = Entropy(S) - \sum_{v \in Values(A)} \frac{S_v}{S} Entropy(S_v),$$

where $Values(A)$ is the set of all possible values of the attribute A and S_v is a subset of S where the attribute A has a value v.

This study used the C4.5 algorithm [26], which allows the management of both the continuous and missing values and is computationally efficient with simple and easily interpretable decision rules.

4.3.1 Implementation Details

We used the J48 algorithm, an implementation of the C4.5 algorithm using a 10-fold cross-validation in Weka. In the data set that we used for our analysis, we selected FALLECIDO as the class attribute. There, the number of samples from the majority class value ("No") exceeded the number of samples from the minority class value ("Si"), thus presenting an imbalance of classes that can produce a significant deterioration in the effectiveness of the classifier, particularly with the patterns of the less represented classes [27]. To treat this problem, we used the random subsampling technique "SpreadSubSample" method included in Weka with default parameters except for "distributionSpread", which we set to 1 to guarantee that there would be the same number of examples of each class.

4.3.2 Results

This study also used the previously cited epidemiological database provided by the Mexican government. We aimed to generate models through DTs that allow us to determine the main factors associated with the risk of dying for patients treated with COVID-19 symptoms in the Mexican health system.

First, we generated a DT with all variables in the database. This analysis resulted in the correct classification of 178,580 out of 195,528, 91.33%, with a sensitivity of 94.76% and a specificity of 87.90%. TIPO_PACIENTE was the most informative variable. However, the size of the DT was 3,612 nodes, making it practically impossible to visualize its graphical representation.

Then we selected seven attributes (TIPO_PACIENTE, INTUBADO, NEUMONIA, DIABETES, HIPERTENSION, RESULTADO, UCI, having FALLECIDO as the class attribute) which were used for the generation of BNs. DT correctly classified 177,196 of 195,528 samples, 90.62%, with a sensitivity of 94.62%, and a specificity of 86.61%.

Some relevant points about DT models are mentioned below, which will be useful for their interpretation:

a) The attribute stemming from the root node is the most informative one.

b) A leaf-rectangle node is the class variable.

c) Each internal node is a variable that can be read as a question, and its possible answers the arcs, which have labels specifying the value or the range of values it can take.

In Fig. 6 we present the DT corresponding to the previous description.

As we can clearly see, TIPO_PACIENTE was identified to be the most informative attribute, and the decision made there is categorical: if the patient is hospitalized, then the probability for him/her to die is high.

On the other hand, if the patient is ambulatory, then a chain of successive tests starts, each one of them considering further attributes, specializing the classification. In this way we can see that at the next level NEUMONIA is tested, having again two possible paths: if the patient did not have pneumonia, then the chances for getting recovered are high. Otherwise, at the next level, the decision depends on the results of the SARS-CoV-2 test. If this is positive, then the probability of dying of the patient is high.

In the tests corresponding to the next two levels of the DT, we can see that being diabetic or hypertensive are the two next successive factors to consider in the computation; if any of these is present, the probability of dying of the patient is high.

In our next experiment, we were interested in working with some other variables generally considered as determining factors of severity, progression, and death due to COVID-19: EDAD, SEXO, DIABETES, HIPERTENSION, OBESIDAD, and TABAQUISMO [28]. To simplify the classification process concerning age, we decided to use the categorized version of this attribute, so we stratified age in groups of 20 years. Here we obtained 152,828 out of 195,528, for 78.16% of the samples correctly classified, a sensitivity of 78.97% and a specificity of 77.35%. The DT for this experiment is presented in Fig. 7, where the class attribute is FALLECIDO.

The main fact that is to be remarked here is that for patients aged 60 and older, their probability of dying is higher, so that for these cases no more conditions are verified. On the other hand, for patients younger than 60, the next attribute to be evaluated is, systematically, DIABETES. For the first two groups of age, if the patient is not diabetic, there is a lower probably of dying, while in the other case, the attribute to be evaluated at the next level is HIPERTENSION. For the first group of ages, the fact of being hypertensive is the determinant factor for the DT in the classification process, while for the second group of ages, sex is the determining factor. One thing that calls our attention, as in the previous examples, is that again people who smoke have a lower risk of dying than non-smokers. For non-hypertensive patients, obesity is the factor that determines the probability of dying. Finally, for the third group of age, being diabetic offers more information than the sex of the patient and the facts of being hypertensive or obese conditions that are tested inversely in the next level of the tree for men and women.

4.3.3 Discussion

One advantage of DTs is that, as they are graphical representations, they are transparent and understandable by medical experts, so that they can validate their usefulness, allowing a better understanding of the phenomenon under study.

The first DT we created obtained the best precision (91.33%), sensitivity (94.76%), and specificity (87.89%), but the model had 3,612 nodes. For this reason, we did not present it here. Patient type was the most informative variable.

The DT considering only seven attributes, as the one of our second example, showed that TIPO_PACIENTE is the most informative attribute, followed by NEUMONIA and RESULTADO.

As for BNs, our DTs yield better results for sensitivity than specificity; that is, they make less

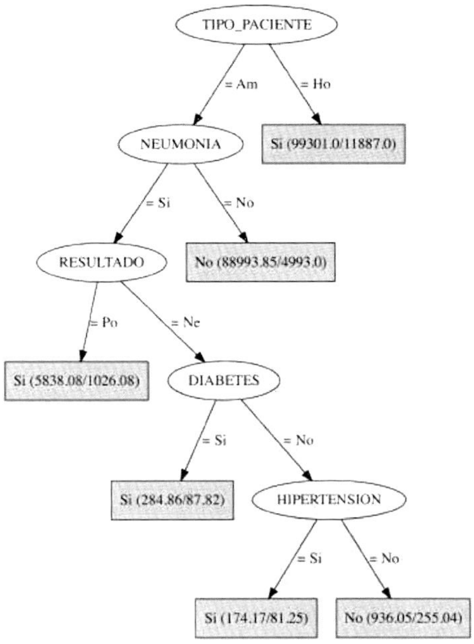

Figure 6: Decision tree for the class variable

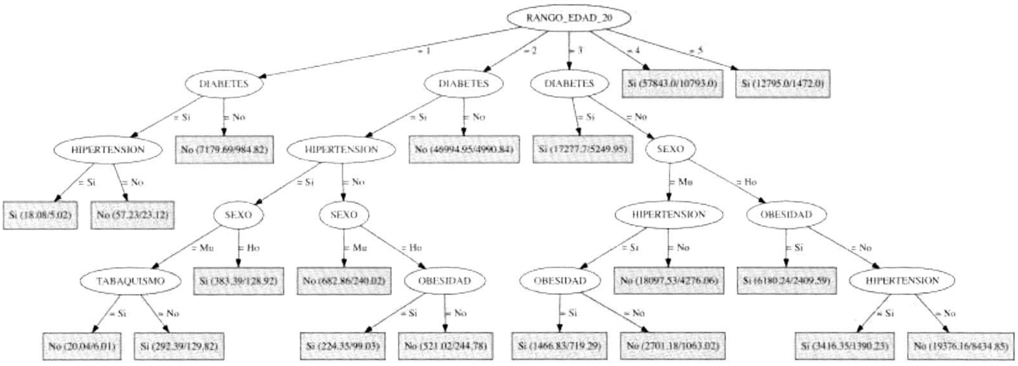

Figure 7: Decision tree for the class variable by 20-year age groups

mistakes for the prediction of the patients who die than for the ones who survive.

In this study, we found that age is the main risk factor for death of COVID-19, which is consistent with the results found in other studies in other countries [28–30]. Results obtained suggest that age, diabetes, hypertension, sex, and obesity are the most important risk factors of death in COVID-19 patients. Interestingly, smoking was not found to be a determinant risk factor for presenting aggravated forms of the disease. In fact, a lower prevalence of active smoking was reported in patients with COVID-19 in Mexico [31]. In another study, active smoking has been linked to a decreased probability of a positive SARS-CoV-2 test result [32]. In a meta-analysis of COVID-19 patients from China, it was suggested that active smoking is not significantly associated with an increased risk of COVID-19 severity [33].

5 CONCLUDING REMARKS

COVID-19 is a health problem of high complexity in several dimensions that are severely touching our lives. One of them is understanding how it propagates, which are its real effects on the human body, which are the factors that increase the risk of death or of other events related to disease progression, and having this as the basic information, how we can prevent its occurrence and/or alleviate its effects.

DS is a good alternative for this, since it allows us to identify correlated variables and to assess and estimate the size of those in either the epidemiological or clinical fields. As in all research enterprise, the quality of the collected data is a key prerequisite.

In the same vein, choosing a set of attributes for systematic collection is of the highest importance, albeit no easy task.

We worked with the original dataset structure, which was modified. We pretend to analyze the new data as soon as enough data will be available.

Results have been presented from an epidemiological point of view, which is the approach adopted by the Mexican government. Eventually, some clinical information could be added to these analyses.

The data collection process should be carefully designed and implemented, and the personnel in charge of doing this must be thoroughly trained to guarantee the quality of data and to minimize the presence of error.

6 CONSENT FOR PUBLICATION

Not applicable.

7 CONFLICT OF INTEREST

The authors declare no conflict of interest, financial or otherwise.

8 ACKNOWLEDGEMENTS

The authors of this text wish to thank the help of José-Clemente Hernández-Hernández, a student of the MSc in Artificial Intelligence, and Emmanuel-Isaac Juárez-Caballero, student at the School of Physics, both in the Universidad Veracruzana, for the technical help that they provided to the development of this work.

References

[1] Bacon F. Meditationes Sacrae. Londini.: Excusum impensis Humfredi Hooper, 1597.

[2] The Merrian-Webster Dictionary. Merrian-Webster Incorporated, [online document], 2021. [cited March 7, 2021] Available from: https://www.merriam-webster.com/

[3] Wiersinga WJ, Rhodes A, Cheng AC, Peacock SJ, Prescott HC. Pathophysiology, Transmission, Diagnosis, and Treatment of Coronavirus Disease 2019 (COVID-19). JAMA [Internet]. 2020 Aug 25 [cited 2021 Oct 2];324(8):782–793. Available from: https://doi.org/10.1001/jama.2020.12839

[4] Struyf T, Deeks JJ, Dinnes J, Takwoingi Y, Davenport C, Leeflang MM, Spijker R, Hooft L, Emperador D, Dittrich S, Domen J, Horn SR, Van den Bruel A. Signs and symptoms to determine if a patient presenting in primary care or hospital outpatient settings has COVID-19 disease. Cochrane Database of Systematic Reviews [Internet]. 2020 Jul 7 [cited 2021 Oct 2]. Available from: https://doi.org/10.1002/14651858.cd013665

[5] Newell A, Shaw JC, Simon HA, Report on a general problem-solving program. In: Proc. International Conference on Information Processing, 1959, pp. 256–264.

[6] McCulloch WS, Pitts W. A logical calculus of the ideas immanent in nervous activity. The

Bulletin of Mathematical Biophysics [Internet]. 1943 Dec [cited 2021 Oct 2];5(4):115–33. Available from: https://doi.org/10.1007/bf02478259

[7] Tale S, Ghosh S, Meitei SP, Kolli M, Garbhapu AK, Pudi S. Post-COVID-19 pneumonia pulmonary fibrosis. QJM: An International Journal of Medicine [Internet]. 2020 Aug 19 [cited 2021 Oct 2];113(11):837–8. Available from: https://doi.org/10.1093/qjmed/hcaa255

[8] Wang F, Kream RM, Stefano GB. Long-Term Respiratory and Neurological Sequelae of COVID-19. Medical Science Monitor [Internet]. 2020 Nov 1 [cited 2021 Oct 2];26. Available from: https://doi.org/10.12659/msm.928996

[9] Datos Abiertos Bases Históricas | Secretaría de Salud | Gobierno | gob.mx [online document], 2021. [cited March 7, 2021] Available from: https://www.gob.mx/salud/documentos/datos-abiertos-bases-historicas-direccion-general-de-epidemiologia/

[10] Pereira RM, Bertolini D, Teixeira LO, Silla CN, Costa YM. COVID-19 identification in chest X-ray images on flat and hierarchical classification scenarios. Computer Methods and Programs in Biomedicine [Internet]. 2020 Oct [cited April 4, 2021];194:105532. Available from: https://doi.org/10.1016/j.cmpb.2020.105532

[11] Datos Abiertos | Secretaría de Salud | Gobierno | gob.mx [online document], 2021. [cited March 7, 2021] Available from: http://datosabiertos.salud.gob.mx/gobmx/salud/datos_abiertos/datos_abiertos_covid19.zip

[12] Datos Abiertos | Secretaría de Salud | Gobierno | gob.mx [online document], 2021. [cited March 7, 2021] Available from: http://datosabiertos.salud.gob.mx/gobmx/salud/datos_abiertos/diccionario_datos_covid19.zip

[13] SNIM: Sistema Nacional de Información Municipal [online document], 2021. [cited March 7, 2021] Available from `http://www.snim.rami.gob.mx/`

[14] Pearl J. Probabilistic Reasoning in Intelligent Systems: Networks of Plausible Inference. San Mateo, Calif: Morgan Kaufmann Publishers; 1988. 552 p.

[15] Cooper GF. An Overview of the Representation and Discovery of Causal Relationships Using Bayesian Networks. In: Computation, Causation, and Discovery [Internet]. [place unknown]: The MIT Press; 1999 [cited 2021 Oct 2]. Available from: `https://doi.org/10.7551/mitpress/2006.003.0002`

[16] Buntine W. A guide to the literature on learning probabilistic networks from data. IEEE Transactions on Knowledge and Data Engineering [Internet]. 1996 Apr [cited 2021 Oct 2];8(2):195–210. Available from: `https://doi.org/10.1109/69.494161`

[17] Cooper GF, Herskovits E. A Bayesian method for the induction of probabilistic networks from data. Machine Learning [Internet]. 1992 Oct [cited 2021 Oct 2];9(4):309–47. Available from: `https://doi.org/10.1007/bf00994110`

[18] Friedman N, Geiger D, et al. Bayesian Network Classifiers. Machine Learning. 1997. pp. 131–163.

[19] Spirtes P. Causation, prediction, and search. New York: Springer-Verlag; 1993. 526 p.

[20] Aguilera-Rueda VJ, Cruz-Ramírez N, Mezura-Montes E. Data-Driven Bayesian Network Learning: A Bi-Objective Approach to Address the Bias-Variance Decomposition. Mathematical and Computational Applications [Internet]. 2020 Jun 20 [cited 2021 Oct 2];25(2):37. Available from: `https://doi.org/10.3390/mca25020037`

[21] Witten IH, Frank E. Data Mining: Practical Machine Learning Tools and Techniques, Second Edition (Morgan Kaufmann Series in Data Management Systems). 2nd ed. Boston, Mass.: Morgan Kaufmann; 2005. 525 p.

[22] Hall M, Frank E, Holmes G, Pfahringer B, Reutemann P, Witten IH. The WEKA data mining software. ACM SIGKDD Explorations Newsletter [Internet]. 2009 Nov 16 [cited 2021 Oct 2];11(1):10–8. Available from: `https://doi.org/10.1145/1656274.1656278`

[23] Darwiche A. Modeling and reasoning with Bayesian networks. Cambridge: Cambridge University Press; 2009.

[24] Geurts P, Irrthum A, Wehenkel L. Supervised learning with decision tree-based methods in computational and systems biology. Molecular BioSystems [Internet]. 2009 [cited 2021 Oct 2];5(12):1593–1605. Available from: `https://doi.org/10.1039/b907946g`

[25] Quinlan JR. Induction of decision trees. Machine Learning [Internet]. 1986 Mar [cited 2021 Oct 2];1(1):81–106. Available from: `https://doi.org/10.1007/bf00116251`

[26] Quinlan JR. C4.5: programs for machine learning. [place unknown]: Elsevier; 2014.

[27] Sun Y, Wong AK, Kamel MS. Classification of imbalanced data: a review. International Journal of Pattern Recognition and Artificial Intelligence [Internet]. 2009 Jun [cited 2021 Oct 2];23(04):687–719. Available from: `https://doi.org/10.1142/s0218001409007326`

[28] Chen Y, Klein SL, Garibaldi BT, Li H, Wu C, Osevala NM, Li T, Margolick JB, Pawelec G, Leng SX. Aging in COVID-19: Vulnerability, immunity and intervention. Ageing Research Reviews [Internet]. 2021 Jan [cited 2021 Oct 2];65:101205. Available from: `https://doi.org/10.1016/j.arr.2020.101205`

[29] Liu Y, Mao B, Liang S, Yang JW, Lu HW, Chai YH, et al. Association between age and clinical characteristics and outcomes of COVID-19. European Respiratory Journal [Internet]. 2020 Apr 20 [cited 2021 Oct 2];55(5):2001112. Available from: `https://doi.org/10.1183/13993003.01112-2020`

[30] Berenguer J, Ryan P, Rodríguez-Baño J, Jarrín, Carratalà J, Pachón J, et al. Characteristics and predictors of death among 4035 consecutively hospitalized patients with COVID-19 in Spain. Clinical Microbiology and Infection [Internet]. 2020 Nov [cited 2021 Oct 2];26(11):1525–36. Available from: https://doi.org/10.1016/j.cmi.2020.07.024

[31] Hernández-Garduño E. Obesity is the comorbidity more strongly associated for Covid-19 in Mexico. A case-control study. Obesity Research & Clinical Practice [Internet]. 2020 Jul [cited 2021 Oct 2];14(4):375–9. Available from: https://doi.org/10.1016/j.orcp.2020.06.001

[32] de Lusignan S, Dorward J, Correa A, Jones N, Akinyemi O, Amirthalingam G, et al. Risk factors for SARS-CoV-2 among patients in the Oxford Royal College of General Practitioners Research and Surveillance Centre primary care network: a cross-sectional study. The Lancet Infectious Diseases [Internet]. 2020 Sep [cited 2021 Oct 2];20(9):1034–42. Available from: https://doi.org/10.1016/s1473-3099(20)30371-6

[33] Lippi G, Henry BM. Active smoking is not associated with severity of coronavirus disease 2019 (COVID-19). European Journal of Internal Medicine [Internet]. 2020 May [cited 2021 Oct 2];75:107–8. Available from: https://doi.org/10.1016/j.ejim.2020.03.014

CHAPTER 6

Epidemic Progression in a Heterogeneously Distributed Population

Malay Banerjee[1], **Samiran Ghosh**[1], **Vitaly Volpert**[*234]

[*] **Corresponding author:** volpert@math.univ-lyon1.fr, Phone: +33 472432765

[1] Indian Institute of Technology Kanpur, Kanpur - 208016, India

[2] Institut Camille Jordan, UMR 5208 CNRS, University Lyon 1, 69622 Villeurbanne, France

[3] INRIA Team Dracula, INRIA Lyon La Doua, 69603 Villeurbanne, France

[4] Peoples Friendship University of Russia (RUDN University), 6 Miklukho-Maklaya St, Moscow, 117198, Russia

Abstract. The chapter is devoted to a compartmental epidemiological model of infection progression in a space-distributed multipatch population with communication between the patches due to the movement of individuals. The subpopulations inside the patches consist of different groups with respect to the intensity of disease transmission both within and between groups. The heterogeneity of the population and its transfer between the patches influence the rate of epidemic progression, the final size of the epidemic, and the number of infected individuals.

Key words: COVID-19 epidemiology, heterogeneous population, multipatch model

1 INTRODUCTION

1.1 Importance

Heterogeneous populations with subpopulations differing in the rate of disease transmission are described with compartmental epidemiological models. Basic reproduction number (BRN), the final size of epidemic, and the maximal current number of infected individuals are determined. It is shown that BRN is not sufficient to determine the epidemic progression in a heterogeneous population. Multipatch models for spatially distributed populations are considered.

1.2 Epidemiological Situation

In the beginning of the second year of the COVID-19 pandemic, we can identify several consecutive stages of its progression. The initial stage with the exponential growth of the number of infected individuals was followed by the next stage characterized by the alternation of more or less strict measures of social distancing and their relaxation, and by the quarantine of the infected individuals. In the absence of vaccines and efficient antiviral drugs against SARS-CoV-2 infection, these were the only available measures to restrain the epidemic progression together with basic sanitary measures such as masks and personal hygiene.

It became clear in early 2020 that a relatively high proportion of severe cases and mortality rates distinguish the coronavirus disease from the annual influenza epidemic for which collective immunity is reached after several weeks after the epidemic peak followed by the epidemic decay. This scenario is impossible for the COVID-19 pandemic because the public health system and, particularly, intensive care units become rapidly saturated and incapable of dealing with the flow of COVID and other patients. Public authorities use measures of social distancing to balance between uncontrolled epidemic growth and economic losses due to reduced activity.

As a result of this strategy accepted throughout the world, according to the official statistics by March 2021, there were about 120 million of total cases of infection, and about 2.6 million of deaths, although these data can be strongly underestimated (at least for infected) due to the large number of asymptomatic and unregistered cases. The total number of cases largely varies between the countries: 5-10% in Europe and USA, and much less in China and some other Asian countries. According to recent estimates, the number of deaths in the USA is about 15% more in 2020 compared to the previous year, with this increase related to the COVID-19 pandemic. A similar death rate increase can be expected in a number of European countries, but, as for the number of infected individuals, it can be substantially less in some Asian countries. There can be many reasons for such large disparities, but it is unclear which of them are the most influential.

The third stage of the epidemic started in January 2021 with the beginning of the vaccination campaign. By the middle of March, the vaccination was barely beginning[1] and the essential decrease in the number of newly infected individuals can only be expected after several months. Since the number of vaccines remains insufficient, the vaccination strategy adopted in many countries consists in the priority vaccination of more vulnerable elderly people and more exposed groups of the population, such as medical workers.

One of the important questions which determines the further evolution of the epidemiological situation concerns the duration of the immunity of the recovered and vaccinated individuals. In the case of recovered individuals, the level of antibodies and their persistence strongly depend on the severity of the disease [1–3]. Secondary coronavirus infections can be related to weak immunity or virus mutations. Reliable statistics on the number of repeated infections is not available, but it remains probably quite limited. The duration of immunity after vaccination is now estimated by 6 months (validity of vaccination certificates), but it can be eventually longer with an inter-individual

[1] `https://www.nytimes.com/interactive/2021/world/covid-vaccinations-tracker.html`

variability.

A limited duration of individual immunity after the disease or vaccination provides a turnover between susceptible and immunized individuals, leading to a possible fourth stage of the epidemic with an equilibrium between susceptible, infected, and immunized classes. This can be considered as a chronic stage of the epidemic which can succeed the previous acute stage. This chronic stage of the epidemic will be discussed below in Section 3.

It was noticed already in the beginning of the epidemic that the severity of the disease and its outcome strongly depends on the age of the patients (see [4] and the references therein). Furthermore, some groups of the population can differ in the intensity of disease transmission because of their social and professional activities, which is the particular case of the so-called superspreaders [5]. Therefore, it is important to take into account the heterogeneity of the population.

Another source of heterogeneity of the population is related to its spatial distribution. Time delay in the epidemic progression in different countries and regions, people exchange, differences in measures of social distancing, and other differences can complicate the evaluation of epidemic progression. We will model the epidemic progression in the distributed population in Section 4.

1.3 Epidemiological Modelling

The COVID-19 pandemic stimulated an unprecedented interest in epidemiological modelling including conventional compartmental models (see [6–11] and the references therein) and more recently agent-based models [12]. The ODE models of epidemic progression were first suggested by D. Bernoulli in the XVIII-th century. He studied the progression of the smallpox epidemic and the efficacy of vaccination on the basis of Halley tables [13]. There is a vast modern epidemiological literature on SIR, SEIR, and their various modifications for homogeneous and heterogeneous populations (see [14–18] and the references therein).

The application of compartmental epidemiological models to the COVID-19 pandemic is to a large extent concentrated on the description of the epidemic evolution in different countries using available data (see, e.g., [3, 19–22]), to the calculation of the basic reproduction number and of the influences of lockdown and quarantine measures on the epidemic progression (see [20, 23–28] and the references therein). These models give a good description of the evolution of the number of infected individuals and the sizes of other classes involved in the epidemiological models in the beginning of the epidemic, and they take into account the influence of the measures of social distancing and some other measures to prevent the rapid epidemic spread. The situation is more complex for the prediction of the future epidemic progression because the parameters of the model are influenced by the measures of social distancing and other behavioural changes, and hence it is impossible to take into account the various scenarios better than to predict in advance.

The role of heterogeneity in the epidemic progression is largely discussed in the existing literature [19, 21, 22, 29, 30]. Different ages and social groups can have different timings in the implementation of the measures of social distancing. Furthermore, the so-called superspreaders, a relatively small group of people with a large number of social interactions, play an important role in the coronavirus epidemic [5]. Consideration of two types of individuals, one having frequent social interactions and the other having restricted/cautious social interactions, together in a single group with an average inactivity can lead to erroneous predictions.

In this work, we study a heterogeneous multipatch population with two subclasses in each patch corresponding to low and high disease transmitting individuals. We begin with a single-patch to recall the main properties of such model, including the basic reproduction number, final size of the epidemic, and the maximum number of infected individuals. Then we study multipatch models and apply them to investigate the epidemic progression in several states in India. A strong second wave of epidemic were observed in India in the spring of 2021. We will discuss it below.

2 MODEL PROBLEM FOR A HETEROGENEOUS POPULATION

We begin the study of epidemic progression in a heterogeneous population with the model problem consisting of susceptible and infected individuals with two subpopulations:

$$\frac{dS_1}{dt} = -\beta_{11}\frac{S_1}{N}I_1 - \beta_{12}\frac{S_1}{N}I_2, \tag{6.1}$$
$$\frac{dS_2}{dt} = -\beta_{21}\frac{S_2}{N}I_1 - \beta_{22}\frac{S_2}{N}I_2, \tag{6.2}$$
$$\frac{dI_1}{dt} = \beta_{11}\frac{S_1}{N}I_1 + \beta_{12}\frac{S_1}{N}I_2 - \sigma_1 I_1, \tag{6.3}$$
$$\frac{dI_2}{dt} = \beta_{21}\frac{S_2}{N}I_1 + \beta_{22}\frac{S_2}{N}I_2 - \sigma_2 I_2, \tag{6.4}$$

where β_{ij} are the rates of disease transmission, σ_j are the clearance rates, and N is the total population. This model is similar to the model recently considered in [31], here we will present a more detailed analysis of the model and extend it to multipatch models. Along with the basic reproduction number and the final size of the epidemic, we will determine the maximal number of infected individuals and will show that for the same value of the basic reproduction number, the populations can strongly differ by their final size and the maximum of infected individuals. This effect is caused by the heterogeneity of the population.

2.1 Basic Reproduction Number

In the beginning of the epidemic, S_1 and S_2 can be considered as constant when the total population is significantly large. We set:

$$\frac{S_1}{N} = k\,, \quad \frac{S_2}{N} = 1 - k, \quad 0 \le k \le 1.$$

The linearized matrix of the system (6.1) - (6.4) evaluated at the disease-free equilibrium point $(kN, (1-k)N, 0, 0)$ is given by

$$J = \begin{pmatrix} 0 & 0 & -k\beta_{11} & -k\beta_{12} \\ 0 & 0 & -(1-k)\beta_{21} & -(1-k)\beta_{22} \\ 0 & 0 & k\beta_{11}-\sigma_1 & k\beta_{12} \\ 0 & 0 & (1-k)\beta_{21} & (1-k)\beta_{22}-\sigma_2 \end{pmatrix}.$$

We find the maximal eigenvalues of J from the equation:

$$\lambda^2-(k\beta_{11}+(1-k)\beta_{22}-\sigma_1-\sigma_2)\lambda+k(1-k)(\beta_{11}\beta_{22}-\beta_{12}\beta_{21})-k\beta_{11}\sigma_2-(1-k)\beta_{22}\sigma_1+\sigma_1\sigma_2=0.$$

To simplify further calculations, we suppose that $\sigma_1=\sigma_2=\sigma$, $\beta_{12}=\beta_{21}=(\beta_{11}+\beta_{22})/2$. Then we obtain (6.5)

$$2\lambda = k\beta_{11}+(1-k)\beta_{22}-2\sigma+\sqrt{k\beta_{11}^2+(1-k)\beta_{22}^2}\,. \tag{6.5}$$

The basic reproduction number $\mathcal{R}_0$ is obtained as follows:

$$R_0=\left(k\beta_{11}+(1-k)\beta_{22}+\sqrt{k\beta_{11}^2+(1-k)\beta_{22}^2}\right)/(2\sigma)\,.$$

Moreover, if, $\beta_{11}=\beta_{22}=\beta$ for some β, then $\lambda=\beta-\sigma$, $R_0=\beta/\sigma$.

2.2 Final Size of the Epidemic

Taking a sum of equations (6.1), (6.3) and (6.2), (6.4), we obtain the equalities (6.6):

$$\frac{dS_1}{dt}+\frac{dI_1}{dt}=-\sigma_1 I_1\,,\quad \frac{dS_2}{dt}+\frac{dI_2}{dt}=-\sigma_2 I_2\,. \tag{6.6}$$

Integrating them from 0 to ∞ and assuming that $I_i(0)=I_i(\infty)=0$, $i=1,2$, we conclude that

$$S_1^0-S_1^f=\sigma_1\int_0^\infty I_1(t)dt\,,\quad S_2^0-S_2^f=\sigma_2\int_0^\infty I_2(t)dt\,.$$

Next, we divide equation (6.1) by S_1, equation (6.2) by S_2 and integrate from 0 to ∞:

$$-\ln\left(\frac{S_1^f}{S_1^0}\right)=\frac{\beta_{11}}{N\sigma_1}\left(S_1^0-S_1^f\right)+\frac{\beta_{12}}{N\sigma_2}\left(S_2^0-S_2^f\right),$$

$$-\ln\left(\frac{S_2^f}{S_2^0}\right)=\frac{\beta_{21}}{N\sigma_1}\left(S_1^0-S_1^f\right)+\frac{\beta_{22}}{N\sigma_2}\left(S_2^0-S_2^f\right).$$

With the notation $x=S_1^f/S_1^0$, $y=S_2^f/S_2^0$, and assumptions $\sigma_1=\sigma_2=\sigma$, $\beta_{12}=\beta_{21}=(\beta_{11}+\beta_{22})/2$, we obtain the system of equations

$$\beta_{11}k(1-x)+\beta_{12}(1-k)(1-y)=-\sigma\ln x, \tag{6.7}$$

$$\beta_{21}k(1-x)+\beta_{22}(1-k)(1-y)=-\sigma\ln y, \tag{6.8}$$

with respect to x and y. If $\beta_{11}=\beta_{22}=\beta$, then this system is reduced to the single equation $R_0(1-x)+\ln x=0$ independent of k. Its solution gives the final size of the susceptible population for the homogeneous population.

In the general case, the solution of this system depends on β_{11},β_{22}, and k. We will let their values vary in such a way that the basic reproduction number does not change (see Table 1), and we will analyze the final size of epidemic.

Consider the following example: $\beta=2.5,\sigma=1$. Then $\lambda=1.5$, $R_0=2.5$. For different values β_{11} and β_{22} such that $(\beta_{11}+\beta_{22})/2=\beta$, we find from (6.5) the value of k for which $\lambda=1.5$:

β_{11}	2.6	3	3.5	4	4.5	4.75	5
β_{12},β_{21}	2.5	2.5	2.5	2.5	2.5	2.5	2.5
β_{22}	2.4	2	1.5	1	0.5	0.25	0
k	0.495	0.475	0.45	0.427	0.403	0.393	3.82

Table 1: Relation between the values of β_{ij} and k

For each of these combinations of parameters, we determine x and y from system (6.7), (6.8), and the corresponding values S_1^f and S_2^f. The results of these calculations are shown in Fig. 1. The final value of the first susceptible subpopulation slowly decreases, while for the second subpopulation it increases. The final value of the total susceptible population increases almost 3 times between the minimal value for the homogeneous population and the maximal value reached for $\beta_{22} = 0$.

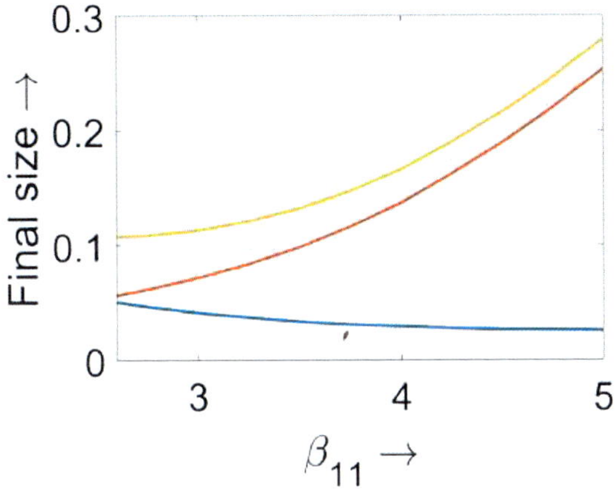

Figure 1: Final value of the total susceptible population and of the two subclasses as functions of β_{11}, S_1^f - lower curve, S_2^f - middle curve, their sum - upper curve. The values of parameters: $\beta_{22} = 5 - \beta_{11}$, $\beta_{12} = \beta_{21} = 2.5$, $\sigma = 1$

In the next example, $\beta = 1.5, \sigma = 1$, $\lambda = 0.5$, $\mathcal{R}_0 = 1.5$. The final susceptible for the homogeneous population is $S^f = 0.417$. The maximal total susceptible for the heterogeneous population is reached for $\beta_{11} = 3$ and equals $S^f = 0.587$. The ratio of the maximal and minimal value decreases with the decrease of $\mathcal{R}_0$, but their difference remains approximately the same as in the previous example.

2.3 Maximum Number of Infected Individuals

2.3.1 Maximum Number of Infected Individuals for a Homogeneous Population

Under the assumption that $\beta_{ij} = \beta$ for all $i, j = 1, 2$ for some β, and $\sigma_1 = \sigma_2$, system (6.1)-(6.4) can be reduced to:

$$\frac{dS}{dt} = -\beta \frac{S}{N} I, \quad \frac{dI}{dt} = \beta \frac{S}{N} I - \sigma I, \tag{6.9}$$

where $S = S_1 + S_2$, $I = I_1 + I_2$. Denote by t_m the time of the maximum of $I(t)$, and by I_m the maximal value, $I_m = I(t_m)$, and $S_m = S(t_m)$. Integrating the sum of the equations

$$\frac{dS}{dt} + \frac{dI}{dt} = -\sigma I$$

from 0 to t_m, we get

$$S_m - S_0 + I_m - I_0 = -\sigma \int_0^{t_m} I(t)dt, \tag{6.10}$$

where $S_0 = S(0) = N$, $I_0 = I(0)$. Next, from the first equation in (6.9),

$$\ln(S_m) - \ln(S_0) = -\frac{\beta}{N} \int_0^{t_m} I(t)dt. \tag{6.11}$$

From equations (6.10), (6.11),

$$I_m - I_0 = S_0 - S_m + \frac{\sigma N}{\beta} \ln\left(\frac{S_m}{S_0}\right). \tag{6.12}$$

From the second equation in (6.9), since the derivative equals 0 at $t = t_m$, we find $S_m = \sigma N/\beta$. Using the notation $\mathcal{R}_0 = \beta/\sigma$, from (6.12), we obtain (6.13):

$$\frac{I_m - I_0}{N} = 1 - \frac{1}{\mathcal{R}_0} - \frac{\ln \mathcal{R}_0}{\mathcal{R}_0}, \quad S_m = \frac{N}{\mathcal{R}_0}. \tag{6.13}$$

If $\mathcal{R}_0 = 1$, then $I_m = I_0$, $S_m = N$. For $\mathcal{R}_0 > 1$, $I_m > I_0$ and $S_m < N$.

2.3.2 Maximum Number of Infected Individuals in a Heterogeneous Population

To find the maximum number of infected individuals in the heterogeneous population, we consider an approximation $t_m^1 = t_m^2$, where t_m^1 is the time of maximum of $I_1(t)$ and t_m^2 of $I_2(t)$. Numerical simulations show that these times to the maximum are close to each other. Integrating equations (6.6) from 0 to t_m, we obtain:

$$S_1^0 - S_1^m + I_1^0 - I_1^m = \sigma_1 \int_0^{t_m} I_1(t)dt, \quad S_2^0 - S_2^m + I_2^0 - I_2^m = \sigma_2 \int_0^{t_m} I_2(t)dt, \tag{6.14}$$

where $S_i^0 = S_i(t_0)$, $S_i^m = S_i(t_m)$, $I_i^0 = I_i(t_0)$, $I_i^m = I_i(t_m)$, $i = 1, 2$. Next, we divide equation (6.1) by S_1, equation (6.2) by S_2 and integrate:

$$-\ln\left(\frac{S_1^m}{S_1^0}\right) = \frac{\beta_{11}}{N} \int_0^{t_m} I_1(t)dt + \frac{\beta_{12}}{N} \int_0^{t_m} I_2(t)dt,$$

$$-\ln\left(\frac{S_2^m}{S_2^0}\right) = \frac{\beta_{21}}{N}\int_0^{t_m} I_1(t)dt + \frac{\beta_{22}}{N}\int_0^{t_m} I_2(t)dt\ .$$

Taking into account (6.14), we obtain

$$-\ln\left(\frac{S_1^m}{S_1^0}\right) = \frac{\beta_{11}}{N\sigma_1}(S_1^0 - S_1^m + I_1^0 - I_1^m) + \frac{\beta_{12}}{N\sigma_2}(S_2^0 - S_2^m + I_2^0 - I_2^m)\ , \tag{6.15}$$

$$-\ln\left(\frac{S_2^m}{S_2^0}\right) = \frac{\beta_{21}}{N\sigma_1}(S_1^0 - S_1^m + I_1^0 - I_1^m) + \frac{\beta_{22}}{N\sigma_2}(S_2^0 - S_2^m + I_2^0 - I_2^m)\ . \tag{6.16}$$

Assuming that $I_1'(t_m) = I_2'(t_m) = 0$, we get from (6.3), (6.4):

$$S_1^m = \sigma_1 N\frac{I_1^m}{\beta_{11}I_1^m + \beta_{12}I_2^m}\ ,\quad S_2^m = \sigma_2 N\frac{I_2^m}{\beta_{21}I_1^m + \beta_{22}I_2^m}\ . \tag{6.17}$$

We suppose that $I_j^0 \ll I_j^m$, $(j = 1,2)$ $\sigma_1 = \sigma_2$. Set $\gamma_{ij} = \beta_{ij}/\sigma$, $(i,j = 1,2)$, $x = I_1^m/N$, $y = I_2^m/N$. With this notation, equations (6.15), (6.16) can be written by using (6.17) in the following form:

$$\ln\left(k\frac{\gamma_{11}x + \gamma_{12}y}{x}\right) = (k - x)\gamma_{11} + (1 - k - y)\gamma_{12} - \frac{\gamma_{11}x}{\gamma_{11}x + \gamma_{12}y} - \frac{\gamma_{12}y}{\gamma_{21}x + \gamma_{22}y}\ , \tag{6.18}$$

$$\ln\left((1-k)\frac{\gamma_{21}x + \gamma_{22}y}{y}\right) = (k - x)\gamma_{21} + (1 - k - y)\gamma_{22} - \frac{\gamma_{21}x}{\gamma_{11}x + \gamma_{12}y} - \frac{\gamma_{22}y}{\gamma_{21}x + \gamma_{22}y}\ . \tag{6.19}$$

Solving this system of equations, we find x and y and, consequently, I_j^m, $j = 1,2$. We then use formula (6.17) to determine S_j^m, $j = 1,2$.

Fig. 2 shows the comparison of the values I_j^m and S_j^m, $j = 1,2$ obtained from direct numerical simulations and found by the approximate analytical method presented above.

The left side of the figure shows the maximum number of infected individuals in direct numerical simulations of system (6.1)-(6.4) (solid lines) and as a solution of system (6.18), (6.19) (dashed lines). The lower curves correspond to the first subpopulation (I_1^m) and the upper curves to the second subpopulation (I_2^m). On the right side are shown the corresponding values of the number of susceptible individuals in numerical simulations of system (6.1)-(6.4) (solid lines) and by formula (6.17). The lower curves correspond to the first subpopulation (S_1^m) and the upper curves to the second subpopulation (S_2^m).

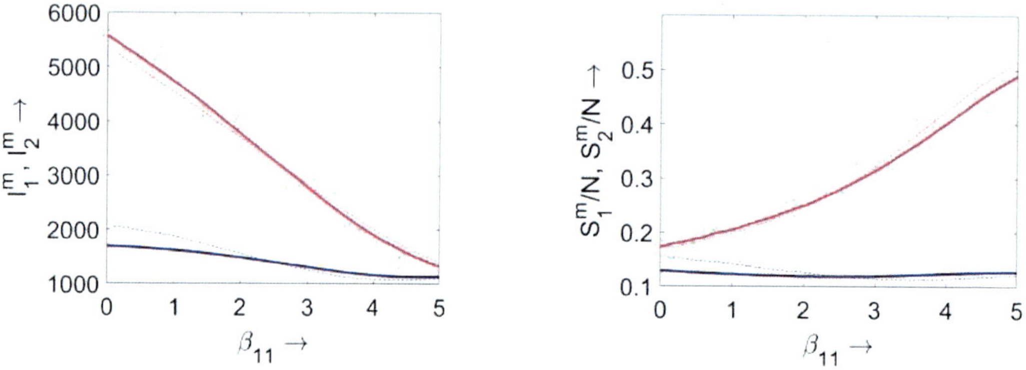

Figure 2: Maximum number of infected individuals (left) and number of susceptible individuals (right). The values of parameters: $\beta_{22} = 5 - \beta_{11}$, $\beta_{12} = \beta_{21} = 2.5$, $\sigma = 0.1$. The value of k is chosen in such a way that the basic reproduction number $\mathcal{R}_0 = 2.5$ is the same in all simulations (see the explanation in the text)

This approximation is more accurate for $\beta_{11} > \beta_{22}$ ($\beta_{11} + \beta_{22} = 5$), which corresponds to our main assumption that the first subpopulation is smaller and spreads infection faster than the second subpopulation. Let us recall that the population is homogeneous if $\beta_{11} = \beta_{22}$. The heterogeneity of the population increases with the increase of β_{11}. The maximum current number of infected individuals decreases with the increase of β_{11}. This effect is especially pronounced for the second subpopulation.

3 MODEL WITH REINFECTION

In this section, we study the epidemic progression in a heterogeneous population with the model problem consisting of susceptible, infected, and recovered individuals with two subpopulations where, after some time, those who recovered can become susceptible again:

$$\frac{dS_1}{dt} = -\beta_{11}\frac{S_1}{N}I_1 - \beta_{12}\frac{S_1}{N}I_2 + b_1R_1, \tag{6.20}$$

$$\frac{dS_2}{dt} = -\beta_{21}\frac{S_2}{N}I_1 - \beta_{22}\frac{S_2}{N}I_2 + b_2R_2, \tag{6.21}$$

$$\frac{dI_1}{dt} = \beta_{11}\frac{S_1}{N}I_1 + \beta_{12}\frac{S_1}{N}I_2 - \sigma_1I_1, \tag{6.22}$$

$$\frac{dI_2}{dt} = \beta_{21}\frac{S_2}{N}I_1 + \beta_{22}\frac{S_2}{N}I_2 - \sigma_2I_2, \tag{6.23}$$

$$\frac{dR_1}{dt} = k_1I_1 - b_1R_1, \tag{6.24}$$

$$\frac{dR_2}{dt} = k_2I_2 - b_2R_2, \tag{6.25}$$

3.1 Basic Reproduction Number

In the beginning of the epidemic, S_1 and S_2 can be considered as constant. We set:

$$\frac{S_1}{N} = k, \quad \frac{S_2}{N} = 1 - k, \quad 0 \leq k \leq 1.$$

The linearized matrix of the system (6.20) - (6.25) evaluated at the disease-free equilibrium (DFE) point $(kN, (1-k)N, 0, 0, 0, 0)$ is given by the equality

$$J = \begin{pmatrix} 0 & 0 & -k\beta_{11} & -k\beta_{12} & b_1 & 0 \\ 0 & 0 & -(1-k)\beta_{21} & -(1-k)\beta_{22} & 0 & b_2 \\ 0 & 0 & k\beta_{11} - \sigma_1 & k\beta_{12} & 0 & 0 \\ 0 & 0 & (1-k)\beta_{21} & (1-k)\beta_{22} - \sigma_2 & 0 & 0 \\ 0 & 0 & 0 & 0 & -b_1 & 0 \\ 0 & 0 & 0 & 0 & 0 & -b_2 \end{pmatrix}.$$

The matrix J has two zero eigenvalues, two negative eigenvalues $-b_1$ and $-b_2$, and two more nonzero eigenvalues of J that can be obtained from the block matrix

$$A = \begin{pmatrix} k\beta_{11} - \sigma_1 & k\beta_{12} \\ (1-k)\beta_{21} & (1-k)\beta_{22} - \sigma_2 \end{pmatrix}.$$

We find the maximal eigenvalue of J from the equation:

$$\lambda^2-(k\beta_{11}+(1-k)\beta_{22}-\sigma_1-\sigma_2)\lambda+k(1-k)(\beta_{11}\beta_{22}-\beta_{12}\beta_{21})-k\beta_{11}\sigma_2-(1-k)\beta_{22}\sigma_1+\sigma_1\sigma_2=0.$$

The largest eigenvalue is given by the expression

$$2\lambda = k\beta_{11} + (1-k)\beta_{22} - 2\sigma + \sqrt{k\beta_{11}^2 + (1-k)\beta_{22}^2},$$

with the assumption that $\sigma_1 = \sigma_2 = \sigma$, $\beta_{12} = \beta_{21} = (\beta_{11} + \beta_{22})/2$. The basic reproduction number around the DFE is given by the formula:

$$\mathcal{R}_0 = \frac{k\beta_{11} + (1-k)\beta_{22} + \sqrt{k\beta_{11}^2 + (1-k)\beta_{22}^2}}{2\sigma}.$$

3.2 Existence of Endemic Equilibrium

To find the endemic equilibrium, we solve the following system of equations (6.26)-(6.31):

$$-\beta_{11}\frac{S_1}{N}I_1 - \beta_{12}\frac{S_1}{N}I_2 + b_1R_1 = 0, \tag{6.26}$$

$$-\beta_{21}\frac{S_2}{N}I_1 - \beta_{22}\frac{S_2}{N}I_2 + b_2R_2 = 0, \tag{6.27}$$

$$\beta_{11}\frac{S_1}{N}I_1 + \beta_{12}\frac{S_1}{N}I_2 - \sigma_1 I_1 = 0, \tag{6.28}$$

$$\beta_{21}\frac{S_2}{N}I_1 + \beta_{22}\frac{S_2}{N}I_2 - \sigma_2 I_2 = 0, \tag{6.29}$$

$$k_1I_1 - b_1R_1 = 0, \tag{6.30}$$

$$k_2I_2 - b_2R_2 = 0. \tag{6.31}$$

Since we consider that the acute stage of the epidemic is finished, we can neglect the disease related death and we can assume that $\sigma_1 = k_1$, $\sigma_2 = k_2$. Then we have, $R_1 = \frac{\sigma_1 I_1}{b_1}$ and $R_2 = \frac{\sigma_2 I_2}{b_2}$. Also we have $S_1 + I_1 + R_1 = S_1^0$ and $S_2 + I_2 + R_2 = S_2^0$. This implies $S_1 = (S_1^0 - I_1 - \frac{\sigma_1}{b_1}I_1)$, and $S_2 = (S_2^0 - I_2 - \frac{\sigma_2}{b_2}I_2)$. Then from (6.28) and (6.29), we get,

$$\frac{\beta_{11}}{N}\left(S_1^0 - I_1 - \frac{\sigma_1}{b_1}I_1\right)I_1 + \frac{\beta_{12}}{N}\left(S_1^0 - I_1 - \frac{\sigma_1}{b_1}I_1\right)I_2 - \sigma_1 I_1 = 0,$$

$$\frac{\beta_{21}}{N}\left(S_2^0 - I_2 - \frac{\sigma_2}{b_2}I_2\right)I_1 + \frac{\beta_{22}}{N}\left(S_2^0 - I_2 - \frac{\sigma_2}{b_2}I_2\right)I_2 - \sigma_2 I_2 = 0.$$

The two equations above can be written as $I_2 = F_1(I_1)$ and $I_1 = F_2(I_2)$, respectively, where

$$F_1(I_1) = \frac{\sigma_1 N}{\beta_{12}}\left(\frac{I_1}{S_1^0 - I_1 - \frac{\sigma_1}{b_1}I_1}\right) - \frac{\beta_{11}}{\beta_{12}}I_1,$$

$$F_2(I_2) = \frac{\sigma_2 N}{\beta_{21}}\left(\frac{I_2}{S_2^0 - I_2 - \frac{\sigma_2}{b_2}I_2}\right) - \frac{\beta_{22}}{\beta_{21}}I_2.$$

Both curves pass through $(0,0)$ and the derivatives of $F_1(I_1)$ and $F_2(I_2)$ at $(0,0)$ are given by the expressions:

$$F_1'(0) = \frac{\sigma_1 - k\beta_{11}}{k\beta_{12}} \qquad F_2'(0) = \frac{\sigma_2 - (1-k)\beta_{22}}{(1-k)\beta_{21}}$$

respectively. Here we used the equalities $S_1^0 = kN$ and $S_2^0 = (1-k)N$. Hence, the condition for the existence of the endemic equilibrium point is given by the inequality:

$$\frac{\sigma_1 - k\beta_{11}}{k\beta_{12}}\frac{\sigma_2 - (1-k)\beta_{22}}{(1-k)\beta_{21}} < 1.$$

It is important to mention here that the existence of the endemic equilibrium point implies that it is unique.

Let us set

$$M_0 = ((\sigma_1 - k\beta_{11})(\sigma_2 - (1-k)\beta_{22}))/(\beta_{12}\beta_{21}k(1-k)).$$

Now, to ease the calculations, we assume that $\beta_{12} = \beta_{21} = \frac{(\beta_{11}+\beta_{22})}{2}$, $\sigma_1 = \sigma_2 = \sigma$. Let, $S_1^0 = kN$ and $S_2^0 = (1-k)N$. Then we have,

$$M_0 = \left(4(\sigma - \beta_{11}k)(\sigma - \beta_{22}(1-k))\right)/\left(k(1-k)(\beta_{11}+\beta_{22})^2\right).$$

Proposition: If $\mathcal{R}_0 < 1$, then $M_0 > 1$, and if $\mathcal{R}_0 > 1$, then $M_0 < 1$.

Proof: Let $\mathcal{R}_0 < 1$. This implies

$$k\beta_{11} + (1-k)\beta_{22} + \sqrt{k\beta_{11}^2 + (1-k)\beta_{22}^2} < 2\sigma,$$

$$\Rightarrow (k\beta_{11}^2 + (1-k)\beta_{22}^2) < (2\sigma - k\beta_{11} - (1-k)\beta_{22})^2.$$

Next,

$$\begin{aligned} & 4(\sigma - \beta_{11}k)(\sigma - \beta_{22}(1-k)) - k(1-k)(\beta_{11}+\beta_{22})^2 \\ = \; & (2\sigma - k\beta_{11} - (1-k)\beta_{22})^2 - ((1-k)\beta_{22} - k\beta_{11})^2 - k(1-k)(\beta_{11}+\beta_{22})^2 \\ > \; & k\beta_{11}^2 + (1-k)\beta_{22}^2 - (1-k)^2\beta_{22}^2 - k^2\beta_{11}^2 + 2k(1-k)\beta_{11}\beta_{22} - k(1-k)(\beta_{11}+\beta_{22})^2 \\ = \; & k\beta_{11}^2 + (1-k)\beta_{22}^2 - (1-k)^2\beta_{22}^2 - k^2\beta_{11}^2 - k(1-k)(\beta_{11}^2+\beta_{22}^2) = 0, \end{aligned}$$

which implies $M_0 > 1$. Similarly, $\mathcal{R}_0 > 1$ implies $M_0 < 1$, this completes the proof.

Consider a specific example for the parameter values $k = 0.2$, $\beta_{11} = 4$, $\beta_{22} = 1$, $\beta_{12} = \beta_{21} = 2.5$, $\sigma_1 = \sigma_2 = 1$, $k_1 = k_2 = 1$, $N = 10M$. As the expressions for $\mathcal{R}_0$ and M_0 are independent of b_1 and b_2, we can calculate $\mathcal{R}_0 = 1.8$ and $M_0 = 0.04$. The following Table 2 shows the components of the endemic equilibrium point for increasing values of b_1 and b_2.

$b_1 = b_2$	S_1^*	I_1^*	R_1^*	S_2^*	I_2^*	R_2^*
0.0001	9.40×10^5	106	1.06×10^6	5.16×10^6	284	2.84×10^6
0.001	9.37×10^5	1062	1.06×10^6	5.16×10^6	2834	2.84×10^6
0.01	9.37×10^5	10524	1.05×10^6	5.16×10^6	28086	2.81×10^6
0.1	9.37×10^5	96632	9.66×10^5	5.16×10^6	257887	2.58×10^6

Table 2: Endemic steady-state levels depending upon b-values

Calculating the relevant quantities from (6.7) and (6.8), we find the following results

$$S_1^f = 3.1 \times 10^5, \; S_2^f = 3.3 \times 10^6.$$

The simulation results for the model under consideration for different values of $b_1 = b_2$ are shown in Fig. 3 and 4. Let us note that the convergence to the endemic equilibrium is oscillating.

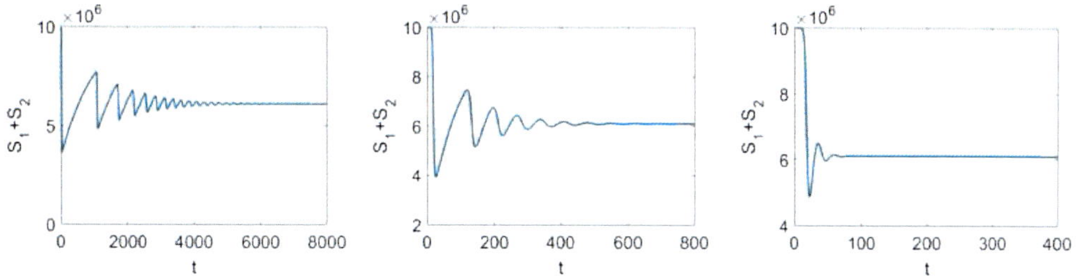

Figure 3: Time evolution of $S_1(t) + S_2(t)$. Left: $b_1 = b_2 = 0.001$; middle: $b_1 = b_2 = 0.01$; right: $b_1 = b_2 = 0.1$

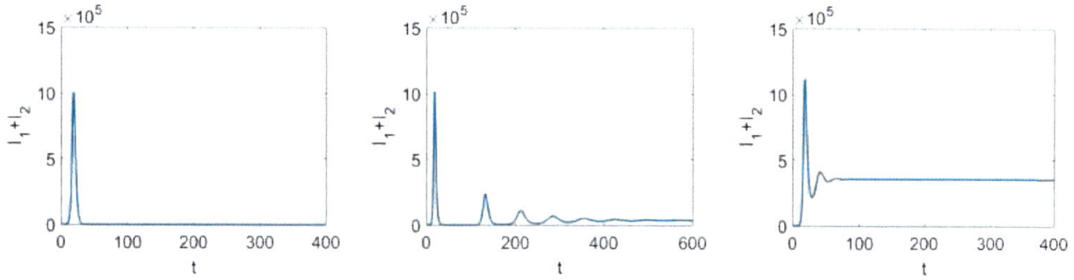

Figure 4: Time evolution of $I_1(t) + I_2(t)$. Left: $b_1 = b_2 = 0.001$; middle: $b_1 = b_2 = 0.01$; right: $b_1 = b_2 = 0.1$

3.3 Final Size of the Epidemic

Suppose that the parametric restriction $\sigma_j > k_j$, $j = 1, 2$ holds. From the numerical simulation it is observed that, if $\sigma_j = k_j$, then $I_j^f = I_j(\infty) = I_j^*$, $R_j^f = R_j(\infty) = R_j^*$, and if $\sigma_j > k_j$, then $I_j^f = 0$, $R_j^f = 0$, for $j = 1, 2$.

Adding equations (6.20), (6.22), (6.24) and (6.21), (6.23), (6.25), we obtain the equalities:

$$\frac{dS_1}{dt} + \frac{dI_1}{dt} + \frac{dR_1}{dt} = (k_1 - \sigma_1)I_1 \,, \quad \frac{dS_2}{dt} + \frac{dI_2}{dt} + \frac{dR_2}{dt} = (k_2 - \sigma_2)I_2.$$

Integrating them from 0 to ∞ and assuming that $I_j(0) = I_j(\infty) = 0$ and $R_j(0) = R_j(\infty) = 0$,

$j = 1, 2$, we conclude that

$$S_1^f - S_1^0 = (k_1 - \sigma_1) \int_0^\infty I_1(t)dt \ , \quad S_2^f - S_2^0 = (k_2 - \sigma_2) \int_0^\infty I_2(t)dt.$$

Integrating (6.7) and (6.8) from 0 to ∞ we get,

$$b_1 \int_0^\infty R_1(t)dt = k_1 \int_0^\infty I_1(t)dt \ , \quad b_2 \int_0^\infty R_2(t)dt = k_2 \int_0^\infty I_2(t)dt.$$

Next, we divide equation (6.20) by S_1, equation (6.21) by S_2 and integrate from 0 to ∞:

$$\ln\left(\frac{S_1^f}{S_1^0}\right) = -\frac{\beta_{11}}{N} \int_0^\infty I_1(t)dt - \frac{\beta_{12}}{N} \int_0^\infty I_2(t)dt + b_1 \int_0^\infty \frac{R_1(t)}{S_1(t)}dt \ ,$$

$$\ln\left(\frac{S_2^f}{S_2^0}\right) = -\frac{\beta_{21}}{N} \int_0^\infty I_1(t)dt - \frac{\beta_{22}}{N} \int_0^\infty I_2(t)dt + b_2 \int_0^\infty \frac{R_2(t)}{S_2(t)}dt \ .$$

We will take an approximation of the integral $b_j \int_0^\infty \frac{R_j(t)}{S_j(t)}dt$, $j = 1, 2$. Then

$$b_j \int_0^\infty \frac{R_j(t)}{S_j(t)}dt \approx \frac{b_j}{p_{1j}S_j^f + p_{2j}S_j^0} \int_0^\infty R_j(t)dt, \quad \text{where,} \quad 0 \leq p_{1j}, p_{2j} \leq 1, \quad j = 1, 2.$$

If we denote $x = S_1^f/S_1^0$, $y = S_2^f/S_2^0$, then we obtain the system of equations

$$-\frac{(\beta_{11}k - \frac{k_1}{p_{11}x+p_{21}})}{(k_1 - \sigma_1)}(x-1) - \frac{\beta_{12}(1-k)}{(k_2 - \sigma_2)}(y-1) = \ln(x), \tag{6.32}$$

$$-\frac{(\beta_{21}k)}{(k_1 - \sigma_1)}(x-1) - \frac{(\beta_{22}(1-k) - \frac{k_2}{p_{12}y+p_{22}})}{(k_2 - \sigma_2)}(y-1) = \ln(y), \tag{6.33}$$

involving the variables x and y. Since we observe numerically that the graphs for S_1, S_2 become almost constant after some transient oscillations, we take $p_{11} = 1$, $p_{21} = 0$ and $p_{12} = 1$, $p_{22} = 0$. The solution of this system of equations gives the final size of the susceptible population.

Fig. 5 (see also Table 3) shows the comparison of the values S_1^f and S_2^f obtained from direct numerical simulations and found by the approximated formula (6.32)-(6.33) presented above. The parameter values are as follows: $N = 10^7$, $k = 0.2$, $k_1 = k_2 = 0.8$, $\sigma_1 = \sigma_2 = 1$, $b_1 = b_2 = 0.01$, $\beta_{22} = 5 - \beta_{11}$, $\beta_{12} = \beta_{21} = 2.5$.

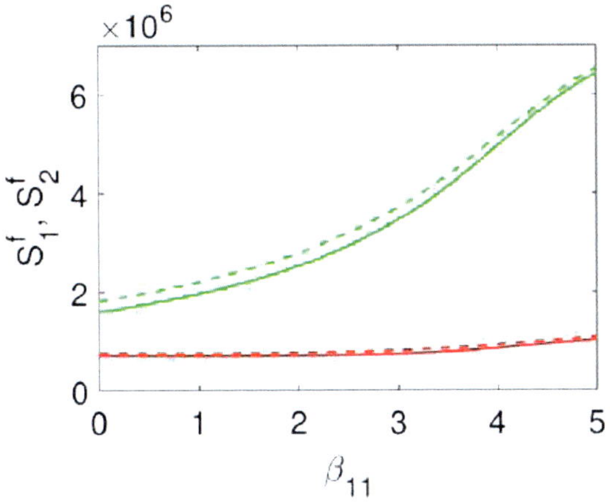

Figure 5: The dashed lines correspond to the direct results from numerical simulation and the solid lines correspond to the approximated formula (6.32)-(6.33). Red lines correspond to S_1^f and green lines correspond to S_2^f. The values of parameters: $\beta_{22} = 5 - \beta_{11}$, $\beta_{12} = \beta_{21} = 2.5$, $b_1 = b_2 = 0.5$, $\sigma_1 = \sigma_2 = 1$, $k_1 = k_2 = 0.8$, $k = 0.2$, $N = 10^7$, $p_{11} = p_{12} = 1$, $p_{21} = p_{22} = 0$

	β_{11}	S_1^f/N	S_2^f/N
Numerical	4	0.094	0.514
	3	0.083	0.371
	2	0.078	0.279
Analytical (formula (6.32) - (6.33))	4	0.087	0.495
	3	0.076	0.346
	2	0.072	0.253

Table 3: Comparison of analytical and numerically approximated values of S_1^f/N and S_2^f/N

4 MULTIPATCH MODEL

In thissection, we will consider the multipatch model for the heterogeneous population. However, we will begin with a single-patch to present another method to calculate the basic reproduction number.

4.1 Two-Group Single-Patch Model

To use the graph theoretic method [15] for finding the basic reproduction number, we consider the single-patch two-group epidemic model (6.34)-(6.39):

$$\frac{dS_1}{dt} = -\beta_{11}\frac{S_1}{N}I_1 - \beta_{12}\frac{S_1}{N}I_2 + b_1R_1, \tag{6.34}$$

$$\frac{dS_2}{dt} = -\beta_{21}\frac{S_2}{N}I_1 - \beta_{22}\frac{S_2}{N}I_2 + b_2R_2, \tag{6.35}$$

$$\frac{dI_1}{dt} = \beta_{11}\frac{S_1}{N}I_1 + \beta_{12}\frac{S_1}{N}I_2 - \sigma_1 I_1, \tag{6.36}$$

$$\frac{dI_2}{dt} = \beta_{21}\frac{S_2}{N}I_1 + \beta_{22}\frac{S_2}{N}I_2 - \sigma_2 I_2, \tag{6.37}$$

$$\frac{dR_1}{dt} = k_1I_1 - b_1R_1, \tag{6.38}$$

$$\frac{dR_2}{dt} = k_2I_2 - b_2R_2, \tag{6.39}$$

Keeping in mind the fact that we want to extend this two-group epidemic model to a multipatch model, we prefer to find the basic reproduction numbers using the graph theoretic method [15]. In the beginning of the epidemic, S_1 and S_2 can be considered as constants, and there are no infected individuals. We set:

$$\frac{S_1}{N} = k\ , \quad \frac{S_2}{N} = 1-k, \quad 0 \leq k \leq 1.$$

The disease-free equilibrium is as follows: $(kN, (1-k)N, 0, 0, 0, 0)$, and

$$F = \begin{pmatrix} k\beta_{11} & k\beta_{12} \\ (1-k)\beta_{21} & (1-k)\beta_{22} \end{pmatrix}, \quad V = \begin{pmatrix} \sigma_1 & 0 \\ 0 & \sigma_2 \end{pmatrix}.$$

The digraph representation of the matrix $F\lambda^{-1} - V$ with nodes $1, 2$ corresponding to I_1, I_2, respectively, is shown in Fig. 6. Using the algorithm in [15], the reduction of the digraph is shown in Fig. 7 and, consequently, $\mathcal{R}_0$ is the largest positive root of the equation

$$-1 + \frac{k(1-k)\beta_{12}\beta_{21}\lambda^{-2}}{((1-k)\beta_{22}\lambda^{-1} - \sigma_2)(k\beta_{11}\lambda^{-1} - \sigma_1)} = 0$$

with respect to λ. Assuming that $\sigma_1 = \sigma_2 = \sigma$, $\beta_{12} = \beta_{21} = (\beta_{11} + \beta_{22})/2$, we get,

$$\mathcal{R}_0 = \frac{k\beta_{11} + (1-k)\beta_{22} + \sqrt{k\beta_{11}^2 + (1-k)\beta_{22}^2}}{2\sigma}.$$

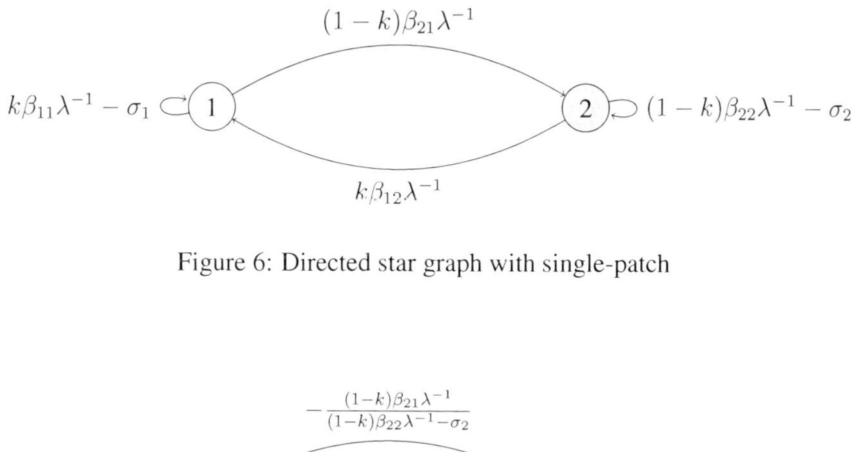

Figure 6: Directed star graph with single-patch

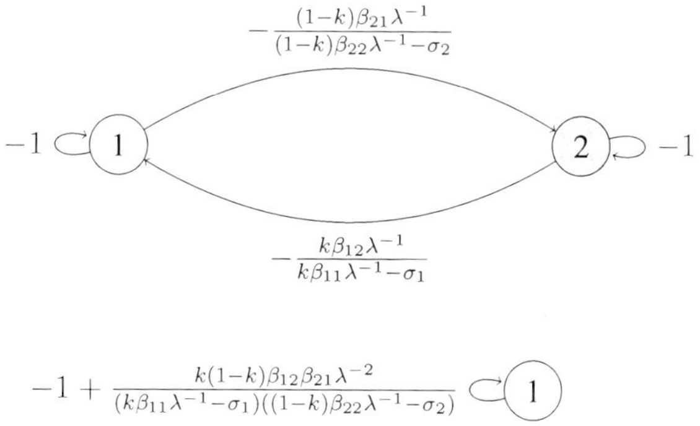

Figure 7: Reduction to node 1

4.2 Two-Group n Patch Model

Now, our goal is to extend the model to n patches. Generally, among some neighbouring patches, one patch is central (e.g., the capital of some state or country). With this hypothesis, we extend our model to n patches where we consider the movement of the first group (S_1, I_1, R_1) through the central patch. We consider the movement of S_1, I_1, R_1 from patch 1 to patch j at the rate l_{1j}, m_{1j}, l_{1j} and from patch j to patch 1 at the rate l_{j1}, m_{j1}, l_{j1}. The model is given by the following equations (6.40)-(6.45):

$$\begin{aligned}
\frac{dS_1^1}{dt} &= -\beta_{11}^1\frac{S_1^1}{N^1}I_1^1 - \beta_{12}^1\frac{S_1^1}{N^1}I_2^1 + b_1^1R_1^1 - \sum_{j=2}^{n} l_{1j}S_1^1 + \sum_{j=2}^{n} l_{j1}S_1^j, && (6.40)\\
\frac{dS_2^1}{dt} &= -\beta_{21}^1\frac{S_2^1}{N^1}I_1^1 - \beta_{22}^1\frac{S_2^1}{N^1}I_2^1 + b_2^1R_2^1, && (6.41)\\
\frac{dI_1^1}{dt} &= \beta_{11}^1\frac{S_1^1}{N^1}I_1^1 + \beta_{12}^1\frac{S_1^1}{N^1}I_2^1 - \sigma_1^1I_1^1 - \sum_{j=2}^{n} m_{1j}I_1^1 + \sum_{j=2}^{n} m_{j1}I_1^j, && (6.42)\\
\frac{dI_2^1}{dt} &= \beta_{21}^1\frac{S_2^1}{N^1}I_1^1 + \beta_{22}^1\frac{S_2^1}{N^1}I_2^1 - \sigma_2^1I_2^1, && (6.43)\\
\frac{dR_1^1}{dt} &= k_1^1I_1^1 - b_1^1R_1^1 - \sum_{j=2}^{n} l_{1j}R_1^1 + \sum_{j=2}^{n} l_{j1}R_1^j, && (6.44)\\
\frac{dR_2^1}{dt} &= k_2^1I_2^1 - b_2^1R_2^1. && (6.45)
\end{aligned}$$

Similarly, for patches $j = 2, ..., n$, we have (6.46)-(6.51):

$$\begin{aligned}
\frac{dS_1^j}{dt} &= -\beta_{11}^j\frac{S_1^j}{N^j}I_1^j - \beta_{12}^j\frac{S_1^j}{N^j}I_2^j + b_1^jR_1^j - l_{j1}S_1^j + l_{1j}S_1^1, && (6.46)\\
\frac{dS_2^j}{dt} &= -\beta_{21}^j\frac{S_2^j}{N^j}I_1^j - \beta_{22}^j\frac{S_2^j}{N^j}I_2^j + b_2^jR_2^j, && (6.47)\\
\frac{dI_1^j}{dt} &= \beta_{11}^j\frac{S_1^j}{N^j}I_1^j + \beta_{12}^j\frac{S_1^j}{N^j}I_2^j - \sigma_1^jI_1^j - m_{j1}I_1^j + m_{1j}I_1^1, && (6.48)\\
\frac{dI_2^j}{dt} &= \beta_{21}^j\frac{S_2^j}{N^j}I_1^j + \beta_{22}^j\frac{S_2^j}{N^j}I_2^j - \sigma_2^jI_2^j, && (6.49)\\
\frac{dR_1^j}{dt} &= k_1^jI_1^j - b_1^jR_1^j - l_{j1}R_1^j + l_{1j}R_1^1, && (6.50)\\
\frac{dR_2^j}{dt} &= k_2^jI_2^j - b_2^jR_2^j. && (6.51)
\end{aligned}$$

In the beginning of the epidemic, S_1^j and S_2^j $(j = 1, 2, \cdots, n)$ can be considered as constants, and there are no infected individuals. We set:

$$\frac{S_1^j}{N^j} = k^j\ , \quad \frac{S_2^j}{N^j} = 1 - k^j, \quad 0 \le k^j \le 1,\ j = 1, ...n.$$

The disease-free equilibrium is $(E_0^1, E_0^2, ..., E_0^n)$, $E_0^j = (k^j N^j, (1-k^j)N^j, 0, 0, 0, 0), j = 1, ..., n,$ and

$$F = \begin{pmatrix} F^1 & \theta_{2\times2} & ... & \theta_{2\times2} \\ \theta_{2\times2} & F^2 & ... & \theta_{2\times2} \\ ... & ... & ... & ... \\ \theta_{2\times2} & \theta_{2\times2} & ... & F^n \end{pmatrix}, \quad V = \begin{pmatrix} V^1 & M^2 & M^3 & M^4 & ... & M^n \\ N^2 & V^2 & \theta_{2\times2} & \theta_{2\times2} & ... & \theta_{2\times2} \\ N^3 & \theta_{2\times2} & V^3 & \theta_{2\times2} & ... & \theta_{2\times2} \\ N^4 & \theta_{2\times2} & \theta_{2\times2} & V^4 & ... & \theta_{2\times2} \\ ... & ... & ... & ... & ... & ... \\ N^n & \theta_{2\times2} & \theta_{2\times2} & \theta_{2\times2} & ... & V^n \end{pmatrix}.$$

where

$$F^i = \begin{pmatrix} k^i\beta_{11}^i & k^i\beta_{12}^i \\ (1-k^i)\beta_{21}^i & (1-k^i)\beta_{22}^i \end{pmatrix}, \quad M^j = \begin{pmatrix} -m_{j1} & 0 \\ 0 & 0 \end{pmatrix}, \quad N^j = \begin{pmatrix} -m_{1j} & 0 \\ 0 & 0 \end{pmatrix},$$

$$V^1 = \begin{pmatrix} \sigma_1^1 + m_{12} + ... + m_{1n} & 0 \\ 0 & \sigma_2^1 \end{pmatrix}, \quad V^j = \begin{pmatrix} \sigma_1^j + m_{j1} & 0 \\ 0 & \sigma_2^j \end{pmatrix}, \quad i = 1, 2, .., n,\ j = 2, 3, .., n.$$

The digraph representation of the matrix $F\lambda^{-1} - V$ with $2n$ nodes representing $I_1^1, I_2^1, ..., I_1^n, I_2^n$, respectively, this is shown in Fig. 8. For a clear visualization of the digraph, we assume that

$$a_i = \beta_{12}^j k^i \lambda^{-1}, \qquad b_i = \beta_{21}^i (1-k^i)\lambda^{-1},$$

$$c_j = \beta_{11}^j k^j \lambda^{-1} - (\sigma_1^j + m_{j1}), \quad d_i = \beta_{22}^i (1-k^i)\lambda^{-1} - \sigma_2^i,$$

$$D = \beta_{11}^1 k^1 \lambda^{-1} - (\sigma_1^1 + m_{12} + ... + m_{1n}), \quad i = 1, ..., n,\ j = 2, ..., n.$$

Using the algorithm in [15], the reduction of the digraph is shown in Fig. 9 and, consequently, $\mathcal{R}_0$ is the largest positive root of the equation (with respect to λ)

$$\beta_{11}^1 k^1 \lambda^{-1} - (\sigma_1^1 + m_{12} + ... + m_{1n}) - \frac{a_1 b_1}{d_1} - \sum_{j=2}^{n} \frac{m_{1j} m_{j1}}{(c_j - \frac{a_j b_j}{d_j})} = 0. \tag{6.52}$$

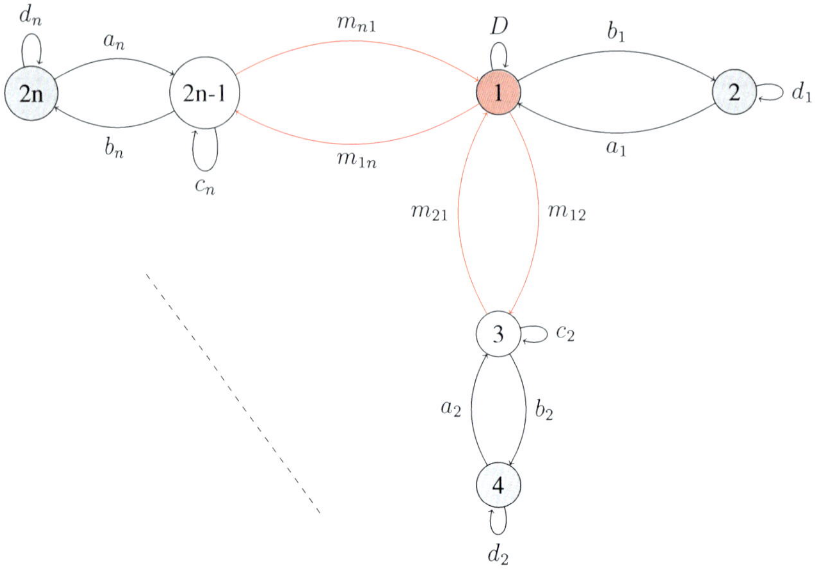

Figure 8: Directed star graph with n patches

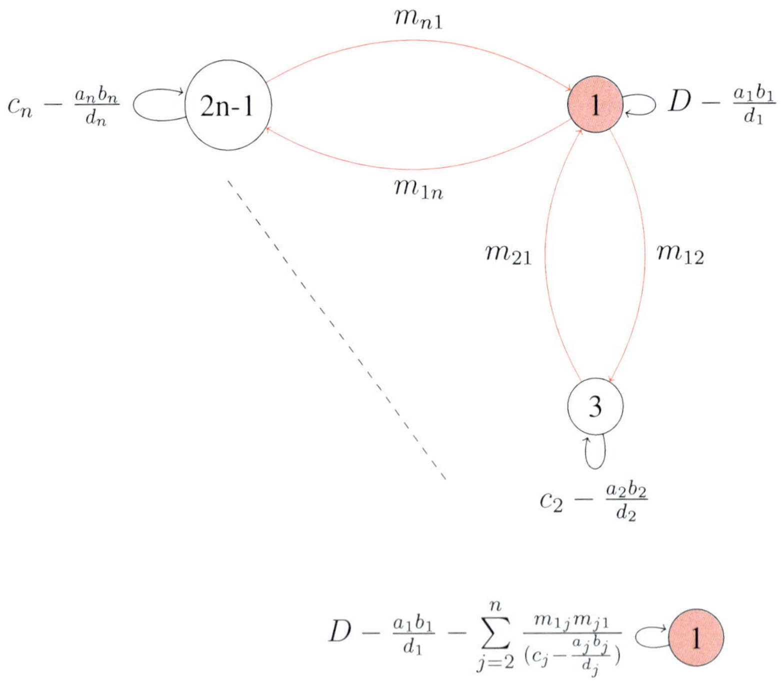

Figure 9: Reduction to node 1

Numerical verification of formula (6.52) for computing the basic reproduction number is shown in Fig. 10 and 11 for two different sets of parameter values with $\mathcal{R}_0 > 1$ for one case and $\mathcal{R}_0 < 1$ for the other case. The numerical simulation is performed for two patches, i.e., $n = 2$. Moreover, in Fig. 10, where $\mathcal{R}_0 > 1$, the epidemic progression for different values of m_{12}, m_{21} is shown.

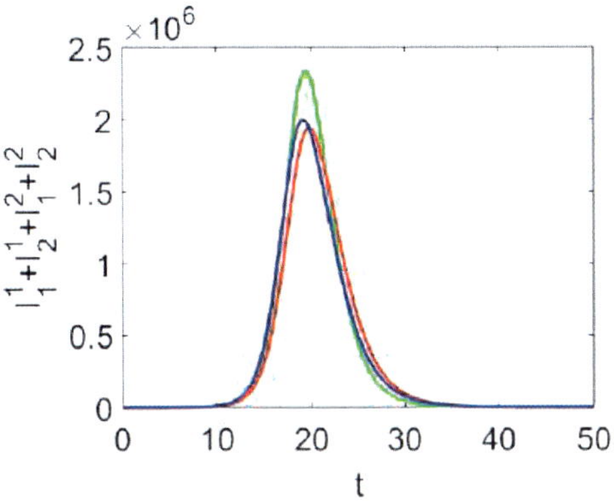

Figure 10: Green color corresponds to $m_{12} = 0.4$, $m_{21} = 0.4$, red color corresponds to $m_{12} = 0.5$, $m_{21} = 0.1$, and blue color corresponds to $m_{12} = 0.1$, $m_{21} = 0.5$. The other parameter values are: $l_{12} = 0.6$, $l_{21} = 0.5$, Patch 1: $\beta_{11}^1 = 2.5$, $\beta_{12}^1 = 2$, $\beta_{21}^1 = 2$, $\beta_{22}^1 = 1.5$, $k^1 = 0.18$, $b_1^1 = 0.001$, $b_2^1 = 0.001$, $\sigma_1^1 = \sigma_2^1 = 0.9$, $k_1^1 = k_2^1 = 0.8$, Patch 2: $\beta_{11}^2 = 2.5$, $\beta_{12}^2 = 2$, $\beta_{21}^2 = 2$, $\beta_{22}^2 = 1.5$, $k^2 = 0.2$, $b_1^2 = 0.001$, $b_2^2 = 0.001$, $\sigma_1^2 = \sigma_2^2 = 1$, $k_1^2 = k_2^2 = 0.8$. The values of $\mathcal{R}_0$ corresponding to green, red, blue curves are 1.83, 1.78, 1.87, respectively

5 EPIDEMIC PROGRESSION IN SOME STATES IN INDIA

In this section, we illustrate the role of multipatch models to describe the disease progression in regions or countries with large populations. As an illustrative example, we consider the epidemic growth in several states in India surrounding the state of Maharashtra, since a large proportion of COVID infected individuals in India are residents of this state. Not only the total number of infected individuals, but also a large proportion of COVID related deaths in India is reported from

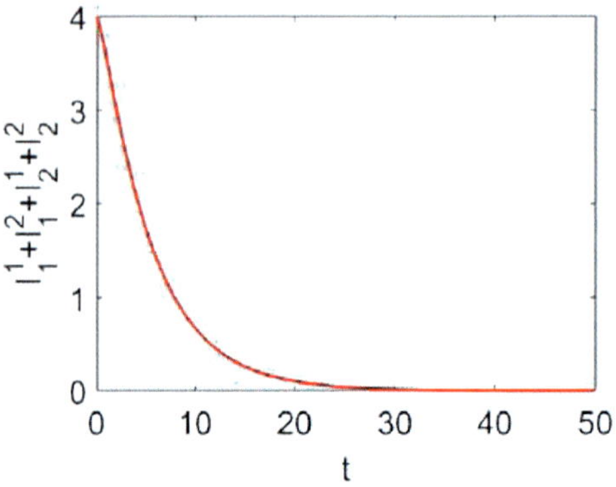

Figure 11: The curve corresponds to $m_{12} = 0.1$, $m_{21} = 0.5$. The other parameter values are: $l_{12} = 0.6$, $l_{21} = 0.5$, Patch 1: $\beta^1_{11} = 1.5$, $\beta^1_{12} = 1$, $\beta^1_{21} = 1$, $\beta^1_{22} = 0.5$, $k^1 = 0.18$, $b^1_1 = 0.001$, $b^1_2 = 0.001$, $\sigma^1_1 = \sigma^1_2 = 0.9$, $k^1_1 = k^1_2 = 0.8$, Patch 2: $\beta^2_{11} = 1.5$, $\beta^2_{12} = 1$, $\beta^2_{21} = 1$, $\beta^2_{22} = 0.5$, $k^2 = 0.2$, $b^2_1 = 0.001$, $b^2_2 = 0.001$, $\sigma^2_1 = \sigma^2_2 = 1$, $k^2_1 = k^2_2 = 0.8$. The corresponding value of $\mathcal{R}_0$ is 0.804

the same state: 25% of the total number of infected individuals in India is from Maharashtra and the death toll there is 34% compared to the total number of deaths in India (data on 12th April, 2021, source [32]). There are six states sharing a part of the border with Maharashtra: Chhattisgarh, Karnataka, Goa, Gujarat, Madhya Pradesh, and Telangana. We consider the epidemic growth in these five neighbouring states around Maharashtra for the period from March 9, 2020 to January 3, 2021, roughly up to the end of the first wave. Daily reported number of infected individuals and 7-days moving average for Maharashtra and its six neighboring states are shown in Fig. 12. We can see that the rate of growth and the day at which the peak has been attended vary significantly between the states. Within a span of 300 days, some of the states have reached more than one peak for the daily number of infected individuals.

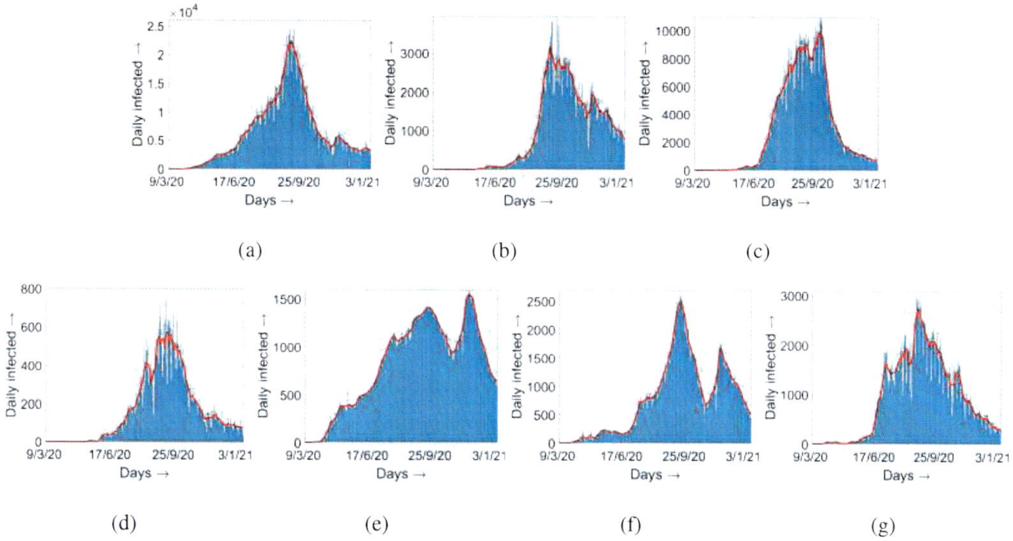

Figure 12: Number of daily infected individuals and their 7-days moving average for seven states. (A) Maharashtra, (B) Chhattisgarh, (C) Karnataka, (D) Goa, (E) Gujarat, (F) Madhya Pradesh, (G) Telangana

5.1 Epidemic Progression in Maharashtra

We begin with the description of epidemic progression in the state of Maharashtra starting with the model for homogeneous population

$$\frac{dS}{dt} = -\beta\frac{SI}{N}, \tag{6.53}$$

$$\frac{dI}{dt} = \beta\frac{SI}{N} - \sigma I, \tag{6.54}$$

$$\frac{dR}{dt} = kI, \tag{6.55}$$

to determine the parameters for the model of heterogeneous population considered below. COVID related death is taken into account through the condition $\sigma > k$, and the effect of lockdown is described through the time-dependent values of β (see [22] for a detailed discussion).

The first infected individual in Maharashtra was reported on March 9, 2020, and lockdown restrictions were imposed 15 days later. There was a complete lockdown during 68 days, followed by gradual uplifting of the restrictions. Fitting the data to the model (6.53) - (6.55) for the first 15 days we find $\beta = 0.4$, $\sigma = 0.05$, and $k = 0.049$, and we determine $\mathcal{R}_0 = 8$. Note that the choice of a relatively simple model to fit the data can increase the basic reproduction number. At the next stage, we estimate the values of parameters fitting the data during the next 68 days: $\beta = 0.106$, $\sigma = 0.05$, $k = 0.045$, and we find $\mathcal{R}_0 = 2.12$. Although the lockdown restrictions were relaxed step by step, most of the people were still confined within their homes since educational institutions (schools, colleges, universities), shops, and restaurants were closed, while the people authorized to go out were under strict surveillance. Therefore, we can assume that all people were following the imposed restrictions till then.

For the next 31 days (unlock-1) and 30 days (unlock-2) we get $\beta = 0.107$, $\sigma = 0.08$, $k = 0.075$ and $\beta = 0.11$, $\sigma = 0.09$, $k = 0.085$; $\mathcal{R}_0 = 1.3375$ and $\mathcal{R}_0 = 1.2222$, respectively. Note that the basic reproduction numbers calculated so far are not based upon the required Jacobian matrix with $S = N$, but with the current size of susceptible compartments.

To describe the third phase of unlock and onward, we use the model for heterogeneous population (6.56)-(6.61):

$$\frac{dS_1}{dt} = -\beta_{11}\frac{S_1}{N}I_1 - \beta_{12}\frac{S_1}{N}I_2, \tag{6.56}$$

$$\frac{dS_2}{dt} = -\beta_{21}\frac{S_2}{N}I_1 - \beta_{22}\frac{S_2}{N}I_2, \tag{6.57}$$

$$\frac{dI_1}{dt} = \beta_{11}\frac{S_1}{N}I_1 + \beta_{12}\frac{S_1}{N}I_2 - \sigma_1 I_1, \tag{6.58}$$

$$\frac{dI_2}{dt} = \beta_{21}\frac{S_2}{N}I_1 + \beta_{22}\frac{S_2}{N}I_2 - \sigma_2 I_2, \tag{6.59}$$

$$\frac{dR_1}{dt} = k_1 I_1, \tag{6.60}$$

$$\frac{dR_2}{dt} = k_2 I_2, \tag{6.61}$$

since there are different population groups with respect to the measures of social distancing.

Beginning from the unlock phase-3 and onward, more people are allowed to go out of their homes, and travel restrictions were partially withdrawn. This results in the fact that some part of the population was not following COVID restrictions in wearing masks, rules of epidemic-related hygiene, and many others. The parts of susceptible and infected individuals that are not following all COVID protocols accurately are denoted now as S_1 and I_1, respectively. If k is the fraction of S joining the class S_1 then $S_2 = (1-k)S$; accordingly, $I_1 = kI$ and $I_2 = (1-k)I$. The parameters of the model for group S_1 are the same as for the model of homogeneous population before lockdown, and for group S_2 as for the same model during the complete lockdown. Therefore, there is only one unknown parameter k that determines the proportion of these two groups. The value k is chosen in such a way that the cumulative number of infected individuals fits the data. Estimation and fitting are done in a periodic manner in accordance with the relaxation of lockdown restrictions phase by phase. During the third phase of unlock (31 days), the estimated parameter values are $\beta_{11} = 0.36$, $\beta_{22} = 0.1$, $\beta_{12} = \beta_{21} = (\beta_{11} + \beta_{22})/2$, $\sigma_1 = 0.09$, $\sigma_2 = 0.09$, $k_1 = k_2 = 0.08$ and the calculated effective reproduction number is $\mathcal{R}_0 = 1.2465$. Fitting the data for the next 30 days during the fourth phase of unlock, we find $\beta_{11} = 0.37$, $\beta_{22} = 0.101$, $\beta_{12} = \beta_{21} = (\beta_{11} + \beta_{22})/2$, $\sigma_1 = 0.13$, $\sigma_2 = 0.13$, $k_1 = k_2 = 0.124$ and $\mathcal{R}_0 = 0.9038$. Next, we set $\beta_{12} = \beta_{21} = (\beta_{11} + \beta_{22})/2$, [22].

At the next stage of epidemic progression, we use the model (6.62)-(6.67) where recovered individuals can become again susceptible due to a finite duration of immunity:

$$\frac{dS_1}{dt} = -\beta_{11}\frac{S_1}{N}I_1 - \beta_{12}\frac{S_1}{N}I_2 + b_1 R_1, \tag{6.62}$$

$$\frac{dS_2}{dt} = -\beta_{21}\frac{S_2}{N}I_1 - \beta_{22}\frac{S_2}{N}I_2 + b_2 R_2, \tag{6.63}$$

$$\frac{dI_1}{dt} = \beta_{11}\frac{S_1}{N}I_1 + \beta_{12}\frac{S_1}{N}I_2 - \sigma_1 I_1, \tag{6.64}$$

$$\frac{dI_2}{dt} = \beta_{21}\frac{S_2}{N}I_1 + \beta_{22}\frac{S_2}{N}I_2 - \sigma_2 I_2, \tag{6.65}$$

$$\frac{dR_1}{dt} = k_1 I_1 - b_1 R_1, \tag{6.66}$$

$$\frac{dR_2}{dt} = k_2 I_2 - b_2 R_2. \tag{6.67}$$

We use this model since the cases of reinfection of a small fraction of those who recovered were reported after approximately six months after the beginning of epidemic. We set $b_1 = b_2 = 0.01$. The values of the other parameters $\beta_{11} = 0.37$, $\beta_{22} = 0.09$, $\beta_{12} = \beta_{21} = (\beta_{11} + \beta_{22})/2$, $\sigma_1 = 0.14$, $\sigma_2 = 0.14$, $k_1 = 0.131$, $k_2 = 0.131$ are adjusted from the values determined above to have a better fit; the calculated value of effective reproduction number is $\mathcal{R}_0 = 0.7991$. This fitting is done up to January 3, 2021, with the total duration 300 days from the beginning of epidemic. Fitting of the cumulative reported cases for Maharashtra according to the method described above is presented in Fig. 13. Seven days moving average of cumulative reported cases is compared with the seven days moving average of the simulation results after estimating the parameters.

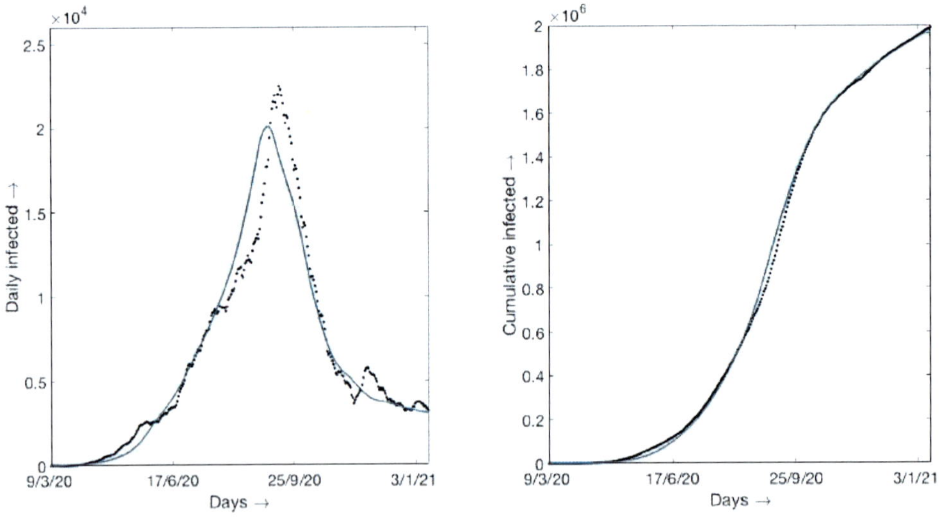

Figure 13: Number of daily infected and 7 days cumulative number of infected individuals in Maharashtra for a duration of 300 days plotted with the simulation results

5.2 Epidemic Progression in the Neighboring States

We have fitted the data from the other six states with the models described above. The values of the parameters are not presented here for the sake of brevity. Simulation results along with the cumulative number of infected individual for the six states are shown in Fig. 14.

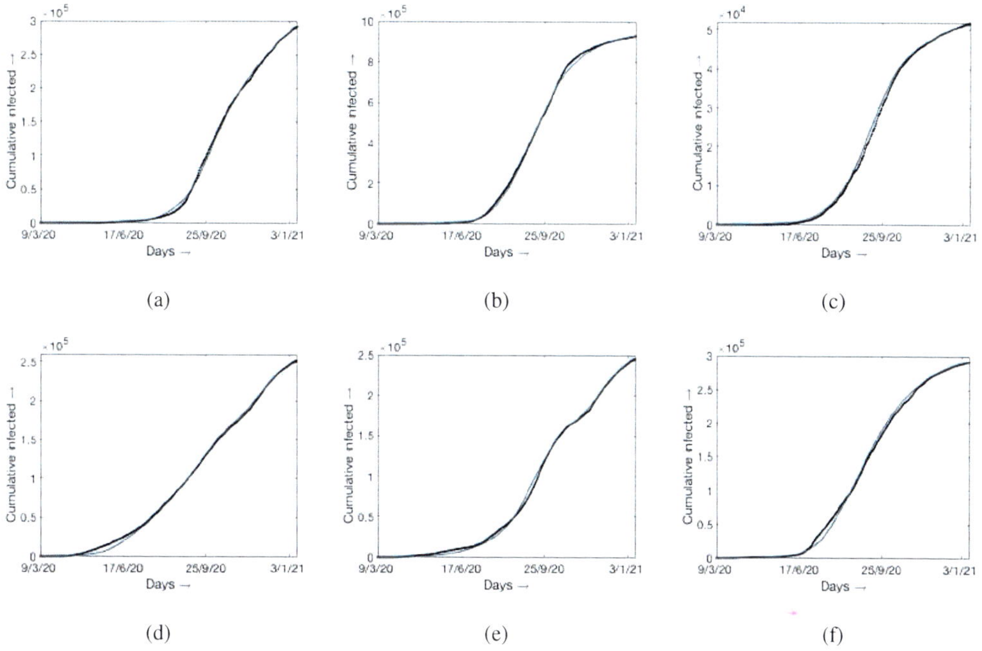

Figure 14: Cumulative number of infected individual is plotted against the corresponding simulated values for six different states. (A) Chhattisgarh, (B) Karnataka, (C) Goa, (D) Gujarat, (E) Madhya Pradesh, (F) Telangana

Finally, we consider the outcome of simulations for the multipatch model. During the fifth phase of unlock and onward, people's displacement between the states was allowed, and travelling through railroads and airplanes was resumed. We now simulate the multipatch model considering

Maharashtra, Gujarat, and Karnataka as the first, second, and third patch, respectively. To simplify the simulations and the interpretation of the results, we consider the movement between the first and second patches, and between the first and the third patches, but not between the second and the third ones. In the absence of available data, we use hypothetical parameter values: $l_{12} = 0.002$, $l_{13} = 0.002$, $l_{21} = 0.005$, $l_{31} = 0.005$, $m_{12} = 0.0003$, $m_{13} = 0.0003$, $m_{21} = 0.0005$ and $m_{31} = 0.0005$. Without the interstate movement, we find that the cumulative number of infected individuals January 3, 2021 equals 1.97×10^6. Once we suppose that susceptible, infected, and recovered people belonging to the first group can travel to and from the states Karnataka and Gujarat to Maharashtra, the cumulative number of infected individuals on the same date becomes 1.99×10^6. A small variation of the parameter values can significantly affect the resulting number of infected individuals. If we choose $l_{21} = 0.01$, $l_{31} = 0.01$ keeping other parameters fixed, we obtain the total number of infected individuals equal 2.09×10^6 on the same date. The simulation results are presented in Fig. 15.

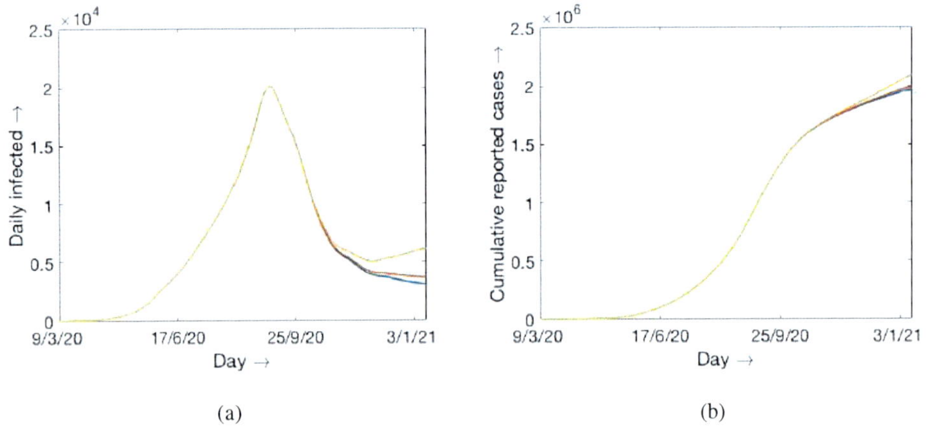

Figure 15: Simulated results for (a) daily number of infected, (b) cumulative number of infected in Maharashtra for no movement between the near-by states (blue) and two different rates of transfer between Maharashtra and neighboring states Gujarat and Karnataka (red & yellow)

Instead of movement between Maharashtra and the two neighboring states Gujarat and Karnataka, we now consider people travelling between Maharashtra and the four other neighboring states: Chhattisgarh, Goa, Madhya Pradesh, and Telangana. We consider the same set of parameter values for all the four neighboring states for the rate of transfer from one state to another: $l_{1j} = 0.002$, $l_{j1} = 0.004$, $m_{1j} = 0.0002$ and $m_{j1} = 0.0003$, $j = 3, 4, 5, 6$ where these subscripts correspond to Chhattisgarh, Goa, Madhya Pradesh and Telangana, respectively. Without movement between the states, the total number of infected individuals January 3, 2021 equal 1.97×10^6. The movement of susceptible, infected, and recovered of the first group results in the total number of infected equal 1.98×10^6. If we assume that only susceptible and recovered individuals are allowed to move between the states, then the total number of infected does not change significantly and remains close to the value 1.97×10^6. From the above simulation, it is clear that the movement of infected individuals plays a crucial role in the epidemic progression.

The outcomes of some other simulations are summarized in the following Table 4. It also includes the effective reproduction number, which determines the epidemic progression rate. Note that these results are obtained for the multipatch model with the movement between Maharashtra and its six neighboring states. In the table, l^r_{1j} with $r = 1$ denotes susceptible individuals of the first group travelling from Maharashtra to other neighboring states, and $r = 2$ indicates the movement of individuals from the second group. Similar notation is used for l^r_{j1}, m^r_{1j}, and m^r_{j1}.

r	l^r_{1j}	l^r_{j1}	m^r_{1j}	m^r_{j1}	Cumulative infected	$\mathcal{R}_0$
-	0	0	0	0	1.97×10^6	0.96
1	0.002	0.006	0	0	2.02×10^6	1.3
1	0.002	0.006	0.0006	0.002	2.07×10^6	1.31
2	0.002	0.006	0	0	2.24×10^6	2.75
2	0.002	0.006	0.0004	0.002	2.24×10^6	2.76

Table 4: Summary of numerical simulation of multipatch model and effective reproduction numbers

6 CONCLUDING REMARKS

Since the beginning of the COVID-19 pandemic, we witness unprecedented modelling efforts aimed to describe various aspects of coronavirus disease and epidemic progression. A large number of epidemiological studies have been devoted to data analysis in different countries and to deal with various related questions. However, many decisions concerning epidemic control (lockdown, social distancing, quarantine, sanitary measures, vaccination) are still adopted empirically on the basis of approximate and intuitive arguments known from the middle age. This is even more surprising considering that epidemiological models confirmed once again their accuracy in the description of epidemic progression.

This large discrepancy between the epidemiological theory and its practical implementation can be explained by several factors. Simple and generic epidemiological models, like SIR, SEIR can describe and predict general tendencies of the epidemic progression such as exponential growth or decay of the number of infected individuals. However, the rates of growth and decay can only be determined by fitting the data and cannot be calculated in advance. More complex models taking into account different age and socio-professional groups are based on contact matrices describing the interactions between these groups. The elements of these matrices are also unknown and depend on various factors which change in time and in different countries. Moreover, people's behavior can differ from what is suggested by the measures of social distancing. Furthermore, fitting the data to epidemiological models is usually strongly underdetermined because the single epidemic growth curve can be fitted by various combinations of parameter values. Altogether, this means that there is no reliable unified modelling approach which is capable to accurately predict the epidemic progression.

The purpose of this study is to work with a relatively simple model without excessive number of parameters which can still take into account the heterogeneity of the population. It is a continuation of our previous work on the model consisting of two subpopulations [22], which allows us to reliably determine the values of parameters fitting to the data before and during lockdown. After that, there is the only free parameter k which determines the ratio between the subpopulations and which can be evaluated from the available data depending upon the information about the implementation and relaxation of lockdown measures. This approach is used in this work to study spatially extended populations with a possible movement of people between countries or regions.

It should be stressed that the basic reproduction number (BRN) is not sufficient to characterize epidemic progression in the case of heterogeneous populations. With the same BRN, the final size of the epidemic and the maximal current number of infected individuals can be essentially different depending on the relative proportions of the different subpopulations. As an illustrative example, we have considered the epidemic growth in Maharashtra, India, and demonstrated the effect of movement of people from the surrounding states. For simplicity of mathematical calculations and numerical simulations, we have not considered the effect of people travelling from and to Maharashtra from distant states and even from abroad. Our analytical results indicate that the movement between patches can alter the BRN and hence affect the epidemic progression - this is validated with illustrative numerical examples. Appropriate estimation of the parameters and fitting the data is a difficult task as the travel data are not available in open sources.

The main limitation of the model is that we consider only two classes of susceptible, infected, and recovered populations. However, as we discussed above, this may be a good compromise allowing us to minimize the number of parameters as well as the number of equations, and to estimate the epidemic-related parameters from the available data. This work opens several interesting directions for future research, including the comparison with more detailed models and the development of immuno-epidemiological models. It will be also an interesting and challenging problem to consider a multigroup and multi-state/multi-city epidemic model with movement between all of them and even from abroad. The model considered will represent a system of stiff differential equations. Analytical derivation of various epidemic indicators will be a challenging task, while the estimation of parameters and related simulations will demand sophisticated computational facilities. Finally, getting appropriate information about various behavioural factors and relevant data is another obstacle. We would like also to remark that the modelling approach discussed here can provide a good understanding of the minute factors which can significantly alter the epidemic spread and provide some guideline to design the control measures.

In this work, we illustrate how the choice of an epidemic model helps to better explain the disease progression. We have started with a two-group epidemic model and then extended it to a multipatch model. The two-group single-patch model is proven to be successful to explain the COVID-19 disease progression in various countries where the movement of individuals in different compartments are uniform and the total population is not too large. However, in the case of a highly populated country like India, the in-flow and outflow of individuals of different compartments varies significantly from one state to another. The rate of change of the daily number of infected individuals, the day on which the daily infected individuals reaches its maximum during the first wave, the rate of decline in the number of daily infected individuals, etc. varies significantly between the neighboring states (see Fig. 12). Here, we have shown that the movement of individuals between the states can lead to the onset of the second wave, although the values of parameters require a more precise estimation. We will further study this issue by constructing a suitable multicomponent two-group model with the mobility of individuals between the neighboring and distant states. It will be a challenging problem to address.

The second wave of COVID-19 epidemic in India started from the middle of February with the epidemic growth rate essentially higher compared to the first wave. The onset of the second wave and the rate of growth of daily cases varies significantly from one state to another. There are several factors which can be responsible for this second wave, but it is quite difficult to identify the key reason. It can be related to large social and political gatherings due to elections in some states, insufficiency of medical facilities, and the lack of implementation of measures of social distancing. As we previously showed in another study [22], a slight change of the coefficient of social interaction, which determines the proportion of different subpopulations, can lead to a sudden and rapid increase in the epidemic growth rate. Appearance of a new virus strain can also be responsible for the rapid growth of the epidemic.

7 CONSENT FOR PUBLICATION

Not applicable.

8 CONFLICT OF INTEREST

The authors declare no conflict of interest, financial or otherwise.

9 ACKNOWLEDGEMENTS

This work is supported by the Ministry of Science and Higher Education of the Russian Federation: agreement no. 075-03-2020-223/3 (FSSF-2020-0018).

References

[1] Hallal PC, Hartwig FP, Horta BL, Silveira MF, Struchiner CJ, Vidaletti LP, Neumann NA, Pellanda LC, Dellagostin OA, Burattini MN, Victora GD, Menezes AM, Barros FC, Barros AJ, Victora CG. SARS-CoV-2 antibody prevalence in Brazil: results from two successive nationwide serological household surveys. The Lancet Global Health [Internet]. 2020 Nov [cited 2021 Oct 2];8(11):e1390–e1398. Available from: https://doi.org/10.1016/s2214-109x(20)30387-9

[2] Le Vu S, Jones G, Anna F, Rose T, Richard JB, Bernard-Stoecklin S, et al. Prevalence of SARS-CoV-2 antibodies in France: results from nationwide serological surveillance. Nature Communications [Internet]. 2021 May 21 [cited 2021 Oct 2];12(1). Available from: https://doi.org/10.1038/s41467-021-23233-6

[3] Wu F, Wang A, Liu M, Wang Q, Chen J, Xia S, Ling Y, Zhang Y, Xun J, Lu L, Jiang S, Lu H, Wen Y, Huang J. Neutralizing Antibody Responses to SARS-CoV-2 in a COVID-19 Recovered Patient Cohort and Their Implications. SSRN Electronic Journal [Internet]. 2020 [cited 2021 Oct 2]. Available from: https://doi.org/10.2139/ssrn.3566211

[4] Gauchon R, Ponthus N, Pothier C, Rigotti C, Volpert V, Derrode S, Bertoglio JP, Bienvenue A, Goard PO, Eyraud-Loisel A, Pageaud S, Loisel S, Roy P, and group CovDyn. Lessons learnt from the use of compartmental epidemic models over the French lockdown period. medRxiv

preprint. 2020 [cited 2021 Oct 2]. Available from: https://doi.org/10.1101/2021.01.11.21249565

[5] Kochanczyk M, Grabowski F, Lipniacki T. Super-spreading events initiated the exponential growth phase of COVID-19 with $\mathcal{R}_0$ higher than initially estimated. Royal Society Open Science [Internet]. 2020 Sep [cited 2021 Oct 2];7(9):200786. Available from: https://doi.org/10.1098/rsos.200786

[6] Arino J, van den Driessche P. Disease spread in metapopulations. In "Nonlinear Dynamics and Evolution Equations", Fields Institute Communications, 48, H. Brunner, X.O. Zhao, X. Zou, (Eds.), AMS, Providence, RI, 1–13, (2006).

[7] Arino J, van den Driessche P. A multi-city epidemic model. Mathematical Population Studies [Internet]. 2003 Jan [cited 2021 Oct 2];10(3):175–93. Available from: https://doi.org/10.1080/08898480306720

[8] Brauer F. Epidemic Models with Heterogeneous Mixing and Treatment. Bulletin of Mathematical Biology [Internet]. 2008 Jul 29 [cited 2021 Oct 2];70(7):1869–85. Available from: https://doi.org/10.1007/s11538-008-9326-1

[9] Castillo-Chávez C, Yakubu AA. Dispersal, disease and life-history evolution. Mathematical Biosciences [Internet]. 2001 Sep [cited 2021 Oct 2];173(1):35–53. Available from: https://doi.org/10.1016/s0025-5564(01)00065-7

[10] Diekmann O, Heesterbeek JA, Metz JA. On the definition and the computation of the basic reproduction ratio R_0 in models for infectious diseases in heterogeneous populations. Journal of Mathematical Biology [Internet]. 1990 Jun [cited 2021 Oct 2];28(4). Available from:https://doi.org/10.1007/bf00178324

[11] Lloyd AL, May RM. Spatial Heterogeneity in Epidemic Models. Journal of Theoretical

Biology [Internet]. 1996 Mar [cited 2021 Oct 2];179(1):1–11. Available from: https://doi.org/10.1006/jtbi.1996.0042

[12] Bouchnita A, Jebrane A. A multi-scale model quantifies the impact of limited movement of the population and mandatory wearing of face masks in containing the COVID-19 epidemic in Morocco. Mathematical Modelling of Natural Phenomena [Internet]. 2020 [cited 2021 Oct 2];15:31. Available from: https://doi.org/10.1051/mmnp/2020016

[13] Bacaër N. Histoires de mathématiques et de populations. [place unknown]: Cassini; 2009.

[14] Brauer F, Castillo-Chávez C, Feng Z. Mathematical Models in Epidemiology [Internet]. New York, NY: Springer New York; 2019 [cited 2021 Oct 3]. Available from: https://doi.org/10.1007/978-1-4939-9828-9

[15] de-Camino-Beck T, Lewis MA, van den Driessche P. A graph-theoretic method for the basic reproduction number in continuous time epidemiological models. Journal of Mathematical Biology [Internet]. 2008 Dec 2 [cited 2021 Oct 3];59(4):503–16. Available from: https://doi.org/10.1007/s00285-008-0240-9

[16] Diekmann O, Britton T, Heesterbeek H. Mathematical Tools for Understanding Infectious Disease Dynamics. [place unknown]: Princeton University Press; 2012. 520 p.

[17] Keeling MJ, Rohani P. Modeling Infectious Diseases in Humans and Animals. [place unknown]: Princeton University Press; 2007. 408 p.

[18] Martcheva M. An Introduction to Mathematical Epidemiology. [place unknown]: Springer; 2015. 467 p.

[19] Ávila-Ponce de León U, Pérez AG, Ávila-Vales E. An SEIARD epidemic model for COVID-19 in Mexico: Mathematical analysis and state-level forecast. Chaos, Solitons & Fractals [Internet]. 2020 Nov [cited 2021 Oct 3];140:110165. Available from: https://doi.org/10.1016/j.chaos.2020.110165

[20] Belgaid Y, Helal M, Venturino E. Analysis of a Model for Coronavirus Spread. Mathematics [Internet]. 2020 May 19 [cited 2021 Oct 3];8(5):820. Available from: https://doi.org/10.3390/math8050820

[21] Kucharski AJ, Russell TW, Diamond C, Liu Y, Edmunds J, Funk S, et al. Early dynamics of transmission and control of COVID-19: a mathematical modelling study. The Lancet Infectious Diseases [Internet]. 2020 May [cited 2021 Oct 3];20(5):553–8. Available from: https://doi.org/10.1016/s1473-3099(20)30144-4

[22] Sharma S, Volpert V, Banerjee M. Extended SEIQR type model for COVID-19 epidemic and data analysis. Mathematical Biosciences and Engineering [Internet]. 2017 [cited 2021 Oct 3];17(6):7562–604. Available from: https://doi.org/10.3934/mbe.2020386

[23] Aguiar M, Ortuondo EM, Bidaurrazaga Van-Dierdonck J, Mar J, Stollenwerk N. Modelling COVID 19 in the Basque Country from introduction to control measure response. Scientific Reports [Internet]. 2020 Oct 14 [cited 2021 Oct 3];10(1). Available from: https://doi.org/10.1038/s41598-020-74386-1

[24] Arino J, Portet S. A simple model for COVID-19. Infectious Disease Modelling [Internet]. 2020 [cited 2021 Oct 3];5:309–15. Available from: https://doi.org/10.1016/j.idm.2020.04.002

[25] Krantz SG, Polyakov P, Rao AS. True epidemic growth construction through harmonic analysis. Journal of Theoretical Biology [Internet]. 2020 Jun [cited 2021 Oct 3];494:110243. Available from: https://doi.org/10.1016/j.jtbi.2020.110243

[26] Sinha S. Epidemiological dynamics of the COVID-19 pandemic in India: an interim assessment. Statistics and Applications. 2020; 18, 333–350.

[27] Supino M, d'Onofrio A, Luongo F, Occhipinti G, Dal Co A. The effects of containment measures in the Italian outbreak of COVID-19. BMC Public Health [Internet]. 2020 Nov 26

[cited 2021 Oct 3];20(1). Available from: https://doi.org/10.1186/s12889-020-09913-w

[28] Zhao S, Lin Q, Ran J, Musa SS, Yang G, Wang W, Lou Y, Gao D, Yang L, He D, Wang MH. Preliminary estimation of the basic reproduction number of novel coronavirus (2019-nCoV) in China, from 2019 to 2020: A data-driven analysis in the early phase of the outbreak. International Journal of Infectious Diseases [Internet]. 2020 Mar [cited 2021 Oct 3];92:214–7. Available from: https://doi.org/10.1016/j.ijid.2020.01.050

[29] Eikenberry SE, Mancuso M, Iboi E, Phan T, Eikenberry K, Kuang Y, Kostelich E, Gumel AB. To mask or not to mask: Modeling the potential for face mask use by the general public to curtail the COVID-19 pandemic. Infectious Disease Modelling [Internet]. 2020 [cited 2021 Oct 3];5:293–308. Available from: https://doi.org/10.1016/j.idm.2020.04.001

[30] Rojas JH, Paredes M, Banerjee M, Akman O, Mubayi A. Mathematical Modeling & the Transmission Dynamics of SARS-CoV-2 in Cali, Colombia: Implications to a 2020 Outbreak & public health preparedness. medRxiv preprint. 2020 [cited 2021 Oct 3]. Available from: https://doi.org/10.1101/2020.05.06.20093526

[31] Dolbeault J, Turinici G. Heterogeneous social interactions and the COVID-19 lockdown outcome in a multi-group SEIR model. Mathematical Modelling of Natural Phenomena [Internet]. 2020 [cited 2021 Oct 3];15:36. Available from: https://doi.org/10.1051/mmnp/2020025

[32] Available from: https://www.covid19india.org/.

CHAPTER 7

Social Inequalities in COVID-19

Jorge Bacallao Gallestey[1], **Alfonso Casado Collado***[2]

* **Corresponding author:** Alfonsojaime.casado@inv.uam.es, Phone: +34 914975486

[1] Atherosclerosis Research and Reference Center. University of Medical Sciences, Havana, Cuba.

[2] Department of Preventive Medicine and Public Health. School of Medicine. Autonomous University of Madrid, Spain.

Abstract. Social inequalities have become an essential component of the health situation analysis. Health statistics are incomplete if its basic indicators are not linked to socioeconomic, sociodemographic, or sociocultural strata. The evaluation of health systems' performance must include global indicators along with their distribution in social strata.

The COVID-19 pandemic has not affected all countries to the same extent. Global statistics of both, confirmed cases and deaths portray wide differences among countries.

Recent reports show wide differences associated with stratification criteria such as skin color or ethnic groups, sex, age, education, socioeconomic condition, and geographic area. The web of interactions between individual and contextual factors also influences the development of the new pandemic.

This chapter lays the conceptual basis for measuring social inequalities in health and presents a basic set of the most common indices. It underscores the fact that a metric choice is not only technical, but to a great extent depends on ethical and political considerations. We document social inequalities in several health indicators associated with COVID-19 using public data or information retrieved from recently published papers.

The first section of this chapter lays the conceptual foundations for measuring health inequalities. The second one exposes selected results and findings in different settings, and a brief analysis of the application of the inequality indices.

Key words: Concentration, COVID-19, dispersion, entropy, health disparity, health indicators, indices, inequities, right to health, social inequality, stratifying variables.

1 INTRODUCTION

1.1 Importance

This chapter provides methodological guidelines to measure social inequalities in the expression of COVID-19 indicators, and general suggestions for the use and interpretation of indices. It also includes illustrative applications and discussion of recent relevant examples. This will encourage the routine inclusion of inequalities to describe and monitor the current pandemic.

1.2 Preamble

The COVID-19 pandemic, which at the time of writing this text - April 1, 2021 - has already claimed the lives of 2.82 million people out of a total of about 129 million cases worldwide, does not affect all countries to the same extent, nor is it homogeneously distributed within a country. This lack of homogeneity has many causes. Some are natural: mortality is much higher in people over 60 years of age, and in those with associated comorbidities, such as high blood pressure and chronic obstructive respiratory disease, regardless of their age. Health personnel in direct contact with patients are at greater risk. There are also recent indications that a certain genetic predisposition could be involved in an increased risk of poor outcome [1]. It is not possible to eradicate these causes.

Other causes, however, are related to unjust orders that imply lack of access to quality health services, precarious living conditions, and low perception of risk. Several of these causes are passed down from one generation to another.

The differences between the two causes, the natural and unavoidable, and the contextual and avoidable, mark a distinction between inequalities (or simple differences) and inequities (or unjust inequalities). This distinction between just and unjust, between avoidable and inevitable, imposes a marked attribute of subjectivity on the study of inequalities, which is added to the intrinsic difficulties of description or analysis, when choosing a metric.

To evaluate the design and implementation of coping strategies, monitoring the classic health indicators of incidence, cumulative incidence, or mortality is not enough. It is necessary to study the distribution of these indicators according to relevant population groups. The performance evaluation of a health system, to put it in statistical language, does not reduce to measures of position, but must also include measures of dispersion. Nor is it possible to limit oneself to negative indicators . Positive indicators such as access to a reliable diagnosis, vaccination, and quality health services that guarantee a better prognosis and better evolution of the disease must be included.

Along with the pandemic, an infodemic has been unleashed in the world that, although it generates considerable benefits in the cognitive order, also carries with it high levels of disinformation and a great danger denounced by the World Health Organization (WHO) itself [2].

The vast theme evoked by the title of this chapter can be considered from three related, but essentially different, approaches. One of them is the impact of social inequality on the severity of the pandemic. This approach would explain at least part of the large gaps between countries and why some have performed better than others. A second focus is on the foreseeable consequences of the pandemic on social inequalities in the world [3]. Gender differences, the gaps between rich and poor and between natives and migrants, to mention just three examples, have increased since the beginning of the pandemic. The third approach, to which this chapter is restricted, consists of describing inequalities in health indicators, both negative and positive, associated with socioeconomic stratification variables.

The chapter has two main objectives. The first is to present a basic typology of indices for measuring social inequalities in health, briefly highlighting the rationality and properties of each index. Second, to illustrate its application to data obtained from public sources of information and to present some examples of recent publications on the inequalities associated with COVID in two countries of the American continent.

2 PRELIMINARIES

2.1 Context and Health in the Life Course

The concept of health has changed remarkably in the last decades. The classic definition of the World Health Organization (WHO), [4] revolutionary at the time because it left behind the obsolete notion of absence of disease, has also been revised and modified [5]. The definition of health as a state of "complete physical, mental, and social well-being, and not simply as the absence of disease" would reduce the universe of healthy people to a tiny minority during a limited stage of their life course, because it implies a qualification of complete well-being that is practically unattainable. This justifies the present emphasis on adaptive capacity in defining health [6–8].

In a more comprehensive view, [9] WHO has defined health as "the measure of the capacity of an individual or a group to fulfill their aspirations and satisfy their needs, on the one hand, and to change and face the challenges of the environment. It conceives of health, therefore, as a resource of daily living and not as the objective of life, as a positive concept that, together with physical capacity, emphasizes personal and social resources".

According to this definition, health risks occur and are reproduced in the midst of physical and social contexts, and their magnitude is directly proportional to socioeconomic inequalities and psychosocial gradients [10, 11]

Health gaps are not reduced with targeted interventions or through the provision of resources to the most vulnerable. It is also imperative to apply strategies oriented to the social factors that generate inequalities in keeping with a broader vision of causality [12].

The determinants of health affect both risk and vulnerability. Socio-economic factors give rise to different exposure profiles, and consequently to different levels of risk, but they also entail greater vulnerability to similar levels of risk.

A fundamental determinant of vulnerability at the population scale is the status of social groups. Social hierarchies generate a network of relatively invariant relationships in the intergenerational transition. Poverty, understood in its broadest sense and not in its simply material side, persists in families from one generation to another, with a social inertia in its distribution and concentration that is only modified as a result of great social movements and great economic transformations [13].

The psychological stress imposed by inequities and social exclusion affects health throughout the life course, through multiple causal paths [14]. Chronic psychosocial stress not only has a great influence on gene expression, modulated by neuroendocrine dysfunction, and is a key concept to understanding the causes of a large number of diseases, especially chronic non-communicable diseases (NCDs), but possibly also plays an important role in shaping the unequal levels of vulnerability to communicable diseases, whether or not they reach epidemic or pandemic dimensions.

The life course approach (LCA) is a causality model that takes into account individual risks caused by factors acting in limited time settings with short-term consequences, together with long-term effects of physical and social exposure factors during critical periods of life [15].

Although genetic factors contribute to the inheritance of certain attributes that predispose humans to health problems, the physical and social environment is of fundamental importance to triggering these genetic mechanisms and modulating them. The LCA tries to identify the components of the physical and social environment responsible for psychophysiological responses. Although the influence of the social environment on health is well-known, the mechanisms that affect health throughout the life course have begun to be revealed only very recently. They include not only the effects of socioeconomic status, but also of physical and social contexts, environmental pollution, violence, and the experience of psychologically traumatic events [16].

Social inequalities appear in all stages of life both as risk determinants and as risk modifiers. The biological response to aggressions from the social environment is cumulative and is not reduced to a series of independent episodes of stress. Some authors have invoked the concept of allostatic load, which refers to the exhaustion of the mechanisms that are activated to cope with environmental stressors. Chronic exposure to these stressors and the adaptive reactions that occur through changes in hormonal levels, generate inflammatory processes during the life course and increase vulnerability to NCDs, while reducing the biological and psychological capacities to cope with communicable diseases [17–19]. Another source of vulnerability is the limited access to quality health services.

Groups with low socioeconomic level, as well as unemployed, marginalized, and discriminated minorities, tend to be more exposed to aggressions from multiple stressors such as environmental pollution, violence, exclusion or limited access to adequate food and quality health services. As a result of these higher levels of exposure, the onset of declining health occurs earlier in life [20]. Structural factors in society influence levels of exposure, risk, and vulnerability through individual experiences and lifestyles, but they also have direct effects, not mediated by individual factors, with a bidirectional causal relationship with social inequalities in health [21].

The influence of the physical and social context from the earliest stages of life generates a sense of belonging and inclusion. Negative experiences such as economic decline, social stigmatization, deprivation of rights and exclusion, suffered by, for example, migrants and a large number of marginalized minorities in all societies, have deleterious effects on health and well-being in multiple components of the causal fabric of health [22]. Less well known and more debatable are the mechanisms that generate a risk gradient associated with this context.

Particularly controversial is the relative contribution of the structural attributes of the space or the attributes added by the populations that inhabit these spaces. This debate in the field of public health and epidemiology has its counterpart in the biomedical sciences in the relative influence of genes and the environment on individual health [23].

In view of the complex synergistic relationships between health and the environment, and the evidence regarding the intergenerational transfer of vulnerabilities to health, it is contradictory that the vast majority of programs and interventions continue to be vertical and focused on factors of isolated exposures even in societies with approaches based on primary health care [24, 25].

2.2 The Right to Health

In the 90s of the last century, health policies were limited to a minimalist model with a delivery of basic services focused on the most vulnerable groups. The failure of this model ignited the debate around the right to health, which has been fought fundamentally on an ethical-legal level, but which in most countries has not crystallized into a defined strategic proposal nor in models of attention that guarantee the state's commitment to fulfill this right.

Until 1990, the concept of human rights was restricted to civil and political rights. From then on, the United Nations began to pay greater attention to other equally important rights, such as those of a social, economic and cultural nature, including the right to have access to the highest attainable standard of health. The United Nations General Assembly, after the proposal of the then Secretary General, Kofi Annan, approved the reform that implied the expansion of the concept of human rights under the aegis of the United Nations (UN).

Until the dawn of this century, there was no clear notion of the scope of the right to health, the foundations of which are rooted in the Universal Declaration of Human Rights. In 2000, General Comment 14 [26] was published, which defined the content of this right and established the obligation of governments to fight discrimination and inequalities. The right to the highest attainable standard of health commits governments to increase access to health for the most vulnerable individuals, groups and communities and to take whatever measures are necessary to provide them with information and encourage their active participation in policies and programs related to their health.

The right to health entails, not only actions to avoid violations of rights, but also proactive actions taken by an effective and accessible health system for all that guarantees:

- Attention to health needs in correspondence with national and local priorities.
- Action on the social determinants of health, such as water and basic sanitation and education, both general and sanitary.
- Active, documented and inclusive participation of the community.
- The development and implementation of a comprehensive plan and not a series of isolated vertical actions.

The right to health is an immanent component of the human condition, and therefore a good in itself that does not require justification. International treaties, which recognize it as an essential component of human rights, provide the binding normative framework for the different actors at national and local levels to design and implement their health policies and strategies and evaluate their results. In this way, human rights guide the public policies of the States, including those in the health field.

The significance of the United Nations (UN) documents that are based on the rights approach and enshrine the right to health, [27] is that they turn into a legal imperative, and not just a moral obligation, the design and implementation of policies based on the social determinants of health, both those with a negative connotation that should be eliminated or reduced to the minimum possible expression, and those that have a positive connotation of health promotion. Thus clearly emerges the link between the rights approach and the social determinants of health approach, and with it, the concepts of "responsibility" and "constructive responsibility" [28, 29] that commit States and Governments to the development of proactive public policies.

By adopting a rights-based approach, States assume the responsibility to include in their legal framework the obligation to promote, respect, protect, and provide universal access to health, and to guarantee that all individuals and human groups, without exclusion, fully enjoy that right. This implies guaranteeing, at the highest level allowed by the prevailing conditions in each country, the following four basic attributes embodied in a comprehensive health system:

- Availability: a sufficient number of public health programs, facilities, goods, and services.
- Accessibility: The establishments, goods and services available to all people, without exclusions. The concept of accessibility comprises three dimensions: (a) physical accessibility, (b) economic accessibility, and (c) accessibility to information.
- Acceptability: The availability of establishments, goods and services that respect the cultural patterns of each scenario, under strict ethical principles.
- Quality: The establishments, goods and services must be equally appropriate from a scientific, technical and good medical practice point of view.

The novelty of the contribution of the rights approach can be summarized in the resolution of several antinomies:

1. Minimum rights vs. universal rights: according to the rights approach, the delivery of a basic basket of health services is only a starting point in the search for the highest attainable levels of satisfaction.
2. Basic benefits vs. maximum delivery of available resources: States are obliged to deliver the maximum of available resources. The link between health and development, and the essential duality of health as a right in itself and as an indispensable means to achieve development, dispel any objection that resources devoted to fulfilling the right to health may undermine other equally basic rights. On the other hand, the principle of maximum available delivery

requires governments to be transparent in the use of resources and grants society as a whole, a legal instrument to demand, in turn, progressive attention to their right to health .

3. Vertical vs. comprehensive approaches to health: The comprehensive approach to health is, on the one hand, the conceptual basis of the approach of social determinants, and on the other, that of the strategic principle of cross-sectorality and intersectorality.

4. Hegemonic vs. democratic relations: Democratic relations imply the right to voluntary admission, privacy, and truthful and objective information, all on an individual level, but also to empowerment and to community participation in health plans and programs.

5. Sector vision vs. intersectoral view of health policies: The sectoral view excludes the possibility of comprehensive coping with health problems. The contribution of the right approach to the intersectoral vision consists of the concepts of integrality, interdependence and indivisibility of rights.

2.3 Conceptual Bases for Measuring Social Inequalities Related to Health

The expression "social inequalities in relation to health" has two similar but essentially different interpretations. The first of them starts from social inequalities as a characteristic of contemporary societies and points to a link that would connect them with health on both an individual and a population scale. Under this interpretation unequal societies should have worse population health indicators. There is broad consensus that, among societies with similar economic development, the less unequal ones perform better in terms of health [30–33]. Much more debated is the impact of inequalities on the health of individuals. The debate has its origins in the difficulty to control the large number of individual factors that could confound the contextual effect of inequality on individual health and lead to the well-known "ecological fallacy" that consists of extrapolating an association from the aggregate to the individual level [32–35].

In the methodological order, the way to verify the influence of inequality on individual health is the application of hierarchical models, which include the contextual effect of inequality, while controlling for other contextual effects and other individual factors. With this approach, several recent works confirm the existence of this contextual effect of social inequalities on individual health [35, 36].

This effect could be due to the fact that in societies with large socioeconomic gaps, substantial segments of the population live in conditions of poverty, which affect health through two mediating variables: insufficient perception of risk, commonly associated with poor sanitary education, and lack of access to quality health services. The other causal trajectory has its origin in the reactions that a relative adverse economic condition triggers in people, when they compare themselves, consciously or not, with others in their milieu. This subjective perception of relative economic condition or social position has a negative impact on health [37, 38].

The second interpretation of the expression "social inequalities in relation to health", which is the subject matter of this chapter, assumes the existence of two leading actors: on the one hand, indicators that describe health, as dependent or response variables; on the other, categorical variables that define a stratification criterion. The expression then makes sense, when the purpose is to measure differences that are expressed in health indicators, and between categories of a social stratifier, which is the generic term that is usually used to refer to cultural, social or economic factors. The link between the these two characters is an index of social inequality in relation to health, which will have to be chosen from a wide range of options.

It should be noted that this choice of a descriptive or analytical resource is not simply - and perhaps not even primarily - technical, as it is in other fields of research or other measurement contexts. Almost always there are underlying value judgments, whether or not the person is aware of them, that distinguish differences that are simple inequalities from those that represent inequities [39].

Inequities are systematic (not random), modifiable (because they have a social origin) and unfair inequalities [40]. Due especially to this last condition, whoever chooses an index implicitly makes an ethical judgment.

The fact that people over 60 have higher death rates from COVID-19 than those aged 20 or less, or people of some blood group higher than those of other blood groups, determines inequalities possibly irreducible, in which no component of justice or injustice intervenes. On the contrary, that it is also higher in some groups and some ethnic minorities [41, 42] is unfair, because they are the product of unjust social conditions or conditions that violate widely shared –although not necessarily unanimous- notions of justice.

Much more controversial is, in fact, whether or not to consider as unfair, the differences in indicators of great relevance and significance such as chronic malnutrition in children under 5 years of age in relation to maternal schooling. The association between these two indicators is well known. The literature collects various experiences about reducing chronic malnutrition by increasing the mother's schooling. Improving the provision of food has a reduced impact on the nutrition of young children, if parallel programs that promote maternal education are not developed [43]. Are these differences clearly the result of an unjust social order or are they structural and therefore irreducible? The question has more practical significance than scientific interest, and the answer, as will be explained in due course, influences the election of an inequality metric.

Indeed, if the problem is attacked through its causes and not through its manifestations, the reduction of chronic malnutrition begins by increasing maternal education. This strategy guarantees, together with progress towards desirable goals of sustainable development in education, the most cost-efficient dividend in terms of reducing chronic malnutrition rates. Its success consists in simultaneously achieving an increase in maternal schooling - an important goal in itself - and a reduction in rates. However, all or almost all the remaining burden of disease from malnutrition (which will not have been reduced to zero) will continue to be concentrated in groups of illiterate mothers or with low education, so that some of the indices, such as the rate ratio of extreme groups, or the measures of concentration of disease burden, would increase.

The fact that these two indices have the attractive attributes of being easy to calculate and interpret could be less important than the goal of revealing what happens with morbidity across all groups of maternal education.

An example, with fictitious data:

School level	Malnourished	Not malnourished	Total
Illiterate	20	80	100
Not illiterate	**20**	**880**	**900**
Total	40	960	1000

Table 1: Maternal illiteracy and chronic malnutrition in children under 5 years of age (time t_0)

School level	Malnourished	Not malnourished	Total
Illiterate	18	32	50
Not illiterate	**10**	**940**	**950**
Total	28	972	1000

Table 2: Maternal illiteracy and chronic malnutrition in children under 5 years of age (time t_1)

Suppose that the strategy of increasing maternal education has the effect described by the change between t_0 and t_1. Maternal illiteracy was reduced by half, from 10% (100/1000) to 5% (50/1000) and in parallel, chronic malnutrition decreased from 4% (40/1000) to 2.8% (28/1000), to a great extent due to literacy programs. However, given the structural relationship between maternal education and malnutrition, much of the chronic malnutrition that prevails is concentrated in the children of illiterate mothers. Indeed, at time t_0, 10% of the population concentrated 50% (20/40) of chronic malnutrition in children under 5 years of age, while at time t_1, 5% of the population concentrated 64% of the chronic malnutrition (18/28).

There is no doubt that the situation described by Table 2 is more favorable than that described by Table 1 (illiteracy was reduced by half and chronic malnutrition to less than half), although it is increasingly concentrated in the illiterate population and although the rate ratio has increased notably: 9 in t_0 ((20/100) / (20/900)) and 34.2 in t_1 ((18/50) / (10/950)).

2.4 Common Contexts and Applications of Inequality Measurement

Inequalities are always measured with a comparative purpose. Like a correlation coefficient, a mean or a variance, an inequality index says very little by itself except in the exceptional cases where it takes extreme values.

Indexes are used for three purposes:

- Comparisons over time to describe the evolution of inequalities. This application, undoubtedly the most consistent with the intention of evaluating the performance of a health system, is problematic in relation to dichotomous variables such as death or illness, because the total variability changes only if the global health indicators change.
- Concurrent comparisons of different scenarios: refers to comparisons that are made routinely between countries or between regions of the same country. The interpretation of these comparisons is complex due to the existence of "confounding" factors of the differences, or measurement biases in the indicators (such as when comparing developing countries, where the sources of information are unreliable, with developed countries, which have reliable sources of information).
- Concurrent comparisons with respect to different socioeconomic stratification criteria or different health indicators: refers to comparisons of inequalities in order to identify the socioeconomic factors to which the largest gaps are associated, or the health indicators in which these gaps are manifested. This application requires the prior standardization of the variables. The greatest difficulty is that information of homogeneous quality is rarely available in relation to stratification factors or health variables.

2.5 Basic Properties and Desirable Attributes for Health Inequality Indices

No index displays all positive attributes nor is unconditionally preferable to all others. Those with the best metric properties are often more difficult to calculate and interpret in practice. The use of any metric resource depends on value judgments, often only implicit at the time of choice. All indices:

1. Must be sensitive to inequalities in health, as this is a basic requirement of validity.
2. Should reflect the social dimension of health inequalities. The link with the social dimension is not always explicit. For example: inequalities in fatality or COVID infection rates between communities or provinces of a country are not strict social inequalities in health, but they become such if these provinces are ordered according to the percentage of the population living in poverty, or some other socioeconomic indicator.
3. Should use all the available information and not only that corresponding to extreme groups of the social hierarchy.
4. Should be sensitive to changes in the distribution of the population. If the composition of the population changes, the ratio of the number of people exposed to those not exposed can vary in a positive or negative sense, and the index should be sensitive to the magnitude and direction of the change. For example, the relative risk of chronic malnutrition among children of poor families with respect to children of non-poor families could remain the same (or even increase), despite the fact that both the prevalence of chronic malnutrition and the percentage of poverty have decreased. There are indices that take into account the distribution of the population and others that ignore it. In general, the former are preferable, but - again - value judgments are involved in this preference.
5. Should be simple to calculate and easy to interpret. Complex and difficult to interpret measurements are not advisable regardless of their analytical properties.
6. Must be sensitive to changes over time. The unweighted metrics and those that do not take into account the entire domain of the classes, are not sensitive to changes over time that do not occur in extreme groups, or that occur at the expense of the population distribution of social groups and not of the magnitude of the health variable in the groups.

Other interesting properties of indices are:

a. That they can be decomposed, either as the sum of a "within groups" and a "between groups", component or as the sum of the contributions of the different dimensions that they comprise. In the first case, the decomposition of inequality would allow estimating what fraction of inequality is attributable to the chosen stratification criterion and what percentage can be considered marginal or residual inequality [44, 45]. In the second case, the decomposition would allow for an ordering of the variables in relation to their contribution to inequality [46–49].

b. That they are sensitive with respect to the average health status of the population. Including the average health of the population in the algorithmic structure of the index, would make it sensitive to this parameter, but at the cost of integrating two notions that are normally evaluated separately.

Some authors [50–52] suggest systematically adding confidence intervals or standard error of the indices to the measurement of inequality. When health indicators are the result of probabilistic surveys, this is possible and desirable; not so, however, when the measurement of inequality is done with population data.

2.6 A Basic Taxonomy of Indices to Measure Inequalities [53]

The measurement of inequalities serves an advocacy purpose, [54]. Advocacy is a key complement to health promotion, whose aims are to raise awareness among decision-makers, and to gain social support and acceptance among the community for health programs and policies. Understanding the role of social determinants has made it essential to measure inequalities as a component in evaluating the performance of health systems. The analysis of inequalities, which goes beyond the purposes of this text, implies the study of the causes and the mechanisms that generate them, through a multilevel approach that includes the influences of the microenvironment (family, work, community) and of the macroenvironment of the individual (physical, cultural, political, and socioeconomic context). All analytical endeavors depend on reliable measurements.

The indices of social inequality in relation to health that are most frequently used in the literature are critically analyzed below. Others that do not satisfy minimum requirements in terms of basic properties or that are too complex and therefore not applicable in practice are not considered.

I. Indices for ordered categories

1. Based on pairwise comparisons
   - **i.** Rate ratio and weighted rate ratio
   - **ii.** Rate difference and weighted rate difference
   - **iii.** Population attributable risk and relative population attributable risk.
2. Indices based on the regression model.
   - **i.** Slope index of inequality
   - **ii.** Pamuk's relative index of inequality.
   - **iii.** Kunst and Mackenbach index.
3. Indices based on the concept of concentration.
   - **i.** Gini index
   - **ii.** Concentration index

II. Indices for unordered categories.

1. Based on pairwisecomparisons
   - **i.** Rate ratio and weighted rate ratio
   - **ii.** Rate difference and weighted rate difference
   - **iii.** Population attributable risk and relative population attributable risk.

2. Dispersion indices

   i. Pearcy-Keppel index

   ii. Between groups variance

   iii. Mean logarithmic deviation

3. Indices based on the comparison of probability distributions

   i. Hoover index

   ii. Theil index

The reason for the first major division of the indices is that the stratification criteria may constitute hierarchies, such as percentiles (eg deciles or quintiles) of income or schooling, or they may simply be nominal categorical variables, such as skin color or geographic areas of a country.

3 INDICES FOR ORDERED CATEGORIES

3.1 Indices Based on Pairwise Comparisons

3.1.1 The Rate Ratio (RR)

The inequality between two groups, according to this index, is defined as the quotient of their respective rates.

$$RR = \frac{t_1}{t_2},$$

where t_1 and t_2 are the rates of groups 1 and 2, respectively. The rate ratio is easy to calculate and interpret, and is invariant to change of scale: if the numerator and denominator are multiplied by a constant, the ratio does not change. Its most common expression is as a quotient of extreme rates in an ordered arrangement according to a health variable or a socioeconomic variable. When the extreme groups of the two rankings do not coincide, the ratio of the extreme rates in the socioeconomic hierarchy underestimates the magnitude of the inequality. Whatever the ordering criterion, the quotient of the extreme rates does not take into account intermediate groups, that may hide a considerable proportion of inequality.

RR is not sensitive to changes in the population structure and takes the same value if the poorest group is much larger than the richest, as if the exact opposite occurs. When comparisons are made over time, it is clear that even when the rates of the best and worst group remain constant, and therefore RR remains invariant, the situation worsens if the proportion of people in the worst group increases. For this reason, the option to weight RR by the quotient of the respective group sizes is suggested.

3.1.2 The Weighted Rate Ratio (WRR)

$$WRR = f * RR,$$

where $f = \frac{n_1}{n_2}$. WRR and RR coincide only when $n_1 = n_2$, n_1 and n_2 are the respective sizes of the classes. WRR is sensitive to a decrease in inequality that occurs not only through a decrease in the ratio of rates, but also through a more favorable distribution of people exposed to class conditions.

3.1.3 The Rate Difference (RD)

$$RD = t_1 - t_2.$$

The limitations indicated with respect to the quotient are also valid in relation to the difference, which is also easy to calculate and interpret, but is not invariant to changes in scale.

3.1.4 The Weighted Rate Difference (WRD)

$$WRD = f * RD.$$

WRD can also decrease not only due to a reduction in RD, but also due to a population redistribution, or to a favorable combination of both factors.

3.1.5 *The Population Attributable Risk (PAR)*

$$PAR = t_{total} - t_{(N)}.$$

In the above expression $t_{(N)}$ represents the rate of the group with the best socioeconomic situation, or the lowest rate of the entire classification, and, t_{total} the rate of the entire population. The PAR is interpreted as the number of events (illnesses or deaths (per 1,000, 10,000, or 100,000 inhabitants, depending on the rate expression) that could be avoided if the population rate were reduced to that of the best group. This index is easy to calculate and formally analogous to another homonymous index frequently used by epidemiologists and health professionals [55].

For the purposes of calculating inequality, PAR only uses the global rate and a benchmark for comparison and ignores the magnitude of the dispersion between the groups, be they classes of a socioeconomic variable or geodemographic units. In this way, attribute 3, already examined, is ignored, by both PAR and its relative version which is defined as:

3.1.6 *Relative Population Attributable Risk (RPAR)*

$$RPAR = 100 * \frac{PAR}{t_{total}}\%$$

3.2 Indices Based on the Regression Model

3.2.1 *The Slope Inequality Index (SII) [53]*

SII is a relative index of inequality because it is based on the association between the health indicator and the relative position with respect to an ordered socioeconomic classification. Once the classes have been ordered (from worst to best) according to the chosen socioeconomic indicator, a regression model is adjusted in which the dependent variable is the health indicator, and the independent variable is the range of the midpoint of each class on a scale between 0 and 1.

If t_i is the value of the health variable and r_i the position of the midpoint of the i-th class in the ordered series of these classes[1], then the SII is defined as the slope β (estimated by the weighted least squares method) of the regression model:

$$t_i = \alpha + \beta * r_i.$$

SII can be interpreted as the difference in rates between the extreme points of the scale that correspond to the values of $r_i = 1$ and $r_i = 0$, which represents the maximum theoretical gap in health. Indeed:

If in the previous expression r_i is replaced by the extreme values of its variation scale, that is, 0 and 1 and then the difference is calculated, the following is obtained:

$$t_{r_i=0} = \alpha, \quad t_{r_i=1} = \alpha + \beta,$$

$$t_{r_i=1} - t_{r_i=0} = \beta.$$

If the t_i are, in effect, rates, the value of β will be negative because the highest rates occur in the groups with the lowest socioeconomic development. If it is a positive health indicator (such as access to services, the value of β will be positive).

SII is not invariant to scale changes in the health variable. If all the rates are multiplied by a constant k, the relative inequality does not change, but the IDP does change, and is multiplied by factor k.

$$kt_i = k\alpha + k\beta * r_i.$$

For this reason, some authors have proposed standardized versions of these indices, which are known as relative indices of inequality:

---

[1] R_i values are known as ridits

3.2.2 The Pamuk Relative Inequality Index ($PRII$) *[50]*

The $PRII$ is defined as:

$$PRII = \frac{SII}{t_{total}},$$

where t_{total} is the overall population rate. Choosing between SII and $PRII$ brings forth the fundamental trade-off between absolute measures and relative measures of inequality. If SII remains constant, relative inequality could increase if the total population rate decreases. This mathematical artifact must be taken into account when evaluating the performance of a health system over time, due to the counterintuitive fact that a decrease in the absolute gap accompanied by a reduction in the overall rate can lead to an increase in relative inequality.

3.2.3 The Kunst and Mackenback Relative Inequality Index (RII_{KM})

Based on the IDP, Kunst and Mackenbach [56] propose the following relative version:

$$RII_{KM} = 1 - \frac{\beta}{t_{r_i=1}},$$

where $t_{r_i=1}$ represents the lowest achievable rate (at the highest end of the socioeconomic hierarchy). The rationality of this index can be better appreciated from the expression

$$RII_{KM} = \frac{\alpha}{\alpha + \beta},$$

which is reached after a minimum algebra in the definition of the RII_{KM}, which is the quotient between the extreme theoretical rates.

SII and RII_{KM} are respectively analogous to the difference and the ratio of extreme rates, but they are based on values estimated from a regression model that takes into account the entire distribution and not only its extremes, thus overcoming a critical shortcoming already noted in indices based on pairwise comparisons.

The three previous indices (SII, $PRII$, IRD_{KM}), particularly the last one, are considered among the best metric options for social inequalities in health. This is due to their properties:

- They explicitly incorporate the socioeconomic dimension of health inequalities.
- They are easy to calculate and interpret.
- They use information for all socioeconomic groups, including their sizes.

These indices can only be used in ordinal classifications such as those generated by income and schooling, or in nominal classifications based on groups characterized and later ordered according to a socioeconomic variable that allows such ordering.

3.3 The Concentration Index (CI)

This index results from comparing two cumulative probability distributions. The categorical variables must be expressed at least on an ordinal scale that allows the construction of a socioeconomic hierarchy.

One of the two cumulative distributions is that of subjects in a population with respect, for example, to a socioeconomic variable; the other, that of a health indicator of interest. The subjects of the first distribution have been previously ordered.

The rationale for the CI is found in the Gini Index, universally used to measure inequalities in income distribution. If the individuals of a population are ordered from poorest to richest on the abscissa axis of a pair of Cartesian axes, the proportion of wealth (goods, resources) accumulated in the lowest strata, given by a curve, known as Lorenz curve, is small and always lies below the bisector of the first quadrant, which corresponds to complete proportionality. The rationality of this index led to its extension to the health field [57–59]. If the cumulative proportion of a health indicator is represented on the ordinate axis, a new Lorenz curve is obtained, which lies below the bisector for positive indicators such as number of vaccinations or access to health services, or above the bisector for negative indicators such as mortality, morbidity and rates of infection.

If from this graphical representation the area between the concentration curve and the diagonal is measured and multiplied by 2, the so-called concentration index is obtained, which takes values between -1 and +1. Normally the concentration curve lies at one side of the diagonal (above or below according to the nature of the health indicator) when there is a monotonous relationship (increasing or decreasing) between the health indicator and the socioeconomic indicator generated by the ordered social hierarchy. If this does not happen, the curve may cross the diagonal, as corresponds to the case in which mortality or morbidity are more frequent at the bottom and at the top of the social scale, and less in the intermediate groups, or to non-linear relationships between the health and the socioeconomic variables.

In data grouped according to socioeconomic classes, the concentration index takes the following form [60]:

$$CI = \frac{2}{t_{total}} \sum_{i=1}^{K} p_i t_i r_i - 1,$$

where K is the number of classes, t_{total} is the overall population rate, t_i is the rate of the i-th class, r_i is the ridit (or average rank) of the i-th class, p_i is the relative size of the i-th class.

The CI and the IDP already exposed can be obtained from each other using the relationship:

$$CI = \frac{2IDP * var(r)}{t_{total}},$$

where $var(r)$ is the variance of the ridits and is given by the expression:

$$var(r) = \sum_{i=1}^{K} p_i \left(r_i - \frac{1}{2} \right)^2 .$$

CI has three fundamental attributes, [53, 61]:

1. It reflects the socioeconomic component of health inequalities.
2. It makes use of the information contained in the whole social hierarchy.
3. It is sensitive to changes, both in the distribution of the health indicator, and in the composition of the population in the groups that make up the socioeconomic scale.

CI is also invariant to changes in scale, that is, if the value of the health indicator in the groups is multiplied by an arbitrary constant $k(k \neq 0)$, the value of the index does not change.

A variant of the CI is the so-called generalized concentration index [62, 63], which is obtained as the product of the CI by the global value of the health indicator in the population (t_{total}).

Despite the good metric properties of the CI [62, 64], its application and interpretation involve some paradoxes, which are not exclusive to this index. One of them is the notion of redistribution, acceptable when it comes to resources or services, but inconceivable in the case of burden of disease. Another, as illustrated by the fictitious example in Tables 1 and 2, if there is a structural relationship - not necessarily unfair - between the health indicator and the stratification criterion, an improvement in global health conditions is always accompanied by a greater concentration in the most vulnerable strata.

4 INDICES FOR NON-ORDERED CATEGORIES

4.1 Indices Based on Pairwise Comparisons

All the definitions, comments, and evaluations already made regarding indices based on pairwisecomparisons in ordinal categories apply to unordered arrangements of classification categories as well.

4.2 Dispersion Indices

These indices reproduce, both formally and conceptually, the notion of variability, essential in the field of Statistics. Despite this intuitive support, they are far from being the most published or the most widely used in practice. In ordered classifications it is preferable to use the indices based on the regression model or the CI.

The indices in this group take into account the entire classification, so they constitute measures of global inequality and not simple pairwise comparisons.

The best known are the Pearcy-Keppel index (PKI), the between groups variance (BGV) and the mean log deviation (MLD).

4.2.1 *Pearcy-Keppel Index* (PKI) *[65]*

$$PKI = \frac{\frac{1}{N}\sum_{i=1}^{N}|t_i - t_{ref}|}{t_{ref}},$$

where N is the number of classes, t_i is the value of the rate in the i-th group, t_{ref} is a reference rate, normally the minimum of the group or class rates[2].

4.2.2 *Between Groups Variance*(BGV) *[66]*

Is defined as:

$$BGV = \sum_{i=1}^{N} W_i(t_i - t_{total})^2,$$

where t_{total} is the global rate of the N groups or classes, t_i is the rate in the i-th group, W_i is the relative size of the i-th class or group (the population of the i-th group divided by the total population).

4.2.3 *Mean Log Deviation* (MLD) *[67]*

It is defined by the expression:

$$MLD = -\sum_{i=1}^{K} W_i\left(\ln(t_i) - \ln(t_{total})\right).$$

Disparity indices do not explicitly incorporate socioeconomic status in their definition. If an arbitrary permutation of the classes is performed, the value of any of these indices does not change.

[2]Other frequent options are the average or global rate or an external reference

If an ordinal socioeconomic indicator like income or schooling is used to define the strata, an indirect link can be obtained. However, for these ordinal rankings, regression-based indices are preferable.

The Pearcy-Keppel index only takes into account the value of the health indicator in the group, and not its size: this implies that small geodemographic strata are assigned the same weight as large strata. The BGV does take into account the size of the stratum. Its worst drawback is that it is not invariant to scale changes [65, 66].

In certain circumstances, however, this property could be an advantage rather than a disadvantage. This occurs when the emphasis is on absolute inequalities, rather than relative ones [66]. Indeed, the relative gap between groups remains invariant if the health indicator is multiplied by a constant k in all groups; however, the absolute gap decreases if $k < 1$, and increases if $k > 1$. From the perspective of its implications in terms of public health, it might be desirable to have an indicator that reflects this fact, and in this case the between groups variance would be a favorable option.

4.3 Indices Based on the Comparison of Two Probability Distributions

In the field of thermodynamics, entropy is a state function that measures the disorder of a physical or chemical system, and therefore its proximity to thermal equilibrium. In information theory, the notion of entropy is used to measure the uniformity in the distribution of information over time [68].

An interesting analogy can be used to construct a measure of inequality. If a disease is uniformly distributed among all classes in a population, there is a maximum entropy, which means that there are no inequalities and that all margin for redistribution has been exhausted.

When inequalities in health conditions decrease, the entropy of the system increases and, conversely. Systems with a high concentration of disease or access to health services are highly redundant systems with a great margin of possibilities to "increase their entropy" or reduce their inequalities. In the field of economics, a system characterized by a high concentration of wealth in some population subgroups, is a redundant system, with a large potential capacity for redistribution [69, 70].

Based on these notions, indicators with good properties have been defined to measure the degree of uniformity (or lack thereof) in the distribution, the burden of disease or access to health services, associated with a classification into social groups [44, 70, 71].

These indicators are based on the comparison of two probability distributions: that of the population in classes given by a socioeconomic variable, and that of their disease burden or their access to resources and services.

The Table 3 represents two probability distributions: that of the population and that of a health variable (available resources or disease burden) in K socioeconomic classes or in K geodemographic units (which may in turn be characterized by a socioeconomic indicator). In each of them, the population is N_i, and the number of patients is S_i[3] so that:

- $N = \sum_{i=1}^{K} N_i$,
- $S = \sum_{i=1}^{K} S_i$,
- $\pi_i = \frac{N_i}{N}$, $P_i = \frac{S_i}{S}$.

The sequences Π_i and S_i are probability functions since

$$\sum_{j=1}^{K} \pi_j = \sum_{j=1}^{K} P_j = 1,$$

and the indices are distances between those functions.

[3]The interpretation of S and SK as the total number of patients in the population and in stratum K, respectively, can be generalized to any non-binary health variable. Argument in terms of a binary variable leads to rates and becomes more intuitive and easy to interpret.

Lessons	Population	Health variable
1	Π_1	Π_2
2	Π_1	Π_2
.	.	.
.	.	.
.	.	.
K	Π_K	P_K
Total	1	1

Table 3: Distribution of the population and disease burden in K groups

4.3.1 *Hoover Index* (HI)

$$HI = \frac{1}{2}\sum_{i=1}^{K} |d_i|,$$

4.3.2 *Theil Index* (THI)

$$HI = \frac{1}{2}\sum_{i=1}^{K} P_i \ln\left(\frac{P_i}{\pi_i}\right),$$

where $d_i = \pi_i - P_i$.

For both indices there are standardized versions that take values in the interval $[0, 1)$

$$Z_{HOOVER} = 1 - \exp(-HI),$$

$$Z_{THEIL} = 1 - \exp(-THI).$$

Indices based on the concept of entropy and distance between distributions lack an explicit link with socioeconomic status. They would take the same value if the strata are ordered in increasing or decreasing order, or if they are assigned a random order. When applied to the study of social inequalities in health, they do not capture the functional relationship between health and socioeconomic conditions (either in an absolute or relative sense), unlike indicators based on regression.

As with several indices to measure inequalities (except those based on direct operations with rates or other health indicators), those based on the notion of entropy are not expressed in known units of measurement, nor do they have a clear-cut interpretation. They are self-referential because there is no reference or threshold of normality that allows making judgments about the magnitude of the inequality that these indices are designed to measure. Its fundamental conditions of application are time comparisons in similar scenarios, or comparisons between different health variables with respect to the same strata, in a single scenario.

The Hoover index has an immediate interpretation in its untransformed expression: the proportion of observations that would have to be redistributed to achieve complete equality. This fact makes it especially applicable to the study of inequalities in the health field, when they refer to access to services or other types of resources. As Schneider and collaborators [53] point out, its application to the analysis of health inequalities, when it comes to negative indicators, such as the classic mortality or morbidity indicators, is questionable because it makes no sense, neither ethically nor practically, to speak of redistributions of illness or death.

The Theil index has several important properties:

1. It is invariant to changes of scale: if the population increases proportionally in all groups or the total burden of disease changes so that the relative burdens of the groups do not change, inequality remains constant [44].

2. It is sensitive to changes in any of the classes or strata and not only in extreme groups [44].

3. Decomposability: The Theil index makes it possible to relate the total inequality in a population with the inequality attributable to social groups, through an additive relationship similar to the one that characterizes the analysis of the variance. If a population P is divided

into k classes, it is possible to show that:

$$THI(total) = THI(\text{“}between\text{''}) + THI(\text{“}within\text{''}).$$

4. In this expression, the term on the left refers to the inequality between all the individuals in the population, which can be deduced from the index formula taking into account that each individual would be a class that represents a population fraction equal to $1/n$, where n is the size of the population in question.

5. On the other hand, THI within groups can be calculated as the weighted average of the THIs of each of the k groups. Normally, the total THI and the THI between groups are calculated by applying the index expression, and the TI within groups is obtained by difference [71, 72][4].

6. The equivalence in entropy: [69] A system of k socioeconomic classes with a level of inequality given by Z (which represents the scaled version $[0, 1]$ of any of the previous indices) can be equated with a system of 2 classes in which one of the classes or strata, which represents $100 * p\%$ of the population, bears $100 * (1 - p)\%$ of the disease burden, while the other, which represents $100 * (1 - p)\%$ bears $100 * p\%$ of the load, where:

$$P = \left(\frac{1}{\pi}\right)\left[\sin^{-1}(1 - Z)^{0.06*Z+0.6}\right].$$

This function is roughly the inverse of:

$$Z = 1 - \left(\frac{1}{1-p}\right)^{2p-1}.$$

7. For example, if $Z_{THEIL} = 0.75$, then $p = 0.13$ (Table 4), which corresponds to a partition into two classes in which 13% of society accumulates 87% of the burden of disease or death

[4]Theil decomposability is applicable at any level of a hierarchical grouping. For example, if the units of analysis are municipalities, and these are grouped into provinces, it is possible to calculate total inequality as the sum of inequality between provinces + inequality within provinces. The latter would be an inequality between municipalities.

(or 87% of health resources), while the remaining 87% accumulates 13% of the burden of disease or death (or 13% of health resources). If $Z_{THEIL} = 0.00$, then $p = 0.50$ and this is equivalent to the complete equality of a society of two classes of equal size in which each bears 50% of the burden of disease or death or owns 50% of the resources. The Table 4 below shows several examples of this equivalence relation in the sense of entropy.

Z index	Transformation p	Equivalence in entropy		Redistribution potential
0	0.5	50	50	0%
		50	50	
0.14	0.36	64	36	14%
		36	64	
0.29	0.30	70	30	20%
		30	70	
0.44	0.24	76	24	26%
		24	76	
0.50	0.22	78	22	28%
		22	78	
0.56	0.20	80	20	30%
		20	80	
0.75	0.13	87	13	37%
		13	87	

Table 4: Entropy equivalence and redistribution potential to eliminate inequality

As the value of Z increases, the distribution becomes more unequal and its redistribution potential increases. A system of socioeconomic classes with an inequality of $Z = 0.56$ (see Table 4) needs a 30% redistribution to eliminate inequality, because the existing level of inequality corresponds to a distribution in which 20% of the population supports 80% of the burden of disease or death (or owns 80% of the resources), while the remaining 80% only experiences 20% of the burden of disease or death (or owns 20% of the resources).

4.4 Options in Measuring Social Inequalities in Relation to Health

Health indicators and stratification criteria are determined by the context, the objectives and the perspective assumed in the face of social inequalities. In the current scenario of a global pandemic of a new coronavirus, the health indicators are, on a negative plane, those that express the levels of transmission and reproduction of the virus, its incidence, and its lethality, and on a positive plane, the health services available, beds in intensive care units, and percentages of the vaccinated population, just to mention a few obvious examples, of both kinds. The stratification criteria can be countries, provinces, communities or regions within countries, ethnic groups, strata according to their migratory status, income quintiles or quartiles, educational level, occupation and others. The taxonomy described in the previous section shows a non-exhaustive, but basic, repertoire of the main and most used indices in the literature and practical applications. The objectives are always linked to highlighting the variability of health indicators between population groups, as a basis for the design of health programs and policies, under the principle of the right to health and the concept that the performance of a system must be measured by both its global health indicators, and the magnitude of health disparities.

Another important choice is to assume a descriptive or an analytical perspective. In the current situation of a global pandemic, which has generated an unprecedented volume of clinical, epidemiological, and basic information and research, often contradictory, and which has stimulated the convergence between science and policy as never before, although not always under optimal conditions of harmony, the perspective is fundamentally descriptive, in order to document the existence of inequalities, rather than explain the processes that generate them.

The choice of one or more indices, which, as we have already commented, is not only technical but also axiological and practical, is crucial, but is not the only one. Other trade-offs, related or not to the selection of the indices, are equally important and briefly discussed below.

4.4.1 How to Choose a Value for the Comparison or Reference Group?

Let us consider k strata (for example, geodemographic units such as municipalities, provinces or countries, income deciles or education levels), and a health variable that characterizes each class.

Normally each group in the classification is compared with a referent. The most common options are the following:

- The population average. It does not refer to any particular group but to the average value of the health variable in the population. The absence of inequality would be given by a zero variance, which would occur only if the health variable took the same value in all groups. For negative indicators such as mortality, morbidity or disease burden, it is not possible to reduce inequality without changing the population health level. Positive indicators such as health services (eg hospital beds, medical personnel or immunizations) can yield less unequal distributions without changing average population levels. Anti-COVID-19 vaccines can be more equally distributed between countries and between population strata within countries. In those cases the population average is a reasonable reference.

- The average of all the groups better than the group in question. With respect to the population average, this option has two advantages. The first is that it does not include the group that is being compared. The second is that the difference represents a gap to be eliminated in order to reduce inequality. In order to describe the trends of a specific group of the population and set goals on an objective basis, the choice of the whole population in a better situation than the group in question may be a preferable option to the population average, because it combines a tendency to reduce the gaps and to improve the population's health indicators.

- The best of the groups. Using the best of groups as a reference implies assuming that all groups in society have the potential to achieve their indicators. If the groups could be characterized by a socioeconomic variable (such as the income deciles, or the average income of the people who make up the group), it could happen that "the best group" in relation to the health indicators, does not coincide with the best group with respect to the socioeconomic variable. When the ordering criterion has a rank correlation unequal to 1 with the health-based criterion, the difference from the best socioeconomic group may underestimate the true magnitude of health inequality. On the other hand, the best group may have a small relative size with respect to the rest, thus the estimates of inequality are unstable, especially when one wishes to describe trends. In practice, however, this is the most common option.

- A fixed external reference. This option gives greater stability to the measurement, particularly in trend studies and when pairwise comparisons are used, but it is contrary to the intuitive idea of inequality as something typical of an internal measurement context.

The dilemma of choosing a reference group occurs mainly in measures based on pairwise comparisons, but it is not exclusive to this type of measure. The most frequent choice is the best group, probably because it corresponds to the epidemiological practice based on the risk ratio with respect to the category to which the lowest risk is associated a priori. For example, in the case of income, an extreme upper percentile of the distribution[5]; in the case of schooling, the college class.

As in all cases, the choice relies on value judgments, whether or not these judgments are made explicit. For example, if any inequality in health levels associated with income is assumed to be unfair and unacceptable, the only consequent reference would be precisely the group with the highest income, and inequality would be eliminated only when the difference with respect to this group was zero, or the quotient was one.

4.4.2 What Variables Should Be Used as Stratification Criteria?

The predominant trend is contextual and subordinated to political ends or value judgments. In some countries the preferred classification criteria are ethnicity or race, gender, urban or rural

[5]Usually the first quintile, the first quartile, or the first decile.

status, and income, while in others occupation and education are used more frequently [61, 73–76]. The choice is usually guided by those criteria that are a priori assumed to exhibit the greatest health gaps. The measurement of inequalities, as part of the evaluation of health systems, has the purpose of highlighting a problem in order to make it visible. For this reason, more than inequalities in relation to health, per se, and their trends, what matters is their covariation with social condition, that can take its maximum values in relation to unusual stratification criteria (for example, regions within a country, native population vs migrants) or latent or non-explicit dimensions of inequality, in which the stratification criterion is a social construct that cannot be directly measured. In practical terms, feasibility is often the determining factor. In the case of inequalities associated with COVID-19, it is understandable that for a long time the approach will be essentially exploratory. It is very common to hear that the pandemic does not recognize classes or social strata, but in one way or another, as in any other health contexts COVID-19 is not immune to the influence of social, economic and cultural factors associated with greater vulnerability, a poorer perception of risk or a lack of access to quality health services.

4.4.3 Are Only Extreme Groups Used or All Groups in the Set?

In any measurement context with k $(k > 2)$ classes, it is always desirable that the inequality measure includes the information contained in all groups. Metrics based on pairwise comparisons, including, for example, only extreme groups, can hide important sources of inequality. The distortion is even greater when groups are unrepresentative, particularly in terms of their population sizes. However, this does not imply disregarding certain specific groups that may have a special meaning when it comes to inequality. This is the case, for example, of marginal groups or geodemographic units with manifest deterioration in health indicators with respect to the rest of the population, whether or not they are representative in terms of the size of their populations.

4.4.4 Is It Important to Weight Classes by Size?

A key question is: should class size be included in the construction of an inequality metric? Some of the best known inequality measures assign identical weights to classes [50]. Again, a value judgment seems to be implicit in the choice of a measure that pays or does not pay attention to the size of the groups. For some, the relative health indicators of a population group or class matter regardless of its size, that is, of the number of people who are exposed to the conditions that prevail in that group. However, it is completely counterintuitive, for example,that the rate ratio between extreme groups in the hierarchy is equally important when the group with the worst rate has twice the population as the group with the best rate, than when the exact opposite happens. From the perspective of their variations over time and their trends, a positive change is not only achieved by reducing the gaps between mortality or morbidity rates, but also by modifying the relative proportions of people exposed to the adverse situation generated, not only poor health conditions, but also by inequalities themselves.

4.4.5 Positive Polarity or Negative Polarity?

A dilemma that is rarely considered as a methodological choice is that of the event that is chosen within a dichotomy for the calculation of the indices. In evaluations of the inequality trend, these options are decisive in judging a change as favorable or unfavorable. In calculating the ratio of rates, although not only in calculating this index, the problem is particularly clear, because every dichotomy, whether it is a positive or a negative indicator, raises such a choice.

Having access to vaccination is a positive event, and dying from a complication, a negative event, but their respective complementary events (not having access to the vaccine or surviving the complication) are just the opposite. Table 5 illustrates this almost unrecognized dilemma in a fictitious example of comparison of Spanish-speakers vs. indigenous population.

Access to vaccination has increased between T_0 and T_1, both in the Spanish-speaking population and in the indigenous population, in the former from 43.1% to 90.9%; in seconds from

35.1% to 88.2%.

Time	Without to vaccination (%)		With acces (%)		Ratio	
	Indigenous population	Spanish speaker	Indigenous Population	Spanish speaker	No access	With access
T_0	64.9	56.9	35.1	43.1	1.14	0.81
T_1	11.8	9.1	88.2	90.9	1.30	0.97

Table 5: Changes in the rate quotient according to polarity

To evaluate the change in the gap between Spanish-speakers and indigenous people over time, what event should be considered: (a) access to vaccination or (b) its complementary event, lack of access? If we consider the lack of access, the relative gap between both subpopulations has grown from 1.14 (64.9 / 56.9) to 1.30 (11.8 / 9.1). However, if we consider access, the gap has narrowed from 0.81 to 0.97. Note, of course, that in the latter case, the gap narrows because the quotient approaches 1.

The usual practice is to always consider the negative side of the event, whatever its polarity.

5 COVID-19 AND INEQUALITIES. SOME SELECTED RESULTS

In the first part of the chapter, three levels were mentioned in which the link between COVID-19 and inequalities is manifested. One is the impact of socioeconomic inequalities on the indicators of incidence, mortality, lethality, levels of contagion, and access to vaccination and other health services. The corresponding question is: do societies with greater socioeconomic gaps have worse indicators? Another, its converse, is the impact that the pandemic could have on the increase in these inequalities through a complex mechanism mediated, among other factors, by the unequal distribution of employment and of family and social loads. The corresponding question is: Have social inequalities increased in the course of, or as a consequence of the pandemic? These two topics are supported by a good number of publications [77, 78]. Although these topics are of great interest, in an initial, essential and basic chapter like this one, we will focus on the uneven distribution of the indicators associated with COVID-19, according to socioeconomic or sociodemographic strata. The question corresponding to this plane of inquiry on social inequalities in health is: are the health indicators X, Y, Z..., distributed homogeneously according to the stratification criteria A, B, C...? We will focus our considerations on the uneven distribution of the indicators associated with COVID-19, according to socioeconomic or sociodemographic strata.

In what follows, several results are presented, some of them derived from public on-line access to information and others taken from the recent literature on the subject.

Example Table 24 in the Appendix shows the approximate population in 2020, the percentage of the vaccinated population until March 22, 2021, and the GDP per capita according to IMF data from September 30, 2020, in 17 Latin American countries with available information for all three variables. A critical look at these data and the application of the indices of the typology presented in the first part of this text yields the following:

There is a high linear correlation coefficient between both variables of 0.59. Chile and Venezuela are clearly two atypical countries in the group. Until the day we took as a reference, Chile had vaccinated a proportion 5 times greater than Uruguay, which is the country that followed in the hierarchy ordered by percentage of vaccination. Similarly, Venezuela had vaccinated 5 times fewer cases than Paraguay, the country that preceded it in the orderly hierarchy. The decision to maintain or eliminate these outliers from the set has a clear impact on the computation of several of the inequality indices and is always an important first step in the analysis. The first thing that stands out is the increase in the correlation coefficient from 0.59 to 0.86, if these two countries are not included in the calculation.

A notable change can be seen, both in the ratios and in the differences, when the outliers are eliminated. In both cases, the countries have been ordered according to the health variable, without taking into account the GDP per capita. Both the ratios and the weighted differences increase when the country has a larger population than the reference (Chile in Table 6 and Uruguay in Table 7). If the socioeconomic variable is taken into account and the countries are ordered according to that variable, the results are as follows (see Table 8).

Group	Quotient	Weighted ratio	Difference	Weighted difference
Chile	1,000	1,000	0,000	0,000
Uruguay	0,203	0,037	35,330	6,473
Panama	0,162	0,036	37,140	8,204
Argentina	0,156	0,336	37,410	87,818
Brazil	0,144	1,577	37,930	415,332
Dominican Rep.	0,140	0,076	38,090	20,602
Costa Rica	0,110	0,029	39,440	10,425
Mexico	0,098	0,469	39,960	264,114
Colombia	0,052	0,133	41,990	106,763
Peru	0,043	0,072	42,420	71,239
Bolivia	0,032	0,019	42,880	25,702
Ecuador	0,017	0,016	43,550	39,394
Honduras	0,010	0,005	43,880	21,059
Guatemala	0,009	0,008	43,930	38,633
Paraguay	0,005	0,002	44,100	16,511
Venezuela	0,001	0,002	44,270	74,599

Table 6: Pairwise comparisons (ratios, weighted ratios, differences and weighted differences) taking Chile as the reference group. Weighted differences are expressed as absolute values

It can be clearly seen that the calculation of the ratio and the difference in rates underestimates the magnitude of the health gap, but guarantees the necessary link with the socioeconomic dimension, which provides the condition of social inequality in health, and not simply health inequality. The percentage of people vaccinated to date, which has been taken as a reference in the countries of the lowest quintile of GDP per capita, was just over 10% (10.6%) of that of the

Group	Quotient	Weighted ratio	Difference	Weighted difference
Uruguay	1,000	1,000	0,000	0,000
Panama	0,798	0,963	1,810	2,182
Argentina	0,768	9,845	2,080	26,652
Brazil	0,710	42,464	2,600	155,401
Dominican Rep.	0,693	2,045	2,760	8,148
Costa Rica	0,542	0,782	4,110	5,930
Mexico	0,484	17,478	4,630	167,057
Colombia	0,258	3,586	6,660	92,431
Peru	0,210	1,929	7,090	64,993
Bolivia	0,159	0,521	7,550	24,702
Ecuador	0,085	0,418	8,220	40,587
Honduras	0,048	0,125	8,550	22,397
Guatemala	0,042	0,203	8,600	41,282
Paraguay	0,023	0,048	8,770	17,923

Table 7: Pairwise comparisons (ratios, weighted ratios, differences and weighted differences) taking Uruguay as the reference group. Weighted differences are expressed as absolute values

Index	% of vaccination
Extreme rate ratio	0.106
Weighted ratio of extreme rates	0.309
Extreme rate difference	6.043
Weighted difference of extreme rates	17.708

Table 8: Extreme rate ratios and differences (weighted and unweighted) for countries ordered according to income quintiles

countries of the highest quintile (see Table 9).

Group	Ratio	Weighted ratio	Difference	Weighted difference
Paraguay	0.023	0.048	8.770	17.923
Guatemala	0.042	0.203	8.600	41.282
Honduras	0.048	0.125	8.550	22.397
Ecuador	0.085	0.418	8.220	40.587
Bolivia	0.159	0.521	7.550	24.702
Peru	0.210	1.929	7.090	64.993
Colombia	0.258	3.586	6.660	92.431
Mexico	0.484	17.478	4.630	167.057
Costa Rica	0.542	0.782	4.110	5.930
Dominican Rep.	0.693	2.045	2.760	8.148
Brazil	0.710	42.464	2.600	155.401
Argentina	0.768	9.845	2.080	26.652
Panama	0.798	0.963	1.810	2.182
Uruguay	1.000	1.000	0.000	0.000

Table 9: Ratios and differences (weighted and unweighted) taking as a reference the country with the highest GDP per capita. Weighted differences are expressed as absolute values

If Uruguay is taken as a benchmark (the country with the highest GDP per capita, in addition to having the highest vaccination rate after eliminating the atypical case of Chile), the values of both ratios and differences are more extreme than when countries are grouped by quintiles.

Let us now look at the indices for groups ordered according to GDP per capita, based on the regression model (see Table 10 and Fig. 1).

The theoretical difference of extreme percentages of vaccination calculated according to the

Index	% of vaccination
Slope inequality index	4.187
Relative index of inequality	0.893
Kunst and Mackenbach Relative Inequality Index	1.618

Table 10: Indices based on the regression model

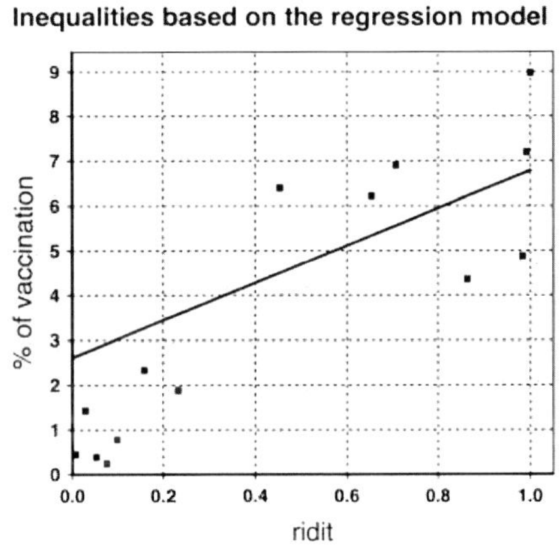

Figure 1: Inequalities based on the regression model

regression model is 4.187, which is obtained by subtracting the value of the intersection of the line at 0 from the value of the intersection at 1, the theoretical limits of the ridits, already defined as a cumulative proportion of the population. This is a difference adjusted by the model, and it takes into account all countries and not only those located at the extremes of the hierarchy. If this difference is expressed in relative terms, as a proportion of the global percentage of people vaccinated in all countries, the value is 0.893. This global percentage is obtained as a weighted average of countries, taking their respective populations as a weighting factor.

Similarly, the extreme percentage ratio adjusted by the model is 1.618 and is represented by the Kunst and Mackenbach index.

The dispersion indices, close to the notion of variance in descriptive statistics, ignore the link with the socioeconomic dimension. They are shown in Tables 11 and 12 and obviously yield very different values depending on whether or not the outliers are included.

Index	% of vaccination
Pearcy-Keppel index	0.581
Weighted Pearcy-Keppel index	1.816
Mean logarithmic deviation	0.211
Variance between groups	4.544

Table 11: Indices based on the notion of dispersion (the extreme values of Chile and Venezuela are excluded)

Index	% of vaccination
Pearcy-Keppel index	0.943
Weighted Pearcy-Keppel index	3.200
Mean logarithmic deviation	0.574
Variance between groups	54.505

Table 12: Indices based on the notion of dispersion (includes the 17 countries)

To finish the analysis of the data in Table 25 of the Annex, the indices based on the distance between the probability distributions of the populations and that of the proportions of vaccinated cases are finally calculated. As already commented in the first part of the chapter, these indices do not take into account the link with the socioeconomic variable. They are included in this text because of the appeal of the notion of entropy equivalence.

The distribution of vaccination percentages is uneven, much more if outliers are included. In this case (Table 13), according to the Theil Index, the distribution of the health variable among the 17 countries would be analogous (in terms of entropy) to one composed of two groups in which, in one group with 73% of the population there are 27% of people vaccinated, and in the other group, with 27% of the population there are 73% of people vaccinated. If Chile and Venezuela are excluded, the distribution becomes more homogeneous (Table 14).

Index	% of vaccination
Kullback-Lieber index	0.258
Hoover index (or dissimilarities)	0.318
Theil index	0.271

Table 13: Entropy equivalence (includes all 17 countries)

Index	% of vaccination
Kullback-Lieber index	0.357
Hoover index (or dissimilarities)	0.348
Theil index	0.375

Table 14: Entropy equivalence (the two countries with extreme values are excluded)

Example Table 24, in the Appendix, shows the percentage of tests performed and the percentage of positive tests for COVID-19 in the week of October 10-19, 2020, chosen haphazardly from a public database. The data for this example also include the proportion of people at risk of poverty and the human development index, as well as the population size of the Spanish communities.

Next, several indices of the typology presented in the first part are applied and the results are analyzed.

The ratio of the percentages of tests carried out in the poorest quintile (with the highest proportion of people at risk of poverty) and the richest quintile is 0.419. Since the size of the population in the worst quintile is also larger, the weighted ratio is higher than the unweighted ratio. The same occurs with the difference and the weighted difference in rates (see Table 15).

Index	Testing rate
Extreme rate ratio	0.419
Weighted ratio of extreme rates	0.730
Extreme rate difference	-15.960
Weighted difference of extreme rates	-27.830

Table 15: Ratios and extreme rate differences (weighted and unweighted) for countries ordered according to income quintiles. Health variable: test rates. Socioeconomic variable: population at risk of poverty

The percentage of positive tests is almost 25% higher in the quintile that corresponds to the communities with the highest risk of poverty (ratio of rates = 1.25). The weighted difference is 5.636 percentage points (see Table 16).

Index	Positivity (%)
Extreme rate ratio	12.249
Weighted ratio of extreme rates	2.178
Extreme rate difference	3.233
Weighted difference of extreme rates	5.636

Table 16: Ratios and extreme rate differences (weighted and unweighted) for countries ordered according to income quintiles. Health variable: test positivity rates. Socioeconomic variable: population at risk of poverty

Obviously, the comparison between the extremes of the hierarchy, both in terms of difference and ratio, yields lower values if the communities are grouped by quintiles (or any other percentile) than when the entire hierarchy is considered. For example, the ratios between Ceuta and Navarra (the communities that occupy the extremes of the hierarchy in relation to the population at risk of poverty), for the percentage of tests carried out and for the positivity of the tests are 0.16 (6.24 / 40.22) and 1.82 (26.57 / 14.6), respectively.

Let us now consider the Concentration Index, with respect to the Human Development Index (see Fig. 2 and Table 17):

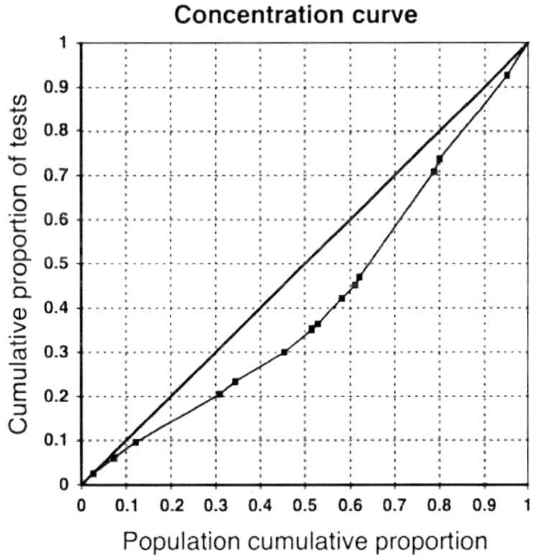

Figure 2: Concentration curve

	Testing rate
Concentration index	0.176

Table 17: Concentration Index for testing rate in Fig. 2

The concentration curve is located below the main diagonal as an expression of the fact that the communities with the lowest HDI carry out a lower proportion of tests. By convention, values below the diagonal have a positive sign and values above it have a negative sign. The CI can vary between -1 and +1, but its values are self-referential, that is, they are always used for a comparative purpose to evaluate changes over time or differences with respect to other stratification criteria.

If we consider the concentration of positivity with respect to the HDI, we obtain the following results (see Fig. 3 and Table 18):

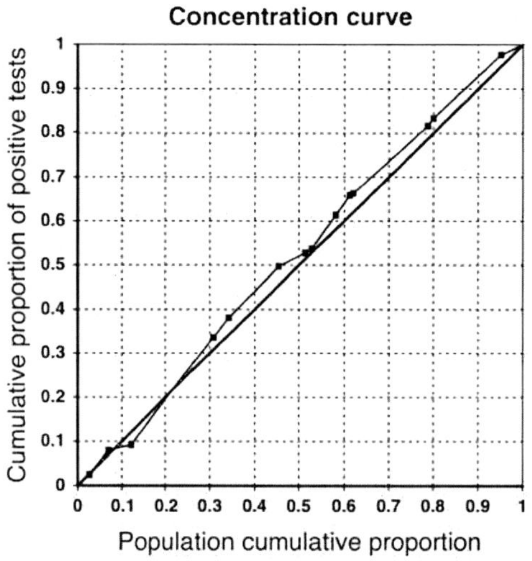

Figure 3: Concentration curve

	Positivity (%)
Concentration index	-0.036

Table 18: Concentration Index for positivity in Fig. 3

Now the index is negative, because the curve is located, albeit slightly, above the main diagonal.

Communities with lower HDI tend to have higher percentages of positivity in tests, although the association is clearly very weak (CI close to 0).

If the link with any of the socioeconomic indicators is ignored and, for example, the Theil index is applied to compare the probability distributions of the health indicators with the population, the entropy equivalence yields the following result (see Table 19):

Index	Testing rate	Positivity (%)
Theil index	0.406	0.420

Table 19: Theil indices for testing rate and positivity

For the test rate, the inequality between Spanish communities is equivalent to that of a society in which 40.6% of the population performs 59.4% of the tests, and 59.4% of the population performs 40.6% of the tests. This implies a redistributive potential of approximately 10% in the tests carried out in the country to achieve full equality. The same interpretation makes little sense for the positivity of the tests, which is not a distributable concept, without changing the population rates.

Finally, the dispersion indices, which ignore the link with the socioeconomic dimension, yield the following results (see Table 20):

Index	Testing rate	Positivity (%)
Pearcy-Keppel index	0.391	0.393
Mean logarithmic deviation	0.074	0.064
Between groups variance	51.469	15.624

Table 20: Dispersion indices for testing rate and positivity

The dispersion of both indicators is equivalent for the PKI and the MLD, but it is greater for the test rate that takes into account the population size of the communities.

Several examples from recent publications are considered in what follows. The first one refers to inequalities associated with skin color and is based on the use of the ratio of incidence and fatality rates, stratified according to poverty conditions in metropolitan areas of 10 large North American cities, which together represented 63.5% of all confirmed cases in the United States as of May 10, 2020, [79]. The study is not limited to measurement, but includes analysis and some simple estimates and inferences using confidence intervals.

The ethnic composition of metropolitan counties has a significant influence on the cumulative incidence, and greater or lesser poverty modifies this influence. If the group of predominantly white counties is taken as a reference, the rate ratio is 7.8 times higher in the mostly non-white counties, in the stratum of the poorest counties, and 2.8 times higher in those with the lowest poverty levels. Poverty acts much more as a modifier of the effect of ethnic composition than as a factor associated with a higher risk of infection (see Table 21).

Counties	**Cumulative incidence of infections per 100 000 residents**			
	Adjusted rates		**Rate ratio (95%)**	
	Counties with less poverty	**Poorest counties**	**Counties with less poverty**	**Poorest counties**
Mainly white	169.3	84.7	1 (Referrer)	1 (Referrer)
With less diversity	321.7	321.7	1.9 (1.4-2.6)	3.8 (2.3-6.1)
With greater diversity	541.8	433.4	3.2 (2.3-4.6)	5.1 (3.3-8.0)
Fundamentally not white	474.0	663.7	2.8 (1.8-4.4)	7.8 (5.1-12.0)

Table 21: Expected rates and ratio of cumulative incidence rates by type of county and poverty level (rates adjusted by models). Adapted from: Adhikari S, Pantaleo N, Feldman J, Olugbenga O, Thorpe L, Troxel A. Assessment of Community-Level Disparities in Coronavirus Disease 2019 (COVID-19). Infections and Deaths in Large US Metropolitan Areas. JAMA Network Open. 2020; 3 (7): e2016938. doi: 10.1001 / jamanetworkopen.2020.16938. [79]

Something very similar happens in relation to mortality. Poverty modifies the rate ratio. The gap between primarily white counties and primarily non-white counties is much larger among counties with high levels of poverty (see Table 22).

Counties	**Cumulative mortality per 100 000 residents**			
	Adjusted rates		**Rate ratio (95% CI)**	
	Counties with less poverty	**Poorest counties**	**Counties with less poverty**	**Poorest counties**
Mainly white	8.2	3.3	1 (Referrer)	1 (Referrer)
With less diversity	14.8	15.4	1.8 (1.1-3.0)	4.7 (2.2-10.0)
With greater diversity	31.2	16.2	3.8 (2.2-6.7)	4.9 (2.4-9.7)
Fundamentally not white	21.3	30.7	2.6 (1.1-6.5)	9.3 (4.7-18.4)

Table 22: Expected rates and ratio of accumulated mortality rates by type of county and poverty level (rates adjusted by models). Adapted from: Adhikari S, Pantaleo N, Feldman J, Olugbenga O, Thorpe L, Troxel A. Assessment of Community-Level Disparities in Coronavirus Disease 2019 (COVID-19). Infections and Deaths in Large US Metropolitan Areas. JAMA Network Open. 2020; 3 (7): e2016938. doi: 10.1001 / jamanetworkopen.2020.16938, [79]

In a study on social inequities in relation to the progression of COVID-19 in Mexico [80], the following percentages of death, hospitalization and intubation or admission to intensive care units are reported according to sociodemographic and clinical indicators, of which only the former are of interest to this text and are summarized in the following Table 23.

For data of this nature, rate ratios are the simplest and most eloquent indices of inequality. For any of the three destinations (death, hospitalization or intubation / admission to the ICU) the risk of indigenous people is higher; something similar happens with people in the lowest quartile of marginalization. The risk of death is lower for the population that uses private services, although the frequency of hospitalization in intensive care units is much higher than the rest of the population, whether it is the open population or the population receiving social security.

	Death (%)	**Hospitalization (%)**	**Int-UCI (%)**
Indigenous			
Do not	13.4	31.2	4.2
Yes	19.9	39.6	7.0
Municipal marginalization (quartiles)			
I	12.1	28.5	3.7
II	14.1	32.4	3.7
III	13.3	30.6	4.3
IV	14.3	33.3	5.2
Institution			
Social security	20.6	43.8	3.1
Open population	8.2	21.3	4.8
Private services	6.3	31.1	9.9

Table 23: Prevalence of severity indicators according to sociodemographic characteristics in Mexican adults infected by SARS-CoV2. Adapted from: Ortiz-Hernández L, Pérez-Sastre MA. Social inequities in the progression of COVID-19 in the Mexican population. Rev Panam Salud Pública 2020; 44: e106. https://doi.org/10.26633/RPSP:2020.106. [80]

6 CONCLUDING REMARKS

The measurement of social inequalities in health is an indispensable task in evaluating the performance of health systems. The components of the measurement are health indicators, stratification factors, and inequality indices. The choice does not rest only on technical criteria, but also on value judgments, the first of which involves distinguishing simple inequalities from unjust, systematic and avoidable inequalities, or inequities. Within a wide repertoire of metric options, the simplicity of calculation and interpretation, the inclusion of the socioeconomic dimension, the inclusion of the entire population hierarchy and of the population's composition together with the health indicators, are relevant attributes.

The current COVID-19 pandemic shows large imbalances and gaps that are and will be the subject of study for a long time. Inequalities are not only manifested between countries, but also within countries. Although the virus does not recognize social classes, those with greater risk perception and with access to quality health services will feel less the impact of the pandemic than those located in the lower strata of the socioeconomic hierarchy.

Although it is not the objective of this study, the gaps in gender, occupation, and other population stratifications associated with socioeconomic and sociocultural status will tend to increase as a consequence of the pandemic, not only as an expression of different degrees of exposure, but also of different levels of vulnerability.

7 CONSENT FOR PUBLICATION

Not applicable.

8 CONFLICT OF INTEREST

The authors declare no conflict of interest, financial or otherwise.

9 ACKNOWLEDGEMENTS

To Dr. Andrés Fraguela, who understood the importance of inequalities associated to this pandemic, and had the kindness of inviting us to participate.

APPENDIX

Countries	% of vaccination	GDP per capita
Chile	44.31	15850
Uruguay	8.98	17820
Panama	7.17	17150
Argentina	6.9	9730
Brazil	6.38	8960
Dominican Republic	6.22	9190
Costa Rica	4.87	12690
Mexico	4.35	10410
Colombia	2.32	6740
Peru	1.89	7320
Bolivia	1.43	3860
Ecuador	0.76	6250
Honduras	0.43	2590
Guatemala	0.38	4810
Paraguay	0.21	5900
Venezuela	0.04	2430

Table 24: Vaccination percentages and GDP per capita of 17 Latin American countries with available data. Data updated to March 22, 2021

CCAA	Population	Poverty Risk	HDI	Tests done (%)	Positivity (%)
Ceuta	84500	40.6	0.847	6.24	26.57
Melilla	84400	35.7	0.871	13.65	28.21
Extremadura	1062900	31.5	0.853	18.87	12.1
Andalucía	8448200	31.3	0.862	10.59	16.5
Canarias	2220100	28.5	0.861	13.73	3.37
Murcia	1495100	27.7	0.873	15.62	16.38
Castilla La Mancha	2038700	26.2	0.859	13.91	15.01
Comunidad Valenciana	4999400	23.7	0.882	10.95	13.23
Asturias	102000	20.7	0.887	24.63	6.59
Galicia	2698900	20.0	0.886	14.92	7.01
Aragón	1324300	17.9	0.898	19.08	20.06
Cantabria	581900	17.3	0.89	15.75	8.84
Madrid	6686400	15.0	0.917	23.49	12.41
Cataluña	7609900	13.9	0.906	25.70	11.65
Castilla y León	2402700	12.9	0.894	20.04	18.15
La Rioja	314400	12.3	0.902	43.91	7.9
País Vasco	2181900	10	0.922	29.41	7.52
Navarra	652500	7.7	0.913	40.22	14.6

Table 25: Socioeconomic variables: Population percentage at risk of poverty, and Human Development Index (HDI)

References

[1] Genomewide Association Study of Severe Covid-19 with Respiratory Failure. New England Journal of Medicine [Internet]. 2020 Oct 15 [cited Sep 29, 2021];383(16):1522–34. Available from: https://doi.org/10.1056/nejmoa2020283

[2] Zarocostas J. How to fight an infodemic. The Lancet [Internet]. 2020 Feb [cited Sep 29, 2021];395(10225):676. Available from: https://doi.org/10.1016/s0140-6736(20)30461-x

[3] El impacto del COVID-19 en América Latina y el Caribe [Internet]. [place unknown]: United Nations Publications; 2020 Jul [cited Sep 29, 2021]. Available from: https://doi.org/10.18356/2d5a2103-es

[4] ONU, Constitution of the World Health Organization, Forty-fifth edition, Supplement, Oct. 2006, Available from: www.who.int/governance/eb/who_constitution_en.pdf

[5] Jadad AR, O'Grady L. How should health be defined? BMJ [Internet]. 2008 Dec 10 [cited Sep 29, 2021];337(dec10 1):a2900. Available from: https://doi.org/10.1136/bmj.a2900

[6] The Lancet. What is health? The ability to adapt. The Lancet [Internet]. 2009 Mar [cited

Sep 29, 2021];373(9666):781. Available from: https://doi.org/10.1016/s0140-6736(09)60456-6

[7] Godlee F. What is health? BMJ [Internet]. 2011 Jul 27 [cited Sep 29, 2021];343(jul27 2):d4817. Available from: https://doi.org/10.1136/bmj.d4817

[8] Huber M, Knottnerus JA, Green L, Horst HV, Jadad AR, Kromhout D, Leonard B, Lorig K, Loureiro MI, Meer JW, Schnabel P, Smith R, Weel CV, Smid H. How should we define health? BMJ [Internet]. 2011 Jul 26 [cited Sep 29, 2021];343(jul26 2):d4163. Available from: https://doi.org/10.1136/bmj.d4163

[9] Young TK. Population health: Concepts and methods. New York: Oxford University Press; 1998. 315 p.

[10] Hertzman C, Power C, Matthews S, Manor O. Using an interactive framework of society and lifecourse to explain self-rated health in early adulthood. Social Science & Medicine [Internet]. 2001 Dec [cited Sep 29, 2021];53(12):1575–85. Available from: https://doi.org/10.1016/s0277-9536(00)00437-8

[11] Singer BH, Ryff CD (eds), New horizons in health: An integrative approach, Washington DC, National Academy Press, 2001.

[12] Halfon N, Hochstein M. Life Course Health Development: An Integrated Framework for Developing Health, Policy, and Research. Milbank Quarterly [Internet]. 2002 Sep [cited Sep 29, 2021];80(3):433–79. Available from: https://doi.org/10.1111/1468-0009.00019

[13] Sampson RJ, Raudenbush SW. Seeing Disorder: Neighborhood Stigma and the Social Construction of "Broken Windows". Social Psychology Quarterly [Internet]. 2004 Dec [cited Sep 29, 2021];67(4):319–42. Available from: https://doi.org/10.1177/019027250406700401

[14] From neurons to neighborhoods: The science of early child development. Washington, D.C: National Academy Press; 2000. 588 p.

[15] Kuh D, Ben-Shlomo Y. A life course approach to obesity. In: A Life Course Approach to Chronic Disease Epidemiology [Internet]. [place unknown]: Oxford University Press; 2004 [cited Sep 29, 2021]. p. 189–217. Available from: https://doi.org/10.1093/acprof:oso/9780198578154.003.0008

[16] Pollitt RA, Kaufman JS, Rose KM, Diez-Roux AV, Zeng D, Heiss G. Early-life and adult socioeconomic status and inflammatory risk markers in adulthood. European Journal of Epidemiology [Internet]. 2007 Jan [cited Sep 29, 2021];22(1):55–66. Available from: https://doi.org/10.1007/s10654-006-9082-1

[17] McEwen BS. Protective and Damaging Effects of Stress Mediators. New England Journal of Medicine [Internet]. 1998 Jan 15 [cited Sep 29, 2021];338(3):171–9. Available from: https://doi.org/10.1056/nejm199801153380307

[18] Chen E, Paterson LQ. Neighborhood, family, and subjective socioeconomic status: How do they relate to adolescent health? Health Psychology [Internet]. 2006 Nov [cited Sep 29, 2021];25(6):704–14. Available from: https://doi.org/10.1037/0278-6133.25.6.704

[19] Gunnar MR, Vázquez DM. Low cortisol and a flattening of expected daytime rhythm: Potential indices of risk in human development. Development and Psychopathology [Internet]. 2001 Sep [cited Sep 29, 2021];13(3):515–38. Available from: https://doi.org/10.1017/s0954579401003066

[20] Geronimus AT, Hicken M, Keene D, Bound J. "Weathering" and Age Patterns of Allostatic Load Scores Among Blacks and Whites in the United States. American Journal of Public

Health [Internet]. 2006 May [cited Sep 29, 2021];96(5):826–33. Available from: https://doi.org/10.2105/ajph.2004.060749

[21] Link BG, Phelan J. Social Conditions As Fundamental Causes of Disease. Journal of Health and Social Behavior [Internet]. 1995 [cited Sep 29, 2021];35:80. Available from: https://doi.org/10.2307/2626958

[22] Sampson RJ, The neighborhood context of investing in children, in Securing the future: investing in children from birth to college, Danziger S, Waldfogel J. (Eds), New York, Russell Sage Foundation, 2000, pp. 205–227.

[23] Macintyre S, Ellaway A. Neighborhoods and Health: An Overview. In: Neighborhoods and Health [Internet]. [place unknown]: Oxford University Press; 2003 [cited Sep 30, 2021]. p. 20–42. Available from: https://doi.org/10.1093/acprof:oso/9780195138382.003.0002

[24] Massey DS. Segregation and stratification: a biosocial perspective. Du Bois Review: Social Science Research on Race [Internet]. 2004 Mar [cited Sep 30, 2021];1(1):7–25. Available from: https://doi.org/10.1017/s1742058x04040032

[25] Acevedo-García D, Lochner KA, Osypuk TL, Subramanian SV. Future Directions in Residential Segregation and Health Research: A Multilevel Approach. American Journal of Public Health [Internet]. 2003 Feb [cited Sep 30, 2021];93(2):215–21. Available from: https://doi.org/10.2105/ajph.93.2.215

[26] UN Committee on Economic, Social and Cultural rights, 2 The right to the highest possible attainable level of health. General Comment 14. E / C.12 / 2000/4.

[27] Primary Health Care: Now more than ever. Geneva, Switzerland: World Health Organization; 2008. Primary Health Care: Now more than ever. Geneva, Switzerland: World Health Organization; 2008.

[28] Potts H, Accountability and the right to the highest attainable standard of health, Essex, University of Essex, 2008.

[29] Freedman LP. Achieving the MDGs: Health systems as core social institutions. Development [Internet]. 2005 Mar [cited Sep 30, 2021];48(1):19–24. Available from: https://doi.org/10.1057/palgrave.development.1100107

[30] Backlund E, Rowe G, Lynch J, Wolfson MC, Kaplan GA, Sorlie PD. Income inequality and mortality: a multilevel prospective study of 521 248 individuals in 50 US states. International Journal of Epidemiology [Internet]. 2007 Mar 15 [cited Sep 30, 2021];36(3):590–6. Available from: https://doi.org/10.1093/ije/dym012

[31] Macinko JA, Shi L, Starfield B, Wulu JT. Income Inequality and Health: A Critical Review of the Literature. Medical Care Research and Review [Internet]. 2003 Dec [cited Sep 30, 2021];60(4):407–52. Available from: https://doi.org/10.1177/1077558703257169

[32] Subramanian S, Kawachi I. Commentary: Chasing the elusive null – the story of income inequality and health. International Journal of Epidemiology [Internet]. 2007 Jun 1 [cited Sep 30, 2021];36(3):596–9. Available from: https://doi.org/10.1093/ije/dym102

[33] Illustrated, Wilkinson RG, Pickett K. The spirit level: why more equal societies almost always do better. [lugar desconocido]: Allen Lane; 2009. 352 p.

[34] Kondo N, Kawachi I, Subramanian SV, Takeda Y, Yamagata Z. Do social comparisons explain the association between income inequality and health?: Relative deprivation and perceived health among male and female Japanese individuals. Social Science & Medicine [Internet]. 2008 Sep [cited Sep 30, 2021];67(6):982–7. Available from: https://doi.org/10.1016/j.socscimed.2008.06.002

[35] Kondo N, Kawachi I, Hirai H, Kondo K, Subramanian SV, Hanibuchi T, Yamagata Z. Relative deprivation and incident functional disability among older Japanese women and men: prospective cohort study. Journal of Epidemiology & Community Health [Internet]. 2009 Feb 12 [cited Sep 30, 2021];63(6):461–7. Available from: https://doi.org/10.1136/jech.2008.078642

[36] Subramanian SV. Income Inequality and Health: What Have We Learned So Far? Epidemiologic Reviews [Internet]. 2004 Jul 1 [cited Sep 30, 2021];26(1):78–91. Available from: https://doi.org/10.1093/epirev/mxh003

[37] Díaz-Perera G, Contextual determinants of diseases associated with atherosclerosis and their risk factors, Thesis presented as an option to the category of Doctor of Health Sciences, Havana. 2011 unpublished.

[38] Díaz-Perera G, Bacallao J, Alemañy E, Relationship between the socioeconomic dimension and the health dimension in Cuban families, Rev Cub Public Health, 38, pp. 403–413, 2012.

[39] Harper S, Rey NB, Meersman SC, Reichman ME, Breen N, Lynch J. Implicit Value Judgments in the Measurement of Health Inequalities. Milbank Quarterly [Internet]. 2010 Mar [cited Sep 30, 2021];88(1):4–29. Available from: https://doi.org/10.1111/j.1468-0009.2010.00587.x

[40] Whitehead M, Dahlgren G, Concepts and principles for tackling social inequalities in health, World Health Organization, Studies on social and economic determinants of population health No. 2, Copenhagen 2007.

[41] Price-Haywood EG, Burton J, Fort D, Seoane L. Hospitalization and Mortality among Black Patients and White Patients with Covid-19. New England Journal of Medicine [Internet]. 2020 Jun 25 [cited Sep 30, 2021];382(26):2534–43. Available from: https://doi.org/10.1056/nejmsa2011686

[42] Baqui P, Bica I, Marra V, Ercole A, van der Schaar M. Ethnic and regional variations in hospital mortality from COVID-19 in Brazil: a cross-sectional observational study. The Lancet Global Health [Internet]. 2020 Aug [cited Sep 30, 2021];8(8):e1018–e1026. Available from: https://doi.org/10.1016/s2214-109x(20)30285-0

[43] Haddad L, Smith LC. Explaining Child Malnutrition in Developing Countries: A Cross-Country Analysis (Research Report (International Food Policy Research Institute)). [lugar desconocido]: Intl Food Policy Research Inst; 1999. 112 p.

[44] Bacallao J, Castillo-Salgado C, Schneider MC, Mujica OJ, Loyola E, Manuel V. Indices based on the notion of entropy for measuring social inequalities in health. Revista Panamericana de Salud Pública [Internet]. 2002 Dec [cited Sep 30, 2021];12(6). Available from: https://doi.org/10.1590/s1020-49892002001200008

[45] Clarke PM, Gerdtham UG, Connelly LB. A note on the decomposition of the health concentration index. Health Economics [Internet]. 2003 [cited Sep 30, 2021];12(6):511–6. Available from: https://doi.org/10.1002/hec.767

[46] Tsui KY. Multidimensional poverty indices. Social Choice and Welfare [Internet]. 2002 Jan 1 [cited Oct 1, 2021];19(1):69–93. Available from: https://doi.org/10.1007/s355-002-8326-3

[47] Gundgaard J, Lauridsen J. Decomposition of sources of income-related health inequality applied on SF-36 summary scores: a Danish health survey. Health and Quality of Life Outcomes [Internet]. 2006 Aug 22 [cited Sep 30, 2021];4(1). Available from: https://doi.org/10.1186/1477-7525-4-53

[48] Yiengprugsawan V, Lim LL, Carmichael GA, Sidorenko A, Sleigh AC. Measuring and decomposing inequity in self-reported morbidity and self-assessed health in Thailand.

International Journal for Equity in Health [Internet]. 2007 Dec [cited Sep 30, 2021];6(1). Available from: https://doi.org/10.1186/1475-9276-6-23

[49] Fernández A, Costa M, Decomposition of the Gini indices and generalized entropy, Spanish Statistics, 40, pp. 233–256, 1998.

[50] Keppel K, Pamuk E, Lynch J, Carter-Pokras O, Insun K, Mays V, Pearcy J, Schoenbach V, Weissman JS, Methodological issues in measuring health disparities, National Center for Health Statistics, Vital Health Stat, 2, 141, pp. 1–16, Jul. 2005.

[51] APHO, Commonly used public health statistics and their confidence intervals, Technical briefing 3, May. 2008. Available from: www.apho.org.uk

[52] Paoli B, Haggard L, Gulzar S, Confidence intervals in public health, Office of Public Health Assessment, Utah Department of Health, 2002

[53] Schneider MC, Castillo-Salgado C, Bacallao J, Loyola E, Mujica OJ, Vidaurre M, Roca A. Methods for measuring inequalities in health. Revista Panamericana de Salud Pública [Internet]. 2002 Dec [cited Sep 30, 2021];12(6). Available from: https://doi.org/10.1590/s1020-49892002001200006

[54] Chapman S. Advocacy in public health: roles and challenges. International Journal of Epidemiology [Internet]. 2001 Dec [cited Sep 30, 2021];30(6):1226–32. Available from: https://doi.org/10.1093/ije/30.6.1226

[55] Schoenbach VJ, Understanding the fundamentals of Epidemiology, (Trans.: Spanish). Chapel Hill, North Carolina, 2000.

[56] Mackenbach JP, Kunst AE. Measuring the magnitude of socio-economic inequalities in health: An overview of available measures illustrated with two examples from Europe. Social Science & Medicine [Internet]. 1997 Mar [cited Sep 30, 2021];44(6):757–71. Available from: https://doi.org/10.1016/s0277-9536(96)00073-1

[57] Silber J, editor. Handbook of Income Inequality Measurement [Internet]. Dordrecht: Springer Netherlands; 1999 [cited Sep 30, 2021]. Available from: https://doi.org/10.1007/978-94-011-4413-1

[58] Le Grand J, Inequalities in health: the human capital approach, Welfare State Program Discussion Paper No. 1, London School of Economics, 1985.

[59] Houweling TA, Kunst AE, Mackenbach JP. World Health Report 2000: inequality index and socioeconomic inequalities in mortality. The Lancet [Internet]. 2001 May [cited Sep 30, 2021];357(9269):1671–2. Available from: https://doi.org/10.1016/s0140-6736(00)04829-7

[60] van Doorslaer E, Wagstaff A, Bleichrodt H, Calonge S, Gerdtham UG, Gerfin M, Geurts J, Gross L, Häkkinen U, Leu RE, O'Donell O, Propper C, Puffer F, Rodríguez M, Sundberg G, Winkelhake O. Income-related inequalities in health: some international comparisons. Journal of Health Economics [Internet]. 1997 Feb [cited Sep 30, 2021];16(1):93–112. Available from: https://doi.org/10.1016/s0167-6296(96)00532-2

[61] Wagstaff A, Paci P, van Doorslaer E. On the measurement of inequalities in health. Social Science & Medicine [Internet]. 1991 Jan [cited Sep 30, 2021];33(5):545–57. Available from: https://doi.org/10.1016/0277-9536(91)90212-u

[62] Kakwani N, Wagstaff A, van Doorslaer E. Socioeconomic inequalities in health: Measurement, computation, and statistical inference. Journal of Econometrics [Internet]. 1997 Mar [cited Sep 30, 2021];77(1):87–103. Available from: https://doi.org/10.1016/s0304-4076(96)01807-6

[63] Erreygers G. Correcting the Concentration Index. Journal of Health Economics [Internet]. 2009 Mar [cited Sep 30, 2021];28(2):504–15. Available from: https://doi.org/10.1016/j.jhealeco.2008.02.003

[64] Koolman X, van Doorslaer E. On the interpretation of a concentration index of inequality. Health Economics [Internet]. 2004 Jul [cited Sep 30, 2021];13(7):649–56. Available from: https://doi.org/10.1002/hec.884

[65] Pearcy JN, Keppel KG. A summary measure of health disparity. Public Health Reports [Internet]. 2002 May [cited Sep 30, 2021];117(3):273–80. Available from: https://doi.org/10.1016/s0033-3549(04)50161-9

[66] Chakravarti MR. The variance as a subgroup decomposable measure of inequality, Soc Indic Res, 53, 79–95, Jan, 2001.

[67] Atuesta B, Mancero X, Tromben V, Tools for the analysis of inequalities and the redistributive effect of public policies, ECLAC, Santiago de Chile, 2018.

[68] García L, Introduction to classical thermodynamics, Mexico DF. Editorial Trillas. 1986.

[69] Atuesta B, Mancero X, Tromben V. Herramientas para el análisis de las desigualdades y del efecto redistributivo de las políticas públicas. CEPAL. 2018. Available from: https://repositorio.cepal.org/bitstream/handle/11362/43678/1/S1800511_es.pdf

[70] Conceiçao PN, Ferreira PM. The Young Person's Guide to the Theil Index: Suggesting Intuitive Interpretations and Exploring Analytical Applications. SSRN Electronic Journal [Internet]. 2000 [cited Sep 30, 2021]. Available from: https://doi.org/10.2139/ssrn.228703

[71] Conceiçao P, Galbraith JK, Bradford P, The Theil index in sequences of nested and hierarchic group structures: implications for the measurement of inequality through time, with data aggregated at different levels of industrial classification, Eastern Economic Journal, 27, pp. 61–74, May. 2000.

[72] Milanović B. Worlds apart: Measuring international and global inequality. Princeton, NJ: Princeton University Press; 2005.

[73] Lynch J. Explaining the social gradient in coronary heart disease: comparing relative and absolute risk approaches. Journal of Epidemiology & Community Health [Internet]. 2006 May 1 [cited Sep 30, 2021];60(5):436–41. Available from: https://doi.org/10.1136/jech.2005.041350

[74] Mackenbach JP, Stirbu I, Roskam AJ, Schaap MM, Menvielle G, Leinsalu M, Kunst AE. Socioeconomic Inequalities in Health in 22 European Countries. New England Journal of Medicine [Internet]. 2008 Jun 5 [cited Sep 30, 2021];358(23):2468–81. Available from: https://doi.org/10.1056/nejmsa0707519

[75] Galobardes B. Indicators of socioeconomic position (part 1). Journal of Epidemiology & Community Health [Internet]. 2006 Jan 1 [cited Sep 30, 2021];60(1):7–12. Available from: https://doi.org/10.1136/jech.2004.023531

[76] Zhang Q, Wang Y. Socioeconomic inequality of obesity in the United States: do gender, age, and ethnicity matter? Social Science & Medicine [Internet]. 2004 Mar [cited Sep 30, 2021];58(6):1171–80. Available from: https://doi.org/10.1016/s0277-9536(03)00288-0

[77] Cevallos Ponce GK, Calle Lino AD, Ponce Cedeño OS. Impacto social causado por la COVID-19 en Ecuador. 3C Empresa. Investigación y pensamiento crítico [Internet]. 2020 Dec 18 [cited Sep 30, 2021]:115–27. Available from: https://doi.org/10.17993/3cemp.2020.edicionespecial1.115-127

[78] Burström B, Tao W. Social determinants of health and inequalities in COVID-19. European Journal of Public Health [Internet]. 2020 Jul 8 [cited Sep 30, 2021];30(4):617–8. Available from: https://doi.org/10.1093/eurpub/ckaa095

[79] Adhikari S, Pantaleo NP, Feldman JM, Ogedegbe O, Thorpe L, Troxel AB. Assessment of Community-Level Disparities in Coronavirus Disease 2019 (COVID-19) Infections and Deaths in Large US Metropolitan Areas. JAMA Network Open [Internet]. 2020 Jul 28 [cited Sep 30, 2021];3(7):e2016938. Available from: https://doi.org/10.1001/jamanetworkopen.2020.16938

[80] Ortiz-Hernández L, Pérez-Sastre MA, Social inequities in the progression of COVID-19 in the Mexican population, Rev Panam Salud Pública, 44, e106, Sep. 2020; https://doi.org/10.26633/RPSP:2020.106. Available from: https://pubmed.ncbi.nlm.nih.gov/32983234

CHAPTER 8

Statistical Approaches to Understand COVID-19 Severity and Fatality

A.H. Seuc[*1], **E. Mertens**[2], **J.L. Peñalvo**[2]

[*] **Corresponding author:** ahseuc@gmail.com, Phone: +53 52595285

[1] National Institute of Hygiene, Epidemiology and Microbiology, Havana 10300, Cuba.

[2] Institute of Tropical Medicine, 2000-Antwerp, Belgium.

Abstract. Statistical methods are essential tools for confronting the current COVID-19 pandemic. These include approaches for quantifying the health impacts of the pandemic, methods for identification of patterns, or risk stratification, for estimating the risk of individuals to become infected, and of patients to die, and important clues on how to approach prediction models in a comprehensive way. The purpose of this chapter is to review basic statistical concepts related to characterization of COVID-19 severity and provide an application of a real scenario related to the identification of predictors of COVID-19 fatality in evolving databases. Some other statistical descriptions and comments are made of problems drawn from real situations.

Andrés Fraguela-Collar (Ed.)

Key words: COVID-19, Statistics, Epidemiology, Prediction models, Health impact, Stratification, Severity, Fatality, Cuba

1 INTRODUCTION

1.1 Importance

Several approaches play an essential role in confronting the COVID-19 pandemic, among them are sociological and mathematical approaches. It is also important to emphasize the role of statistics in helping countries, societies, and the international community to understand and confront this pandemic in an efficient and sustainable manner.

1.2 Preliminaries

Statistics is a methodological discipline with roots in probability and mathematics. Statistics focuses on the variability of data, aiming to explaining it with statistical concepts and based on the knowledge of a particular context. The analysis of individual units (e.g. only one country) or situations (e.g. only developing countries) only offer a limited description of the issue. Statistics needs to use data from different units and from different situations so that inferences can be made from what has been observed, although with a certain level of uncertainty. Solutions to problems like the COVID-19 pandemic are in general based on comparisons.

Statisticians must understand well the context (e.g. biomedicine, sociology) on which statistical methods will be applied, as well as the complementary methodological disciplines that are available for a particular discipline. For example statistics often coincide with epidemiological methods to address medical research, such as the COVID-19 pandemic. Statistical thinking is key in facing the COVID-19 pandemic, and a correct calculation and interpretation of statistical and epidemiological indicators is necessary when characterizing the evolution of the outbreak, the prediction of future outcomes, and to inform the efficient allocation of healthcare resources to mitigate current and future COVID-19 related burdens.

The purpose of this chapter is to review the basic statistical concepts related to the characterization of COVID-19 severity, and provide an application of a real scenario related to the identification of predictors of COVID-19 fatality in evolving databases.

2 BASIC STATISTICS APPLIED TO COVID-19 SEVERITY

2.1 Confirmed Cases, Severity, and Recovery or Death

When dealing with an outbreak of a new infectious agent it is priority to understand its severity as a main indicator of fatality. While at the individual level, severity is assessed by the gravity of signs and symptoms, at the population level, fatality ratios are calculated to assess the severity of disease and, when calculated for specific population subgroups, identify vulnerable groups and prioritize healthcare allocation of resources. Fatality rates can be calculated accounting for deaths among all infected individuals (infection fatality ratio, IFR) or deaths among confirmed cases (case fatality ratio, CFR). At the onset of the COVID-19 outbreak, only CFR could be calculated as only cases derived from surveillance systems and/or severe cases from reporting hospitals were available. Mild cases not seeking healthcare attention are common, and so is the proportion of asymptomatic individuals. These unaccounted cases introduce an important bias in CFR estimates stemming from the preferential ascertainment of severe cases, and delayed reporting, [1], and hinder the comparison of the infection severity across populations.

Underreporting is a particularly important issue in COVID-19 due to the magnitude of the crisis and the overloaded testing capacity of the health systems across the world [2]. As the pandemic evolves and testing becomes more available, CFR estimates will be more reliable but, especially when comparing populations, the limitations of the use of CFR should be acknowledged and methods to increase comparability should be applied, for example, by introducing time in the calculation by using a lag-time since first case reported in the country to avoid insufficient testing and delayed reporting [3]. Furthermore, it is advisable to report the period during which deaths are counted to calculate the CFR (e.g. the 1-month CFR of COVID-19) to obtain an estimate as reliable as possible [1].

$$CFR = (num\ deaths\ from\ COVID - 19)/(num\ confirmed\ cases) \times 100,$$

$$IFR = (num\ deaths\ from\ COVID - 19)/(num\ infested\ cases) \times 100.$$

The calculation of CFR implies the use of a case definition (diagnosis for confirmed cases), and this also varies across countries despite overall guidance available in the WHO interim guidance on Global surveillance for COVID-19 [4]. Reliable CFR estimates can be used to assess the severity of an epidemic towards the end of the outbreak once all cases have recovered or died. However, this calculation may not be reliable in an ongoing epidemic, where the outcome of the disease (whether cases have recovered or died) might not be known at the moment of the calculation. Outcome prediction among active cases using modified Kaplan-Meier survival analyses has been proposed to circumvent this limitation, however this approach increases the complexity of the calculation, and requires individual data which is often not available [1].

In summary, when estimating the severity of an outbreak using CFR, caution must be applied in the interpretation, particularly when comparing populations or countries. Case definitions vary widely, and so do testing strategies. This together with the demographic structure and the patient's profile in a particular country should be taken into consideration.

2.2 Burden of COVID-19

The measures of severity discussed earlier, and the mortality rate of COVID-19 characterize the dimension of the public health issue. To complement these indicators, other summary measures of population health have been established to further characterize the burden of disease. Among these measures, the disability-adjusted life year (DALY) is one of the most frequently used and has been central in the development of the Global Burden of Disease study [5].The DALY provides an estimation of the years of healthy life years lost due a particular disease or risk factor by combining the number of years of life lost due to premature mortality (YLL) and the number of years lost due to disability (YLD) caused by the disease or risk factor [6].

$$DALY = YLL + YLD.$$

YLL is calculated as the product of the number of deaths and the remaining life expectancy at the time of death. YLD is the product of the number of incident cases, and the average duration until disease resolution (recovery or death), further adjusted by the disability originated from the disease measured as the reduction in health from 0 (no effect) to 1 (death) in what is better known as the disability weight.

Disease (COVID-19) burden estimates are intended to allow comparisons across countries or among population strata to infer potential subgroup vulnerabilities. For relevant comparisons, DALYs should be presented per 100,000 persons. Moreover, for COVID-19 in particular, DALYs per case in addition to the absolute burden of disease could be calculated for additional comparisons with other infectious agents.

Beside the calculation of COVID-19-related DALYs as a direct impact of the pandemic in the population, indirect impacts should be also estimated. The consequence of overloaded health systems worldwide has resulted in an increased morbidity and mortality in other diseases/conditions such as cancer, and cardiometabolic diseases; this is usually carried out by comparing the observed morbidity/mortality with the expected one, for the reference time period, and for the studied disease [7].

2.3 Cluster Analysis for Patient Stratification

Cluster analysis is an exploratory multivariate technique that identify groups (clusters) of units (subjects/patients) with a particular pattern within a selected and relevant set of variables.

There are several approaches to cluster analysis, and the hierarchical approach is one of the most popular one. This hierarchical approach considers that, at the beginning, each of the n units is a cluster. In the initial step, the two most similar n units in relation to the preselected set of variables, are clustered, and as a result n-1 clusters remain. In a second step, the two most similar within the n-1 units are subsequently clustered, and as a result there aren-2 clusters. This process is reiterated until all units are assigned to just one cluster [8]. This clustering process is only useful for stratification when the optimal step for stopping is identified. Stopping rules are subjective and data-dependent. In the case of the COVID-19 pandemic, clustering (stratifying) countries according to the patterns of evolution of the epidemic curves (rates of active cases, rates of daily incidence, rates of cumulative confirmed cases, etc.) as relevant variables for each country and the particular time period of interest, the average, the (linear, quadratic, etc.) time trend, and number of "peaks" and/or variability, in the curve of rates of active cases, could be a useful tool to group country areas with similar characteristics. The results of this clustering exercise would provide groups/clusters of countries with "similar" patterns of the pandemic in terms of the mentioned variables, and "labels" could be assigned to these patterns according to the particular behaviour of the variables in each cluster.

At the individual-level, COVID-19 patients could be also grouped according to for example age, sex, co-morbidities, time (month) of diagnosis, etc. In this case, if the CFR is calculated in each cluster, patients could be identified with particular patterns that are associated with high risk of death (and vice-versa). The focus could also be on large clusters (independently of their risks of death), which would allow to identify the patterns in the population that are more at risk of becoming infected.

2.4 Prediction Models for Severity and Fatality

The wealth of data accumulated from months of patient's encounters with the health care system, offers an opportunity to understand the impact of COVID-19 in people's health and lives as well as to identify the role of comorbidities, among other factors, in determining COVID-19 progression into severe or critical stages, and subsequent recovery or death. Identifying predicting factors for an accurate risk prediction of COVID-19 progression would be of added value for efficient patient care management and relieving the pressure on the health care systems. Towards this need, more than a hundred prognostic models for patients diagnosed with COVID-19 have been developed from the early phases of the pandemic, as summarized in the living systematic review of Wynants and co-workers, [9]. Frequent classical statistical tools to identify COVID-19 predictors include logistic regression models, and to a lesser extent Cox proportional hazard models, and only one competing risk model [9]. Also, machine learning approaches, such as random forests, neural networks and K-Nearest Neighbour, are being increasingly used in prediction [9]. This section will focus on discussing the application of classical tools in the context of predicting COVID-19 fatality.

To develop a risk prediction model, the following steps need to be taken: 1) Selecting variables, 2) Building the prediction model, and 3) Measuring performance of the prediction model.

2.4.1 Selecting Variables

2.4.1.1 Pre-Screening of Variables

For the identification of predictor variables and the construction of the risk prediction model, it is recommended to screen variables in advance to consider their usefulness for inclusion as candidate predictors. This selection of candidate predictors is preferably built upon previous literature and expert option rather than in a purely data-driven manner [10], and this, in particular, should be done for datasets with limited sample size [11]. In practice it is however likely that some of the potential important candidate predictors identified needed to be excluded because of missingness, and for categorical variables also because of imbalances (like $> 90\%$ or $< 10\%$ yes). In model building, only the observations with complete data will be used, either by omitting the observations with incomplete data or the variable with missing values from the list of candidate predictors. This decision is likely to be dependent, not only on the number of missing values, but also on the pattern of missingness (e.g. variables collected only after a certain time point, related to certain characteristics, etc.). For continuous variables, non-linearity and different dimensionality among variables which require standardisation, are two of the problems one is frequently confronted with. Another one is the option or transforming them into categorical ones and the choice of a categorisation rule.

Predictors frequently identified for prognosis after COVID-19 diagnosis are: age, sex, comorbidities, vital signs (such as body temperature), image features, lymphocyte count, and C-reactive protein, [9]. When building a new prediction model, it is recommended to consider these in the list of potential very important candidate predictors, when appropriate, i.e. they are available and accurately measured in patients included in the hospital data under study.

2.4.1.2 Regularization Methods for Selection of Predictors

The underlying concept of regularization is to improve the generalization of the prediction model to new, unseen data, related to the accuracy of predictions, which is exactly the goal of predictive modelling. Intuitively, regularization can be seen as a penalty against complexity: imposing such a penalty will reduce (i.e. shrink) some coefficient values towards zero, allowing less contributing variables to be omitted so that picking up peculiarities and noise is prevented. In other words, regularization aims to minimize bias and variance by imposing a shrinkage factor that determines the amount of shrinkage, referred as tuning parameter lambda. The higher the value of lambda, the more coefficients are shrunken towards zero. Lambda is preferably selected by k-fold cross-validation that leads to estimation of the optimal lambda that minimised the mean cross-validated prediction error (lambda min) and the lambda within 1 standard error from the optimal lambda (lambda 1se). The latter leads to a more parsimonious model with less predictors, preferable for large datasets, while the optimal lambda is often used for small datasets. This k-fold cross-validation for lambda selection is a random process, thus a seed should be set in order to generate reproducible results.

Generally, there are three types of penalized regression: Ridge [12], Least Absolute Shrinkage and Selection Operator (LASSO) [13] and Elastic Net [14]. In Ridge regression, the regression coefficients are shrunk, by penalizing the regression model with the L2-norm penalty term, i.e. the sum of the squared coefficients. In this way, variables with minor contribution to the outcome will have their coefficients close to zero, but all predictors will still be included in the final model, hence no variable selection. LASSO regression shrinks the regression coefficients towards zero by penalizing the regression model with the L1-norm penalty term, i.e. the sum of the absolute coefficients. This penalty term forces some of the regression coefficients, with a minor contribution, to be exactly zero, which amounts to selecting variables and reducing model complexity. LASSO regression tends to perform well when the number of significant parameters is low, i.e. only a few parameters influence the response, and tends to select only one of a group of highly correlated predictors. The variable selection using LASSO regression can, however, be very dependent on the data, and thus unstable. Elastic Net regression combines the penalties of Ridge and LASSO regression in order to get the best of both and is done by setting the mixing parameter alpha between 0 (Ridge) and 1 (LASSO). Mixing parameter alpha can be set arbitrarily (Often 0.5 is chosen), or selected via k-fold cross-validation as done for estimating lambda min and lambda 1se.

2.4.2 Building the Prediction Model

The prediction model should be built using the appropriate statistical tool to predict the outcome of interest with variable selection by using the parameters lambda and alpha, as described above. Of the existing COVID-19 prognostic models, outcomes to predict have been: in-hospital death, progression to a severe or critical disease, as well as single or composite outcomes that include recovery, length of hospital stay, intensive care unit admission, intubation or extracorporeal membrane oxygenation, (duration of) mechanical ventilation, acute respiratory distress syndrome, amongst others [9].

2.4.2.1 *Advanced Classical Regression Models*

When it is of interest to predict non-fatal intermediate events (such as progression to severe disease, e.g. rapid clinical deterioration, ICU-admission, enhanced respiratory support treatment) and exclusive endpoints (e.g. recovery or in-hospital death) after hospital admission, prediction models should be built using time-to-event data in a multi-state setting. This multi-state setting would fit the COVID-19 hospital setting when time-to-event data are available, as documented in several recent papers [15–18]. In such a multi-state time-to-event framework, hospitalization is followed by either recovery or death, with or without experiencing an intermediate severe disease state. The state-occupation probabilities for intermediate and final events at a future time t, for example 30 days after hospital admission, can be modelled indirectly via the transition hazards using Cox proportional hazard regression and directly using pseudo-value regression. In brief, the multi-state models are regarded as an extension of competing risks models by also describing transitions to intermediate events when time-to-intermediate events is available [19].

A competing risk is the occurrence of an event that prevents the observation of another event and/or modifies the probability that this event occurs. For example, in a time-to-event analysis of hospital data, if death is the event of interest, then discharged alive or recovery should be considered as a competing event, and the same holds when recovery or discharged alive is the event of interest with death as the competing event [20]. Prediction models, where the probability of observing the reference event in the presence of competing risks is of interest, are built by the Fine & Gray regression model for the cumulative incidence functions, also called sub-distribution hazard, as applied in one study aimed at predicting progression to severe COVID-19 [21].

2.4.2.2 *Time-to-Event Regression Models*

Standard survival analysis i.e. time-to-event models, allows censoring of patients who are still hospitalised at last follow-up date, i.e. a special type of missing data that occurs because patients did not experience the event during follow-up time. Excluding these patients with incomplete follow-up data that are still in the hospital yields a selected study sample, and hence might introduce selection bias that in turn possibly nullifies the effect of important predictors [20]. That is why, time-to-event models, that account for censoring, are preferred for identifying patient-level predictors for the event of interest [20].

In the analysis for predicting for example in-hospital death after COVID-19 diagnosis, the methodological considerations on time-to-event can be described as follows: "days" is used as time-scale where date of hospital admission is the time origin, i.e. the point at which the follow-up starts, and patients exit at their event (i.e. date of discharged (recovery) or date of death) or censoring days (i.e. in case a patient has not yet experienced the event by the end of the study or was lost to follow-up during the study). The main assumption underlying time-to-event data is that of non-informative censoring, i.e. patients that are censored have the same probability of experiencing an event as patients that remain in the study. Of course, sufficient follow-up time and number of events are also needed for adequate statistical power. The outcome of interest includes not only whether or not the event occurred, but also when it occurred.

Time-to-event data are commonly analysed with the multi-variate approach of Cox Proportional regression model that describes the relation between the event incidence, as expressed by the Hazard function given in terms of time t, covariate vector x (explanatory variables), and coefficient vector β:

$$\lambda(t) = \lambda_0(t)e^{x^T\beta},$$

where λ_0 is the baseline hazard (an arbitrary function of time).

A key assumption underlying the Cox model is the proportional hazard assumption, i.e. a constant relationship between the outcome and covariates, or in other words the hazard ratios are proportional at any point in time and do not vary with time. The Cox model is considered a semi-parametric approach as it contains a non-parametric component, i.e. the baseline hazard corresponding to the value of the hazard when all predictors equal zero, and the parametric component, i.e. predictors and associated regression coefficients, [22]. In the setting of predicting survival probabilities, the risk function could be derived from using the regression coefficients and the baseline hazard rates, as commonly estimated using Breslow estimator, [23]. The Breslow estimator uses the profile likelihood approach by extending the Nelson-Aalen estimator [24] which estimates the baseline survival function as an exponential function of the cumulative baseline hazard function [25, 26].

A limited number of studies with available time-to-event data employed Cox models to predict in-hospital death after COVID-19 within a pre-specified period of time [27, 28]), progression to severe COVID-19 operationalized by composite measures of rapid clinical deterioration or worsening of imaging features, also within a pre-specified number of days [29, 30] or length of hospital stay [31], while accounting for censoring.

2.4.2.3 Logistic Regression Model

Logistic regression is an appropriate tool if patient data are available until discharge, and commonly used to identify predictors for the event of interest, for example, in-hospital death. In its basic form, the logistic regression uses a logit function to model a binary dependent variable, for example recovery and in-hospital death, labelled as 0 and 1, respectively. The logarithm of the odds (log-odds) for the variable labelled "1", i.e. the probability of having the outcome of interest, varies between 0 and 1, and is a linear combination of one or more predictors (explanatory variables x_i) which can be categorical or continuous.

$$\log\left(\frac{p}{1-p}\right) = \beta_0 + \beta_i x_i$$

Several studies employed logistic regressions to predict in-hospital death after COVID-19 without specifying when death occurred after diagnosis [32–39], but also to predict COVID-19 disease severity, operationalized, for example, by severe symptoms three days after admission, [40] acute respiratory distress syndrome [41], mechanical ventilation $>$ 96 hours [38], hospital stay longer than 10 days [42], amongst composite measures of rapid clinical deterioration features [43], and of transfer to ICU and death [44, 45], often occurring within a period of 15 days or unspecified.

In short, logistic regression is widely used as an exploratory model for the probability of an event, such as discharged alive or recovered versus death, to identify potential risk factors, with the advantage that only a binary outcome variable and patient characteristics as exploratory variables are needed. This makes this classical statistical technique very appropriate for developing countries where reliable available data are far from perfect.

2.4.3 Measuring Performance of the Prediction Model

Performance statistics can be ranked in order of strength of the validation approach: external (i.e. evaluation in an independent dataset), internal (including bootstrapping, cross-validation and random Training-Testing split) and apparent validity (i.e. evaluation in the same data used for development). Assessing the predictive accuracy of the model should involve quantifying the utility of the prediction model to identify subjects at increased risk for the outcome (i.e. discrimination) as well as how close predictions are to the actual outcome (i.e. calibration)[46], both preferably measured in new, unseen data, like an independent external dataset or otherwise in a testing set when applying any of the internal performance statistics mentioned above. Briefly, with bootstrapping or cross-validation, multiple models on resampled samples with replacements, or multiple subsets, respectively, are fitted and evaluated for their performance on average. The Training-Testing split is a procedure to divide the dataset randomly into two subsets: the first subset to fit the model, referred as the training set, and the second subset referred to as Testing set in which the predictions are made using the fitted model and compared with the observed values.

Conditional on the true outcome status, the discriminating ability of the model measures how well a prediction model distinguished between patients with and without the outcome of interest, as given by the Receiver Operating Characteristics (ROC)-curve that plots sensitivity against 1-specificity with varying threshold values for the probability of having the outcome. Sensitivity is the true positive fraction and 1-specificity is the false positive fraction, and both are measured by comparing the actual observations with the predictions made by the regression model. These predicted outcomes, in turn, depend on the relative position of the estimated probabilities with respect to pre-specified thresholds. The ROC-curve and associated summary measures of area under the curve (AUC) and the concordance index (c-index) are relevant to the rank order of the prediction, but not to the actual predictions themselves, i.e. they ignore calibration.

In practice, clinicians are, however, more interested in the benefits and harms of the decision based on the prediction model, also referred to as clinical utility or the Net Benefit, [47]. The Net Benefit is calculated as

$$Sensitivity * Prevalence - (1 - Specificity) * (1 - Prevalence) * w$$

where w is a varying threshold probability value for having the outcome of interest, and often plotted in a decision curve, [48]. Such a decision tool facilitates the clinical judgement of the relative value of benefits and harms associated with the prediction model, and indeed, a prediction model would only be recommended for clinical use if it has the highest level of benefits across a range of clinically reasonable preferences.

Calibration refers to the agreement between observed and predicted outcomes, and is graphically assessed by plotting the predictions on the x-axis and the observed outcomes on the y-axis with a 45° line indicating perfect predictions, [49]. This calibration plot can be further characterised by an intercept and a calibration slope. The intercept that has a target value of 0 indicates the extent of calibration-in-the-large (i.e. systematically too high (negative) or too low (positive values for in the intercept) predictions), and the calibration slope having a target value of 1 evaluates the spread of the prediction outcomes. A slope > 1 suggests that the predictions are too moderate, whereas a slope < 1 reflects overfitting or, in other words, that the predictions are too extreme, i.e. too high for patients who are at high risk and too low for patients who are at low risk, hence the need for shrinkage of regression coefficients in a prediction model, [50].

Alternatively, a commonly used measure to assess predictive accuracy by capturing both discrimination and calibration aspects at the same time is the prediction error. The prediction error is a measure for the difference between the predicted probability and the observed event, and most commonly operationalized by the Brier score (or quadratic loss function), [51].

In the context of COVID-19, available prediction models were often built with a limited sample size, in particular a median of 338 (interquartile range (IQR) 134-707) patients and a median number of events of 69 (IQR 37-160) [9], which might increase the risk of overfitting, [52]. To partly overcome this risk, most studies employed a 5-fold cross-validation, with a 80/20 or 70/30 Training-Testing split, and to a lesser extent bootstrapping for measuring prediction performance, and in this way using all available, although limited, data for model building, [9]. Up till now, the majority of studies have not yet carried out an external validation that assesses not only discrimination, but also calibration as well as clinical utility (net benefit) in large datasets collected by means of appropriate study designs and representative of the target population, [9].

3 CASE-EXAMPLE: PREDICTORS OF COVID-19 FATALITY IN CUBA

3.1 Background

One of the important problems related to COVID-19 is to identify risk factors for severity and fatality. Data on clinical characteristics and prognostic factors in hospital settings are scarce, however, particularly in low and middle-income countries. The evidence based on potential predictors of death/recovery among COVID-19 cases is very limited. Many studies conducted around the world so far use less than 200-300 patients, usually from a single institution [53–60], with few studies having up to 3000 patients, [61]. A meta-analysis was identified involving seven studies and more than 26000 patients [62]; another study was a systematic review, but using country as the unit of analysis, [63].

A preliminary database, dated Feb 15th, 2021, was obtained from the Cuban Ministry of Public Health, with socio-demographic and clinical data of all COVID-19 cases since March 11th , 2020, when the first case was detected/reported, until Feb 15th, 2021; all data leading to eventual identification of patients were deleted before any analyses. The COVID-19 pandemic puts great pressure on medical resources worldwide and makes healthcare professionals wonder which patients are in imminent need of special/intensive care. With appropriate data on each patient, hospitals could decide whether or not a patient requires immediate special/intensive care.

Not many countries, particularly low and middle-income ones, have a database of all COVID-19 cases, with socio-demographic and clinical characteristics for each of them. Exploring potential risk factors should facilitate early screening and identification of patients, allowing timely intervention, optimization of scarce resources, and reductions in lethality.

Taking into account the above considerations, a study was done to illustrate the application of multilevel logistic regression to identify risk factors for death from COVID-19, using a dataset with all COVID-19 cases in Cuba with socio-demographic and clinical variables. Some studies have used machine learning methods [53, 57, 59], which are out of the scope of this manuscript and chapter; some have used survival analysis techniques [55], but since the time period usually involved from diagnosis to final clinical outcome in the case of COVID-19 patients is relatively short (2-3 weeks), logistic regression (as used in [54, 56, 60, 61]) could be more useful at this stage of the pandemic.

3.2 Materials and Methods

A preliminary database was used with cases diagnosed from the onset of the epidemic of COVID-19 in Cuba on March 11, 2020, until February 15, 2021. Socio-demographic and clinical variables were collected for each patient. This is a preliminary database because not all data were checked and validated at the moment of this analysis, particularly information about comorbidities; it contains information from 39,004 patients from the whole country.

Our objective was to identify risk factors for case fatality, with final outcome "death/recovery"; information on the final clinical outcome was missing in 23,800 patients at the time these data were collected, so just 15,204 patients were available and the outcome variable known with certainty. Data from 2,339 patients was revised/checked , and they were identified with a specific code in a quality filter variable and were used for a "First Analysis"; all patients (n=15,204), independently of the value of the filter variable, were used for an alternative "Second Analysis" which is not reported in this text. See Fig. 1, Flow Diagram.

Patients diagnosed in February 2021 were excluded from all analyses because data for this month were not complete. Twenty eight cases from Feb 2021 were excluded from those with reliable information (First Analysis), and 36 from the 15,204 available for the Second Analysis.

Finally, 71 cases were excluded from the First Analysis due to missing values in the potential predictor variables, and 1,738 for the same reason from the Second Analysis. See Fig. 1, Flow Diagram.

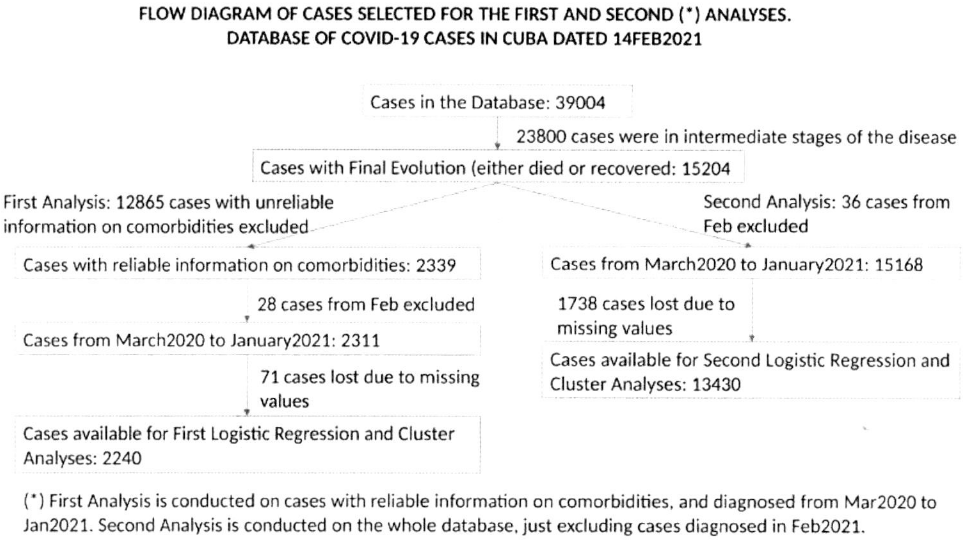

Figure 1: Flow Diagram

All COVID-19 cases were diagnosed using RT-PCR tests. The outcome variable was "Final Outcome or Evolution of patient" (died/recovered), and 18 potential predictor variables were considered for the analyses. Age, sex, and comorbidities, have been usually included as potential risk factors in previous studies [55, 56, 60, 62]. In this study comorbidities (a total of 10: HTA (Hypertension), Cancer, CKD (Chronic Kidney Disease), Obesity, Dementia, IHD (Ischemic Heart

Disease), DM (Diabetes Mellitus), COPD (Chronic Obstructive Pulmonary Disease), HIV, and Asthma)) were self-reported by patients, and "obesity" was assessed subjectively by the clinician.

The other potential predictors considered in this study were: "ANAC" (Average Number of Active Cases at month of diagnosis); "MUNI_LC" (Living Conditions of the Municipality where diagnosis was made, categorized as High, Medium and Low); PROTOCOL (one of 4 protocols used for the treatment of COVID-19 patients, and "SYMPTOMS" (delay between date of diagnosis and isolation, with four categories: "no symptoms at diagnosis", "≤ 3 days", "4-7 days", and "8+ days"). Finally, variables "PROVINCE" (province where diagnosis occurred), and "MONTH" (month of diagnosis) were considered as random effects.

In a previous section, we underscored the importance of validating a prediction model. However, in this case-example, due to the preliminary and rapidly evolving nature of the database we decided just to explore potential risk factors and not to formally validate the resulting model.

Univariate associations between each of the potential predictors and the response variable were calculated, and statistical significance was considered when $p < 0.05$ in the corresponding chi-square tests. These univariate analyses did help us to identify relevant predictors for inclusion in the multivariate logistic regression model. To avoid important multicollinearity, Spearman correlation coefficients were computed for the 18 potential predictor variables, which allowed us to eventually exclude some variables from the multilevel logistic regression models. For the sake of consistency, correlation coefficients of variable "province" were included, though they are not relevant as the provinces' codes do not follow any COVID-19 related criterion. The event "Death" is rather rare, meaning the odds ratios from the logistic regression are quite close to the corresponding relative risks, and for this reason we label them on the tables as RR. The R statistical environment v.4.0.2 and IBM SPSS v21.0 were used for all analyses.

A model with two levels was used. Level one model was:

$$\ln\left(\frac{p_{ij,k}}{1-p_{ij,k}}\right) = b_{ij,0} + b_{ij,1}EDAD\_C_{ij,k} + b_{ij,2}DM_{ij,k} + \dots,$$

and level two model:

$$
\begin{aligned}
b_{ij,0} &= B_0 + u_{ij} + v_{ij},\\
b_{ij,1} &= B_1,\\
b_{ij,2} &= B_2,\\
&\cdots
\end{aligned}
$$

where random effect / error terms at level two are assumed to follow independent normal distribution, i.e. error terms associated to provinces are independent from those associated to months:

$$
\begin{aligned}
u_i &\sim N(0, \sigma_u^2),\\
v_i &\sim N(0, \sigma_v^2).
\end{aligned}
$$

We could include terms that vary by "province" and by "month", but often adjusting for these random effects on the intercept is sufficient.

With this model we are able to estimate the odds of COVID-19 case fatality, adjusting for several potentially predictor variables, and controlling for the two crossed random effects (province and month).

Three two-level models were compared:

- fm11: no random effects included.
- fm12: "PROVINCE" random effect included.
- fm13: "PROVINCE" and "MONTH" random effects included.

3.3 Results and Discussion

Tables 1, 2, 3, 4, 5 and 6 present univariate associations between the potential predictors and the final outcome. HIV, Protocol, and MUNI_LC were not significantly associated with the final outcome, and they were excluded from the logistic regression models. Asthma was significantly but inversely associated, so it was also excluded. MONTH and ANAC were both significantly associated with the Final Outcome, but they were highly correlated (Spearman correlation coefficient 0.67, see Tables 7 and 8); finally ANAC was included as a fixed effect, and MONTH as a random effect. Then, a total of 12 potential predictors, as fixed effects, were included in the multilevel models: 8 comorbidities, Age, Sex, ANAC, and SYMPTOMS; two random effects were considered, "PROVINCE" and "MONTH".

The three models mentioned in the previous section were compared using functions glm and glmer in R:

fm11

```
> ## In model fm11 (using function glm), no random effects are included.
> fm11 <- glm(EVOLU_N ~ 1+HTA2020+Cancer2020+IRC2020+Obesidad2020+
+ demencia2020+CI2020+DM2020+EPOC2020+EDAD_C+SEXON+
+ SINTOMAS+ANAC1, cf_cuba_01,family=binomial)
```

fm12

```
> ## In model fm12, the random effect of MONTH is included.
> fm12 <- glmer(EVOLU_N ~ 1+HTA2020+Cancer2020+IRC2020+Obesidad2020+
+ demencia2020+CI2020+DM2020+EPOC2020+EDAD_C+SEXON+
+ SINTOMAS+ANAC1+(1|MONTH), cf_cuba_01,binomial)
```

fm13

```
> ## In model (fm13), the random effect of PROVINCE (provinces in Cuba) is
> # introduced, in addition to the random effect of MONTH.
> # The effect "PROV" and "MESC" are crossed random effect
```

Recovery Outcome (Death/Recovery)						
Variable	Death		Recovery		Total	
Age	n	%	n	%	n	%
0-39	5	0.8	634	99.2	639	100.0
40-64	51	4.8	1001	95.2	1052	100.0
65+	144	23.3	475	76.7	619	100.0
Total	200	8.7	2110	91.3	2310	100.0
$p < 0.001$						
Sex	n	%	n	%	n	%
Male	118	9.9	1076	90.1	1194	100.0
Female	82	7.3	1035	92.7	1117	100.0
Total	200	8.7	2111	91.3	2311	100.0
$p = 0.03$						
Dementia	n	%	n	%	n	%
No	177	7.9	2054	92.1	2231	100.0
Yes	23	28.8	57	71.3	80	100.0
Total	200	8.7	2111	91.3	2311	100.0
$p < 0.001$						
Obesity	n	%	n	%	n	%
No	182	8.2	2047	91.8	2229	100.0
Yes	18	22.0	64	78.0	82	100.0
Total	200	8.7	2111	91.3	2311	100.0
$p < 0.001$						

Table 1: Absolute and relative frequencies of final outcome (death/recovery) by potential predictors

Asthma	n	%	n	%	n	%
No	187	9.5	1786	90.5	1973	100.0
Yes	13	3.8	325	96.2	338	100.0
Total	200	8.7	2111	91.3	2310	100.0
$p = 0.001$						
CKD	n	%	n	%	n	%
No	171	7.7	2057	92.3	2228	100.0
Yes	29	34.9	54	65.1	83	100.0
Total	200	8.7	2111	91.3	2311	100.0
$p < 0.001$						
HTA	n	%	n	%	n	%
No	63	5.4	1113	94.6	1176	100.0
Yes	137	12.1	998	87.9	1135	100.0
Total	200	8.7	2111	91.3	2311	100.0
$p < 0.001$						
DM	n	%	n	%	n	%
No	122	6.4	1784	93.6	1906	100.0
Yes	78	19.3	327	80.7	405	100.0
Total	200	8.7	2111	91.3	2311	100.0
$p < 0.001$						

Table 2: Absolute and relative frequencies of final outcome (death/recovery) by potential predictors. Continued

COPD	n	%	n	%	n	%
No	171	7.7	2038	92.3	2209	100.0
Yes	29	28.4	73	71.6	102	100.0
Total	200	8.7	2111	91.3	2311	100.0
$p < 0.001$						
IHD	n	%	n	%	n	%
No	142	6.9	1924	93.1	2066	100.0
Yes	58	23.7	187	76.3	245	100.0
Total	200	8.7	2111	91.3	2311	100.0
$p < 0.001$						
CANCER	n	%	n	%	n	%
No	179	8.1	2032	91.9	2211	100.0
Yes	21	21.0	79	79.0	100	100.0
Total	200	8.7	2111	91.3	2311	100.0
$p < 0.001$						
HIV	n	%	n	%	n	%
No	199	8.7	2092	91.3	2291	100.0
Yes	1	5.0	19	95.0	20	100.0
Total	200	8.7	2111	91.3	2311	100.0
$p = 0.559$						

Table 3: Absolute and relative frequencies of final outcome (death/recovery) by potential predictors. Continued

	Final Outcome (Death/Recovery)					
Variable	Death		Recovery		Total	
ANAC	n	%	n	%	n	%
[0-200]	13	6.0	203	94.0	216	100.0
]200-400]	17	10.2	150	89.8	167	100.0
]400-600]	84	6.6	1182	93.4	1266	100.0
]600-800]	19	6.9	257	93.1	276	100.0
]800-1000]	9	3.5	249	96.5	258	100.0
]1000-...]	58	45.3	70	54.7	128	100.0
Total	200	8.7	2111	91.3	2311	100.0
$p < 0.001$						
MONTH	n	%	n	%	n	%
Mar-20	10	10.3	87	89.7	97	100.0
Apr-20	57	10.0	511	90.0	97	100.0
May-20	17	10.2	150	89.8	167	100.0
Jun-20	2	4.0	48	96.0	50	100.0
Jul-20	1	1.4	68	98.6	69	100.0
Aug-20	15	6.8	205	93.2	220	100.0
Sep-20	19	6.9	257	93.1	276	100.0
Oct-20	8	3.1	251	96.9	259	100.0
Nov-20	4	1.8	215	98.2	210	100.0
Dec-20	9	3.5	249	96.5	258	100.0
Jan-20	58	45.3	70	54.7	129	100.0
Total	200	8.7	2111	91.3	2311	100.0
$p < 0.001$						

Table 4: Absolute and relative frequencies of final outcome (death/recovery) by potential predictors. Continued

PROVINCE	n	%	n	%	n	%
LH	104	9.2	1028	90.0	1132	100.0
AR	3	5.9	48	94.1	51	100.0
CA	18	13.3	117	86.7	135	100.0
CF	3	6.3	45	93.8	48	100.0
CM	2	2.2	88	97.8	90	100.0
GR	0	0.0	20	100.0	20	100.0
GT	6	30.0	14	70.0	20	100.0
OH	5	12.8	34	87.2	39	100.0
IJ	1	5.0	19	95.0	20	100.0
LT	2	6.9	27	93.1	29	100.0
MT	12	15.8	64	84.2	76	100.0
MY	0	0.0	31	100.0	31	100.0
PR	10	4.6	207	95.4	217	100.0
SC	11	14.5	65	85.5	76	100.0
SS	8	4.7	162	95.3	170	100.0
VC	15	9.6	142	90.4	157	100.0
Total	200	8.7	2111	91.3	2311	100.0
$p < 0.001$						
MUNI_LV	n	%	n	%	n	%
HIGH	93	9.2	923	90.8	1016	100.0
MEDIUM	65	7.6	791	92.4	856	100.0
LOW	40	9.2	396	90.8	436	100.0
Total	198	8.6	2110	91.4	2308	100.0

Table 5: Absolute and relative frequencies of final outcome (death/recovery) by potential predictors. Continued

SYMPTOMS	n	%	n	%	n	%
NO SYMPTOMS	46	4.0	1104	96.0	1150	100.0
$\leq$ 3 DAYS	77	9.8	705	90.2	782	100.0
4-7 DAYS	36	16.7	179	83.3	215	100.0
8+ DAYS	17	18.1	77	81.9	94	100.0
Total	176	7.9	2065	92.1	2241	100.0
$p < 0.001$						
PROTOCOL	n	%	n	%	n	%
P2	10	10.3	87	89.7	97	100.0
P3	30	11.5	231	88.5	261	100.0
P4	47	9.4	455	90.6	502	100.0
P5	113	7.8	1338	92.2	1451	100.0
Total	200	8.7	2111	91.3	2311	100.0
$p = 0.195$						

Table 6: Absolute and relative frequencies of final outcome (death/recovery) by potential predictors. Continued

	AGE	SEX	DEMENTIA	OBESITY	ASTHMA	CDK	HTA	DM	COPD
AGE	1.000	.024	.137*	.015	-.144**	.122**	.360**	.238**	.194**
SEX		1.000	.002	.034	.046*	-.052	.018	.037	.003
DEMENTIA			1.000	-.036	-.018	.014	-.035	.012	.063**
OBESITY				1.000	-.007	.026	.074**	.096**	.004
ASTHMA					1.000	-.060**	-.137**	-.081**	-.023
CDK						1.000	-.076**	.095**	.060**
HTA							1.000	.239**	.033
DM								1.000	.045**
COPD									1.000
IHD									
CANCER									
HIV									
ANAC									
MOTH									
PROVINCE									
MUNI_LC									
SYMPTOMS									
PROTOCOL									
** Correlation is significant at level 0.01 (bilateral)									
* Correlation is sifnificant at level 0.05 (bilateral)									

Table 7: Spearman correlation coefficients for the 18 predictor variables

	IHD	CANCER	HIV	ANAC	MONTH	PROVINCE	MUNI_LC	SYMPTOMS	PROTOCOL
AGE	.278**	.123**	-043*	.071**	.076**	.002	-.035	.053*	.045*
SEX	-.018	-.023	-.044	.019	-.006	.031	-.001	.034	.003
DEMENTIA	.035	-.017	-.018	-.024	-.042	.006	-.020	-.007	-.052
OBESITY	-.005	-.006	-.018	.017	.036	-.034	-.021	.028	.030
ASTHMA	-.079	-.058	.014	.025	.030	-.056**	.022	.002	.062**
CDK	.017**	.073**	-.018	-.006	-.045*	.004	-.001	-.052*	-.055**
HTA	.157**	.025	-.026	.106**	.138**	.027	-.032	.038	.128**
DM	.207**	.031	-.018	.072**	.059**	.021	.004	.052*	.033
COPD	.083**	.079**	.003	.048*	.010	-.011	-.005	.088**	-.008
IHD	1.000	.051*	-.017	.035	.011	.039	-.016	.030	-.025
CANCER		1.000	.003	-.050*	-.030	-.008	.002	.030	-.025
HIV			1.000	-.008	.008	-.030	-.007	.026	.004
ANAC				1.000	.669**	.089**	-.091**	-.094**	.514**
MOTH					1.000	.214**	-.087**	-.202**	.852**
PROVINCE						1.000	-.249**	-.018	.082**
MUNI_LC							1.000	-.032	-.025
SYMPTOMS								1.000	-.178**
PROTOCOL									1.000
** Correlation is significant at level 0.001 (bilateral)									
* Correlation is sifnificant at level 0.05 (bilateral)									

Table 8: Spearman correlation coefficients for the 18 predictor variables (continued)

```
> # (assuming we are not interested in effects for specific provinces);
> # This is so because each month (each category of MESC) does appear
> # in different provinces; MESC levels are not specific to PROV levels.
> # Variables PROV and MESC are, both at the same level (second level).
> # The first level units are the patients, and the second level units are
> # months and provinces. Months are second level units, and provinces are also 2nd level units.
> fm13 <- glmer(EVOLU_N ~ 1+HTA2020+Cancer2020+IRC2020+Obesidad2020+
+ demencia2020+CI2020+DM2020+EPOC2020+EDAD_C+SEXON+
+ SINTOMAS+ANAC1+(1|MONTH)+(1|PROVINCE), cf_cuba_01,binomial).
```


```
> # The first level units are the patients, and the second level units are
> # months and provinces. Months are second level units, and provinces are also 2nd level units.
> fm13 <- glmer(EVOLU_N ~ 1+HTA2020+Cancer2020+IRC2020+Obesidad2020+
+ demencia2020+CI2020+DM2020+EPOC2020+EDAD_C+SEXON+
+ SINTOMAS+ANAC1+(1|MONTH)+(1|PROVINCE), cf_cuba_01,binomial).
```


Results of the comparison are shown in Table 9. The goodness of fit in terms of the Akaike Information Criterion (AIC) is similar for the three models; model fm13 was kept as the final model, as it includes PROVINCE and MONTH as crossed random effects. As a result of the inclusion of random effects for MONTH (fm12) and MONTH and PROVINCE (fm13) the standard errors of fixed effects are larger than when no random effects are included (fm11), as expected (see Table 10).

In Table 11, estimations of the RRs for the categories of each of the 12 predictors are presented. Among comorbidities, statistically significant results are observed for CKD, Obesity, Dementia, and DM; particularly, Obesity increases the risk of death almost 4 times, adjusting for the other 11 covariates. Age is one of the strongest predictors of death: belonging in the age group 65+ increases the risk of death 29 times with respect to belonging in the age group < 34. The other strong predictor of death is "Average Number of Active Cases" at month of diagnosis; a patient diagnosed in a month where this average is above 1000 increases the risk of death 30 times with respect to a patient diagnosed in a month where this average is less than 200, adjusting for all other 11 covariates.

When compared with previous studies, there was coincidence for age [54–56, 58–62], and CKD [56, 60, 62], which are among the predictors most frequently reported as statistically significant. In the cases of dementia [56], and obesity [60], our results are not usually reported as statistically significant.

With respect to methodological issues, it is worth mentioning the inclusion of predictor SYMPTOMS, categorized as "NO SYMPTOMS" and three categories for delays between first symptoms and diagnosis; this is because it allows to use all the information available, while preserving the possibility of important comparisons between "no symptoms" vs. "symptoms" on one hand, and between different delays in diagnosing patients with symptoms.

Also, considering the Average Number of Active Cases at (month of) Diagnosis (ANAC) as a potential predictor is methodologically important, as it does show the general impact of flattening the curve of active cases on reducing case fatality. Although this is not useful in the management of patients arriving at hospitals.

Classifying Municipalities according to Living Conditions allowed us to assess the potential impact of this social factor on case fatality; it was relevant to include it within the list of potential predictors, allowing the data to confirm its impact in the Cuban context. The classification of Cuban Municipalities according to Living Conditions can be found in [64].

Although not presented in this report, a second analysis was conducted with the full/global dataset to assess the consistency of the results under the assumptions of high quality data vs. routine quality data.

Several studies have included laboratory indicators as predictors of death or recovery [53–56, 58]. Not having laboratory variables in our dataset, as well as genetic indicators, is a limitation of our models, as regards prognostic capacity. About 30% of deaths in the first analysis and 29% in the second analysis, were correctly predicted by the logistic regression models.

Variables	fm11 Coefficients:				fm12 Fixed effects:				fm13 Fixed effects:			
	Stimate	Std. Error	*p*		Stimate	Std. Error	*p*		Stimate	Std. Error	*p*	
(Intercept)	-6.490	0.640	< 0.001	* * *	-6.510	0.653	<0.001	* * *	-6.631	0.667	<2e-16	* * *
HTA	-0.045	0.208	0.827		-0.032	0.209	0.878		-0.045	0.210	0.832	
Cancer	0.563	0.335	0.093		0.550	0.337	0.103		0.559	0.338	0.098	
CKD	1.169	0.306	<0.001	* * *	1.137	0.309	<0.001	* * *	1.164	0.311	<0.001	* * *
Obesity	1.369	0.393	<0.001	* * *	1.372	0.397	0.001	* * *	1.366	0.400	0.001	* * *
IHD	0.436	0.236	0.065	.	0.426	0.237	0.072	.	0.462	0.240	0.054	
DM	0.596	0.213	0.005	**	0.589	0.215	0.006	**	0.587	0.215	0.006	**
COPD	0.441	0.308	0.153		0.435	0.309	0.159		0.446	0.312	0.153	
AGE_C2	1.670	0.546	0.002	**	1.684	0.546	0.002	**	1.669	0.548	0.002	**
AGE_C3	3.362	0.546	0.002	* * *	3.371	0.546	<0.001	* * *	3.347	0.548	<0.001	* * *
SEX_2	-0.595	0.196	0.002	**	-0.602	0.197	0.002	**	-0.591	0.198	0.003	**
SYMPTOMS2	1.525	0.250	<0.001	* * *	1.501	0.252	<0.001	* * *	1.501	0.252	<0.001	* * *
SYMPTOMS3	2.128	0.310	<0.001	* * *	2.097	0.314	<0.001	* * *	2.097	0.317	<0.001	* * *
SYMPTOMS4	2.064	0.401	<0.001	* * *	2.032	0.403	<0.001	* * *	1.993	0.410	<0.001	* * *
ANAC_2	0.800	0.456	0.079	.	0.827	0.512	0.106		0.775	0.496	0.118	
ANAC_3	0.085	0.342	0.804		0.023	0.384	0.952		0.056	0.378	0.883	
ANAC_4	0.359	0.417	0.390		0.380	0.477	0.425		0.229	0.493	0.643	
ANAC_5	-0.356	0.485	0.464		-0.340	0.537	0.527		-0.291	0.522	<0.001	
ANAC_6	3.395	0.473	<0.001	* * *	3.412	0.526	<0.001	* * *	3.529	0.526	<0.001	* * *
	AIC: 834.81				AIC: 836				AIC: 837.1			
* ≤ 0.05; ** ≤ 0.005; * * * ≤ 0.001												

Table 9: Comparison of models fm11, fm12, and fm13 (Coefficients, standard errors and p values)

Cluster Size (N)	% with respect to whole sample (=2240)	Case Fatality m	%	% Deaths with respect to total Deaths (=200)	Label/Descrition of the cluster
14	0.6	8	57.14	4.00	Men 65+, symptomatic, IHD
11	0.5	5	45.45	2.50	Women 65+, symptomatic, Dementia, some IHD
15	0.7	6	40.00	3.00	Men 65+, symptomatic, DM and IHD
7	0.3	2	28.57	1.00	Persons 65+, symptomatic, CKD
30	1.3	8	26.67	4.00	Women 65+, symptomatic, DM
16	0.7	4	25.00	2.00	Women 65+, symptomatic, IHD
8	0.4	2	25.00	1.00	Men < 65, symptomatic, Cancer and Obesity
69	3.1	17	24.64	8.50	Men 65+, symptomatic, some Dementia
17	0.8	4	23.53	2.00	Women symptomatic, IHD
49	2.2	11	22.45	5.50	Women 65+, symptomatic, no comorbidities

Table 10: Results of Cluster Analysis to identify patterns with highest case fatality. Note: Hierarchical cluster analysis based on 10 binary variables, with squared Euclidean distance was applied, to data already described

Final estimates and 95% Cis for model fm13			
	Estimate	95%CI	
(Intercept)	0.00	0.00	0.00
HTA	0.97	0.63	1.44
Cancer	1.73	0.90	3.39
CKD	3.12	1.74	5.90
Obesity	3.94	1.79	8.58
Dementia	3.02	1.56	6.02
IHD	1.53	0.99	2.54
DM	1.80	1.18	2.74
COPD	1.55	0.85	2.88
AGE_C2	5.39	1.81	15.54
AGE_C3	29.11	9.72	83.15
SEX_2	0.55	0.38	0.82
SYMPTOMS2	4.53	2.74	7.35
SYMPTOMS3	8.14	4.37	15.16
SYMPTOMS4	7.63	3.29	16.37
ANAC_C2	2.29	0.82	5.74
ANAC_C3	1.02	0.50	2.22
ANAC_C4	1.46	0.48	3.30
ANAC_C5	0.71	0.27	2.08
ANAC_C6	30.33	12.16	95.63

Table 11: Estimation of RRs for the "Final" model, fm13. First category as reference: Age (< 34, 35-64, 65+), Sex (Male,Female), SINTOMAS (1:No, 2:≤ 3, 3:4-7, 4$>$7), ANAC1 (0-199, 200-399, 400-599, 600-799, 800-1000, $>$1000)

However, in low and middle-income countries and communities, where expensive laboratory tests and other tests cannot be afforded, the results of this study based on socio-demographic and clinical variables could provide useful guides about risk factors for COVID-19 case fatality, and on how to optimize the management of patients.

The results of this case-example are a first look into the problem, not only because potentially relevant indicators were not available, but also because of the rapidly changing characteristics of the epidemic and the virus itself.

However, it is important to draw as many lessons as possible from the data currently available, acknowledging that this learning is a continuous and evolving process.

Age, and average number of active cases at (month of) diagnosis, seem to be the two most important predictors of case fatality. Among comorbidities, our results suggest the most important risk factors are CKD, obesity and dementia.

As far as methods are concerned the chosen approach might be useful for other researchers dealing with this problem in their specific contexts.

3.4 Further Applications of Statistical and Epidemiological Techniques

In this section we briefly describe some other statistical and/or epidemiological techniques that have been applied to the study of the COVID-19 pandemic.

3.4.1 Meta-Analysis

One of these applications is the use of meta-analysis to summarize available evidence on the presence and/or persistence (14+ days) of the SARS-Cov-2 virus in bodily fluids involved in the sexual act: saliva, semen, vaginal and rectal. This is an ongoing study coordinated by the Department of Sexual and Reproductive Health and Research, WHO, and registered in the PROSPERO database (CRD42020204741). Meta-analysis is a quantitative review and synthesis of the results of related but independent studies, which allows the research to have more statistical power to detect an effect (or more precision to estimate a parameter) than an analysis based on only one study. In a meta-analysis an overall treatment effect is calculated as a weighted average of the individual summary statistics. Greater weights are given to the results from studies that provide more and/or better information. The weights are often the inverse of the variance (the square of the standard error) of the treatment effect, which is a function of the sample size.

For this study, "presence" of the virus in the fluid was defined as "presence at the time of diagnosis", and "persistence" was defined as "presence 14 days or more after diagnosis"; from each study the two corresponding proportions were obtained and used. A total of 8 meta-analyses were conducted, 4 for presence and 4 for persistence, using the R package METAFOR. Although the study has not yet been published, we can say in advance that presence and persistence of the virus is higher in saliva and rectal, than in semen and vaginal.

3.4.2 Stratification of COVID-19 Risks

Stratification of COVID-19 cases can be conducted using cluster analysis. In cluster analysis, the multidimensional distance between every two observational units is calculated and used to join those that are similar. With cluster analysis, homogeneity within clusters and heterogeneity between clusters are maximized; in hierarchical cluster analysis, at the beginning, each unit is a cluster, and during the clustering process, the units that are similar according to the chosen distance are put together; thus, until the end, all units belong to the same cluster. Following the whole process, it is possible to find a subjective intermediate solution that satisfies approximately the purpose of the study. Using the database of COVID-19 cases described in a previous section above, a hierarchical cluster analysis with squared Euclidean distance and "between average" agglomeration method was conducted using 10 binary variables: 6 comorbidities (DM, IHD, Cancer, CKD, Obesity, Dementia), Age (< 65, 65+), Sex (male/female), ANAC (< 1000, 1000+), and SYMPTOMS (asymptomatic, symptomatic). The solution with 130 clusters allowed to identify clusters of patients with particular patterns in these 10 variables, with the highest case fatality. The 10 clusters with highest case fatality are presented in Table 10, together with a general description/label that succinctly characterizes each of them.

3.4.3 Is Transmission Mainly Affecting a Particular Subgroup of the Population According to Age and Sex?

It is natural to be concerned when reports are issued about children and adolescents getting infected with COVID-19, and eventually dying from this disease. The human and health impacts of any disease tend to be higher in these groups. But sometimes these reports might mislead one into thinking that COVID-19 is particularly affecting them. At least until January 2021 in Cuba, cases aged 65+ had a much higher risk of dying (approximately 29 times) than cases aged < 34. Table 12 shows that differences between "observed" and "expected" cases is relatively small, indicating that the progression of the disease is proceeding quite uniformly in the different age by sex subgroups of the Cuban population, until January 2021.

3.4.4 An Example of (Mis-)Using a Good Technique for the Wrong Purpose

The misuse of sampling techniques to identify COVID-19 cases seems to have occurred in some circumstances during this COVID-19 pandemic. The early detection of cases has become a priority for different reasons: one is that in doing so the "basic reproductive number" is reduced, as a case is prevented from transmitting the disease to more susceptibles via its early isolation, and also because treatment can be initiated earlier, reducing the risk of case fatality. Some authors believe that selecting subjects at random from the population and testing them for the disease is a satisfactory way of flattening the epidemic curve. Sampling approaches have indeed been used in relation to COVID-19, particularly for estimating the incidence and prevalence of the disease at a particular point in time in a particular population.

But estimating a parameter in a population by probabilistic sampling, is quite different from early detection of cases, which requires active search either by testing among population usually

COMPARATIVE TRASMITION OF COVID-19 VIRUS IN POPULATION GROUPS BY AGE AND SEX. CUMULATIVE CASES UP TO 21 JANUARY 2021						
AGE GROUPS	0-9	10-19	20-39	40-59	60+	Total
A) STRUCTURE OF THE CUBAN POPULATION 2019, BY AGE AND SEX						
MALE(N)	620394	637097	1473460	1753139	1080083	5564173
FEMALE(N)	580515	600839	1397050	1802632	1248261	5629297
TOTAL(N)	1200909	1237936	2870510	3555771	2328344	11193470
MALE(%)	5.5	5.7	13.2	15.7	9.6	49.7
FEMALE(%)	5.2	5.4	12.5	16.1	11.2	50.3
B) STRUCTURE OF COVID-19 CASES IN CUBA UP TO 21 JANUARY 2021						
MALE(N)	301	420	2136	2300	976	6133
FEMALE(N)	273	425	1911	2012	938	5559
TOTAL(N)	574	845	4047	4312	1914	11692
MALE(%)	2.6	3.6	18.3	19.7	8.3	52.5
FEMALE(%)	2.3	3.6	16.3	17.2	8.0	47.5
C) PERCENTAGE DIFFERENCES (CASES -GENERAL POPULATION)						
MALE	-3.0	-2.1	5.1	4.0	-1.3	2.7
FEMALE	-2.9	-1.7	3.9	1.1	-3.1	-2.7

Table 12: Transmission of COVID-19 virus in the Cuban population, by age and sex

at high risk of contagion (health workers and other public services workers), or by sensible and timely epidemiological enquiries, looking for contacts of recently detected cases.

4 CONCLUDING REMARKS

Statistical and epidemiological basic concepts, thinking, and methods, are necessary to obtain important information from the volumes of data that are being generated by the COVID-19 pandemic, both at the country level and globally; and for sound interpretation and communication of results to public health decision makers.

The need for careful consideration in the selection and calculation of basic indicators, and in their proper interpretation, have been discussed; we have also discussed some statistical procedures that have been used at different levels around the world, to find plausible answers to right questions, related to the monitoring of the pandemic curves, the health impact of the pandemic, the identification of patterns for infection among the population, and for death among infected, the identification of potential predictor factors for outcomes at the country level and patient level, etc.

Finally, the application of a particular statistical technique, multilevel logistic regression, to the exploration of risk factors for COVID-19 fatality in Cuba, has been illustrated using as much as possible statistical and epidemiological thinking, and common sense.

It is hoped that this chapter has contributed to make clear that statistics should be an essential component in the set of tools to confront the current and potential future pandemics.

5 CONSENT FOR PUBLICATION

Not applicable.

6 CONFLICT OF INTEREST

The authors declare no conflict of interest, financial or otherwise.

7 ACKNOWLEDGEMENTS

To the group of experts and scientists who collaborated with the Cuban government and kindly provided all the information for this study.

References

[1] Lipsitch M, Donnelly CA, Fraser C, Blake IM, Cori A, Dorigatti I, Ferguson NM, Garske T, Mills HL, Riley S, Van Kerkhove MD, Hernán MA. Potential Biases in Estimating Absolute and Relative Case-Fatality Risks during Outbreaks. PLOS Neglected Tropical Diseases [Internet]. 2015 Jul 16 [cited Oct 01, 2021];9(7):e0003846. Available from: https://doi.org/10.1371/journal.pntd.0003846

[2] Lau H, Khosrawipour T, Kocbach P, Ichii H, Bania J, Khosrawipour V. Evaluating the massive underreporting and undertesting of COVID-19 cases in multiple global epicenters. Pulmonology [Internet]. 2020 Jun [cited Oct 01, 2021]. Available from: https://doi.org/10.1016/j.pulmoe.2020.05.015

[3] Mertens E, Peñalvo JL. The Burden of Malnutrition and Fatal COVID-19: A Global Burden of Disease Analysis. Frontiers in Nutrition [Internet]. 2021 Jan 21 [cited Oct 01, 2021];7. Available from: https://doi.org/10.3389/fnut.2020.619850

[4] World Health Organization. Global surveillance for COVID-19 caused by human infection with COVID-19 virus: interim guidance, 20 March 2020. Geneva: World Health Organization; 2020 2020. Contract No.: WHO/2019-nCoV/SurveillanceGuidance/2020.6.

[5] Global Burden of Disease (GBD). Available from: http://www.healthdata.org/gbd

[6] Murray CJL. Quantifying the burden of disease: The technical basis for disability-adjusted life years. Bull World Health Organization. 1994;72:429–45.

[7] Aburto JM, Kashyap R, Schöley J, Angus C, Ermisch J, Mills MC, Dowd JB. Estimating the burden of the COVID-19 pandemic on mortality, life expectancy and lifespan inequality in England and Wales: a population-level analysis. Journal of Epidemiology and Community Health [Internet]. 2021 Jan 19 [cited Oct 01, 2021];75(8):735–40. Available from: https://doi.org/10.1136/jech-2020-215505

[8] Everitt BS, Landau S, Leese M, Stahl D. Cluster Analysis. [place unknown]: Wiley & Sons, Incorporated, John; 2011. 346 p.

[9] Wynants L, Van Calster B, Collins GS, Riley RD, Heinze G, Schuit E, et al. Prediction models for diagnosis and prognosis of covid-19: systematic review and critical appraisal. BMJ [Internet]. 2020 Apr 7 [cited Oct 01, 2021]:m1328. Available from: https://doi.org/10.1136/bmj.m1328

[10] Steyerberg EW. Clinical prediction models: A practical approach to development, validation, and updating. New York, NY: Springer; 2009. 497 p.

[11] van Smeden M, Moons KG, de Groot JA, Collins GS, Altman DG, Eijkemans MJ, Reitsma JB. Sample size for binary logistic prediction models: Beyond events per variable criteria. Statistical Methods in Medical Research [Internet]. 2018 Jul 3 [cited Oct 02, 2021];28(8):2455–74. Available from: https://doi.org/10.1177/0962280218784726

[12] Hoerl AE, Kennard RW. Ridge Regression: Biased Estimation for Nonorthogonal Problems. Technometrics [Internet]. 1970 Feb [cited Oct 02, 2021];12(1):55–67. Available from: https://doi.org/10.1080/00401706.1970.10488634

[13] Tibshirani R. Regression Shrinkage and Selection Via the Lasso. Journal of the Royal Statistical Society: Series B (Methodological) [Internet]. 1996 Jan [cited Oct 02, 2021];58(1):267–88. Available from: https://doi.org/10.1111/j.2517-6161.1996.tb02080.x

[14] Zou H, Hastie T. Regularization and variable selection via the elastic net. Journal of the Royal Statistical Society: Series B (Statistical Methodology) [Internet]. 2005 Apr [cited Oct 02, 2021];67(2):301–20. Available from: https://doi.org/10.1111/j.1467-9868.2005.00503.x

[15] Burn E, Tebé C, Fernández-Bertolín S, Aragón M, Recalde M, Roel E, et al. The natural history of symptomatic COVID-19 in Catalonia, Spain: a multi-state model including 109,367 outpatient diagnoses, 18,019 hospitalisations, and 5,585 COVID-19 deaths among 5,627,520 people. medRxiv. 2020:2020.07.13.20152454.

[16] Hazard D, Kaier K, von Cube M, Grodd M, Bugiera L, Lambert J, Wolkewitz M. Joint analysis of duration of ventilation, length of intensive care, and mortality of COVID-19 patients: a multistate approach. BMC Medical Research Methodology [Internet]. 2020 Aug 11 [cited Oct 02, 2021];20(1). Available from: https://doi.org/10.1186/s12874-020-01082-z

[17] von Cube M, Grodd M, Wolkewitz M, Hazard D, Lambert J. Harmonizing heterogeneous endpoints in COVID-19 trials without loss of information - an essential step to facilitate decision making. medRxiv. 2020:2020.03.31.20049007.

[18] Deschepper M, Eeckloo K, Malfait S, Benoit D, Callens S, Vansteelandt S. Prediction of hospital bed capacity during the COVID–19 pandemic. BMC Health Services Research [Internet]. 2021 May 18 [cited Oct 02, 2021];21(1). Available from: https://doi.org/10.1186/s12913-021-06492-3

[19] Putter H, Fiocco M, Geskus RB. Tutorial in biostatistics: competing risks and multi-state models. Statistics in Medicine [Internet]. 2007 [cited Oct 02, 2021];26(11):2389–430. Available from: https://doi.org/10.1002/sim.2712

[20] Wolkewitz M, Lambert J, von Cube M, Bugiera L, Grodd M, Hazard D, White N, Barnett A, Kaier K. Statistical Analysis of Clinical COVID-19 Data: A Concise Overview of Lessons Learned, Common Errors and How to Avoid Them. Clinical Epidemiology [Internet]. 2020 Sep [cited Oct 02, 2021];Volume 12:925–8. Available from: https://doi.org/10.2147/clep.s256735

[21] Zeng L, Li J, Liao M, Hua R, Huang P, Zhang M, et al. Risk assessment of progression to severe conditions for patients with COVID-19 pneumonia: a single-center retrospective study. medRxiv. 2020:2020.03.25.20043166.

[22] Wang J, Lee ET. Statistical Methods for Survival Data Analysis. [place unknown]: Wiley & Sons, Incorporated, John; 2003. 534 p.

[23] Rodríguez G. Non-parametric estimation in survival models: Spring; 2005. 20 p.

[24] Breslow NE. Discussion on Professor Cox's Paper. Journal of the Royal Statistical Society: Series B (Methodological) [Internet]. 1972 Jan [cited Oct 02, 2021];34(2):202–20. Available from: https://doi.org/10.1111/j.2517-6161.1972.tb00900.x

[25] Nelson W. Theory and Applications of Hazard Plotting for Censored Failure Data. Technometrics [Internet]. 1972 Nov [cited Oct 02, 2021];14(4):945–66. Available from: https://doi.org/10.1080/00401706.1972.10488991

[26] Aalen O. Nonparametric Inference for a Family of Counting Processes. The Annals of Statistics [Internet]. 1978 Jul [cited Oct 02, 2021];6(4):701–26. Available from: https://doi.org/10.1214/aos/1176344247

[27] Lu J, Hu S, Fan R, Liu Z, Yin X, Wang Q, et al. ACP Risk Grade: A Simple Mortality Index for Patients with Confirmed or Suspected Severe Acute Respiratory Syndrome Coronavirus 2 Disease (COVID-19) During the Early Stage of Outbreak in Wuhan, China. SSRN Electronic Journal [Internet]. 2020 [cited Oct 02, 2021]. Available from: https://doi.org/10.2139/ssrn.3543603

[28] Bello-Chavolla OY, Bahena- López JP, Antonio-Villa NE, Vargas-Vázquez A, González-Díaz A, Márquez-Salinas A, Fermín-Martínez CA, Naveja JJ, Aguilar-Salinas CA. Predicting Mortality Due to SARS-CoV-2: A Mechanistic Score Relating Obesity and Diabetes to COVID-19 Outcomes in Mexico. The Journal of Clinical Endocrinology & Metabolism [Internet]. 2020 May 31 [cited Oct 02, 2021];105(8):2752–61. Available from: https://doi.org/10.1210/clinem/dgaa346

[29] Guo Y, Liu Y, Lu J, Fan R, Zhang F, Yin X, et al. Development and validation of an early warning score (EWAS) for predicting clinical deterioration in patients with coronavirus disease 2019. medRxiv. 2020:2020.04.17.20064691.

[30] Ji D, Zhang D, Xu J, Chen Z, Yang T, Zhao P, Chen G, Cheng G, Wang Y, Bi J, Tan L, Lau G, Qin E. Prediction for Progression Risk in Patients With COVID-19 Pneumonia: The CALL Score. Clinical Infectious Diseases [Internet]. 2020 Apr 9 [cited Oct 03, 2021];71(6):1393–9. Available from: https://doi.org/10.1093/cid/ciaa414

[31] Wang S, Zha Y, Li W, Wu Q, Li X, Niu M, Wang M, Qiu X, Li H, Yu H, Gong W, Bai Y, Li L, Zhu Y, Wang L, Tian J. A fully automatic deep learning system for COVID-19 diagnostic and prognostic analysis. European Respiratory Journal [Internet]. 2020 May 22 [cited Oct 03, 2021];56(2):2000775. Available from: https://doi.org/10.1183/13993003.00775-2020

[32] Caramelo F, Ferreira N, Oliveiros B. Estimation of risk factors for COVID-19 mortality–preliminary results. medRxiv. 2020.

[33] Xie J, Hungerford D, Chen H, Abrams ST, Li S, Wang G, Wang Y, Kang H, Bonnett L, Zheng R, Li X, Tong Z, Du B, Qiu H, Toh CH. Development and External Validation of a Prognostic Multivariable Model on Admission for Hospitalized Patients with COVID-19. SSRN Electronic Journal [Internet]. 2020 [cited Oct 03, 2021]. Available from: `https://doi.org/10.2139/ssrn.3562456`

[34] Pourhomayoun M, Shakibi M. Predicting mortality risk in patients with COVID-19 using machine learning to help medical decision-making. Smart Health [Internet]. 2021 April [cited Oct 03, 2021];20:100178. Available from: `https://doi.org/10.1016/j.smhl.2020.100178`

[35] Hu C, Liu Z, Jiang Y, Shi O, Zhang X, Xu K, et al. Early prediction of mortality risk among patients with severe COVID-19, using machine learning. International Journal of Epidemiology [Internet]. 2020 Sep 23 [cited Oct 03, 2021]. Available from: `https://doi.org/10.1093/ije/dyaa171`

[36] Levy TJ, Richardson S, Coppa K, Barnaby DP, McGinn T, Becker LB, et al. Development and Validation of a Survival Calculator for Hospitalized Patients with COVID-19. medRxiv. 2020:2020.04.22.20075416.

[37] Liu Q, Fang X, Tokuno S, Chung U, Chen X, Dai X, Liu X, Xu F, Wang B, Peng P. Prediction of the clinical outcome of COVID-19 patients using T lymphocyte subsets with 340 cases from wuhan, china: a retrospective cohort study and a web visualization tool. SSRN Electronic Journal [Internet]. 2020 [cited Oct 3, 2021]. Available from: `https://doi.org/10.2139/ssrn.3557995`

[38] Guillamet CV, Guillamet RV, Kramer AA, Maurer PM, Menke GA, Hill CL, et al. Toward a COVID-19 score-risk assessments and registry. medRxiv. 2020:2020.04.15.20066860.

[39] Zhang H, Shi T, Wu X, Zhang X, Wang K, Bean D, Dobson R, Teo JT, Sun J, Zhao P, Li

C, Dhaliwal K, Wu H, Li Q, Guthrie B. Risk Prediction for Poor Outcome and Death in Hospital In-Patients with COVID-19: Derivation in Wuhan, China and External Validation in London, UK. SSRN Electronic Journal [Internet]. 2020 [cited Oct 03, 2021]. Available from: https://doi.org/10.2139/ssrn.3590468

[40] Huang H, Cai S, Li Y, Li Y, Fan Y, Li L, Lei C, Tang X, Hu F, Li F, Deng X. Prognostic Factors for COVID-19 Pneumonia Progression to Severe Symptoms Based on Earlier Clinical Features: A Retrospective Analysis. Frontiers in Medicine [Internet]. 2020 Oct 5 [cited Oct 03, 2021];7. Available from: https://doi.org/10.3389/fmed.2020.557453

[41] Jiang X, Coffee M, Bari A, Wang J, Jiang X, Huang J, Shi J, Dai J, Cai J, Zhang T, Wu Z, He G, Huang Y. Towards an Artificial Intelligence Framework for Data-Driven Prediction of Coronavirus Clinical Severity. Computers, Materials & Continua [Internet]. 2020 [cited Oct 03, 2021];62(3):537–51. Available from: https://doi.org/10.32604/cmc.2020.010691

[42] Yue H, Yu Q, Liu C, Huang Y, Jiang Z, Shao C et al. Machine learning-based CT radiomics method for predicting hospital stay in patients with pneumonia associated with SARS-CoV-2 infection: a multicenter study. Annals of Translational Medicine [Internet]. July 2020 [cited Octubre 03, 2021];8(14):859. Available from: https://doi.org/10.21037/atm-20-3026

[43] Gong J, Ou J, Qiu X, Jie Y, Chen Y, Yuan L, Cao J, Tan M, Xu W, Zheng F, Shi Y, Hu B. A Tool for Early Prediction of Severe Coronavirus Disease 2019 (COVID-19): A Multicenter Study Using the Risk Nomogram in Wuhan and Guangdong, China. Clinical Infectious Diseases [Internet]. 2020 Apr 16 [cited Oct 03, 2021];71(15):833–40. Available from: https://doi.org/10.1093/cid/ciaa443

[44] Carr E, Bendayan R, Bean D, Stammers M, Wang W, Zhang H, et al. Evaluation and improvement of the National Early Warning Score (NEWS2) for COVID-19: a multi-hospital

study. BMC Medicine [Internet]. 2021 Jan 21 [cited Oct 03, 2021];19(1). Available from: https://doi.org/10.1186/s12916-020-01893-3

[45] Colombi D, Bodini FC, Petrini M, Maffi G, Morelli N, Milanese G, Silva M, Sverzellati N, Michieletti E. Well-aerated Lung on Admitting Chest CT to Predict Adverse Outcome in COVID-19 Pneumonia. Radiology [Internet]. 2020 Aug [cited Oct 03, 2021];296(2):E86–E96. Available from: https://doi.org/10.1148/radiol.2020201433

[46] Steyerberg EW, Vickers AJ, Cook NR, Gerds T, Gonen M, Obuchowski N, Pencina MJ, Kattan MW. Assessing the Performance of Prediction Models. Epidemiology [Internet]. 2010 Jan [cited Oct 03, 2021];21(1):128–38. Available from: https://doi.org/10.1097/ede.0b013e3181c30fb2

[47] Vickers AJ, Van Calster B, Steyerberg EW. Net benefit approaches to the evaluation of prediction models, molecular markers, and diagnostic tests. BMJ [Internet]. 2016 Jan 25 [cited Oct 03, 2021]:i6. Available from: https://doi.org/10.1136/bmj.i6

[48] Vickers AJ, van Calster B, Steyerberg EW. A simple, step-by-step guide to interpreting decision curve analysis. Diagnostic and Prognostic Research [Internet]. 2019 Oct 4 [cited Oct 03, 2021];3(1). Available from: https://doi.org/10.1186/s41512-019-0064-7

[49] Hilden J, Habbema JD, Bjerregaard B. The Measurement of Performance in Probabilistic Diagnosis. Methods of Information in Medicine [Internet]. 1978 Oct [cited Oct 03, 2021];17(04):227–37. Available from: https://doi.org/10.1055/s-0038-1636442

[50] Harrell FE, Lee KL, Mark DB. Multivariable prognostic models: issues in developing models, evaluating assumptions and adequacy, and measuring and reducing errors. Statistics in Medicine [Internet]. 1996 Feb 29 [cited Oct 03, 2021];15(4):361–87. Available from:

https://doi.org/10.1002/(sici)1097-0258(19960229)15:4%3C361::aid-sim168%3E3.0.co;2-4

[51] Brier GW. Verification of forecasts expressed in terms of probability. Monthly Weather Review [Internet]. 1950 Jan [cited Oct 03, 2021];78(1):1–3. Available from: https://doi.org/10.1175/1520-0493(1950)078%3C0001:vofeit%3E2.0.co;2

[52] Riley RD, Ensor J, Snell KI, Harrell FE, Martin GP, Reitsma JB, Moons KG, Collins G, van Smeden M. Calculating the sample size required for developing a clinical prediction model. BMJ [Internet]. 2020 Mar 18 [cited Oct 03, 2021]:m441. Available from: https://doi.org/10.1136/bmj.m441

[53] Ryan L, Lam C, Mataraso S, Allen A, Green-Saxena A, Pellegrini E, Hoffman J, Barton C, McCoy A, Das R. Mortality prediction model for the triage of COVID-19, pneumonia, and mechanically ventilated ICU patients: a retrospective study. Annals of Medicine and Surgery [Internet]. 2020 Nov [cited Oct 03, 2021];59:207–16. Available from: https://doi.org/10.1016/j.amsu.2020.09.044

[54] Yang HJ, Zhang YM, Yang M, Huang X. Re: Predictors of mortality for patients with COVID-19 pneumonia caused by SARSCoV-2: a prospective cohort study. European Respiratory Journal [Internet]. 2020 Aug 3 [cited Oct 03, 2021]:2002439. Available from: https://doi.org/10.1183/13993003.02439-2020

[55] Liu J, Liu Z, Jiang W, Wang J, Zhu M, Song J, Wang X, Su Y, Xiang G, Ye M, Li J, Zhang Y, Shen Q, Li Z, Yao D, Song Y, Yu K, Luo Z, Ye L. Clinical predictors of COVID-19 disease progression and death: Analysis of 214 hospitalised patients from Wuhan, China. The Clinical Respiratory Journal [Internet]. 2020 Nov 8 [cited Oct 03, 2021]. Available from: https://doi.org/10.1111/crj.13296

[56] Bellan M, Patti G, Hayden E, Azzolina D, Pirisi M, Acquaviva A, et al. Fatality rate and

predictors of mortality in an Italian cohort of hospitalized COVID-19 patients. Scientific Reports [Internet]. 2020 Nov 26 [cited Oct 03, 2021];10(1). Available from: https://doi.org/10.1038/s41598-020-77698-4

[57] Li Y, Horowitz MA, Liu J, Chew A, Lan H, Liu Q, Sha D, Yang C. Individual-Level Fatality Prediction of COVID-19 Patients Using AI Methods. Frontiers in Public Health [Internet]. 2020 Sep 30 [cited Oct 03, 2021];8. Available from: https://doi.org/10.3389/fpubh.2020.587937

[58] Ruan Q, Yang K, Wang W, Jiang L, Song J. Clinical predictors of mortality due to COVID-19 based on an analysis of data of 150 patients from Wuhan, China. Intensive Care Medicine [Internet]. 2020 Mar 3 [cited Oct 03, 2021];46(5):846–8. Available from: https://doi.org/10.1007/s00134-020-05991-x

[59] Yadaw AS, Li YC, Bose S, Iyengar R, Bunyavanich S, Pandey G. Clinical features of COVID-19 mortality: development and validation of a clinical prediction model. The Lancet Digital Health [Internet]. 2020 Oct [cited Oct 03, 2021];2(10):e516–e525. Available from: https://doi.org/10.1016/s2589-7500(20)30217-x

[60] van Halem K, Bruyndonckx R, van der Hilst J, Cox J, Driesen P, Opsomer M, Van Steenkiste E, Stessel B, Dubois J, Messiaen P. Risk factors for mortality in hospitalized patients with COVID-19 at the start of the pandemic in Belgium: a retrospective cohort study. BMC Infectious Diseases [Internet]. 2020 Nov 27 [cited Oct 03, 2021];20(1). Available from: https://doi.org/10.1186/s12879-020-05605-3

[61] Das AK, Gopalan SS. Epidemiology of COVID-19 and Predictors of Recovery in the Republic of Korea. Pulmonary Medicine [Internet]. 2020 Jul 30 [cited Oct 03, 2021];2020:1–6. Available from: https://doi.org/10.1155/2020/7291698

[62] Kim W, Han JM, Lee KE. Predictors of Mortality in Patients with COVID-19: A Systematic

Review and Meta-analysis. Korean Journal of Clinical Pharmacy [Internet]. 2020 Sep 30 [cited Oct 03, 2021];30(3):169–76. Available from: https://doi.org/10.24304/kjcp.2020.30.3.169

[63] Mehraeen E, Karimi A, Barzegary A, Vahedi F, Afsahi AM, Dadras O, Moradmand-Badie B, Seyed Alinaghi SA, Jahanfar S. Predictors of mortality in patients with COVID-19–a systematic review. European Journal of Integrative Medicine [Internet]. 2020 Dec [cited Oct 03, 2021];40:101226. Available from: https://doi.org/10.1016/j.eujim.2020.101226

[64] Corral A. Desigualdades en la carga global de enfermedad según condiciones de vida. Cuba 2013. Horizonte Sanitario. 2019;18(3).

CHAPTER 9

Understanding the Impact of Cuban Immunotherapy Protocols During COVID-19 Disease: Contributions from Mathematical Modeling and Statistical Approaches

K. García-Martínez[*1], **P. L. Luaces-Álvarez**[1], **L. Sánchez-Valdés**[1]
K. León-Monzón[1], **T. Crombet-Ramos**[1] **and R. Pérez-Rodríguez**[1]

[*] **Corresponding author:** karina@cim.sld.cu, Phone: +53 7 2717933
[1] Center of Molecular Immunology, Havana, Cuba

Abstract. Cuban protocols to treat patients with COVID-19 include interferon alpha 2B and anti-inflammatory therapy at different moments of the progression of the disease. Here, we present the results obtained using a mathematical model to study the immunopathology associated with COVID-19. Model simulations reproduce the clinical observations for the antiviral and anti-inflammatory therapies and provide explanations for their efficacy from an immunological point of view. In addition, we present new data and statistical analysis of the clinical use of itolizumab, a humanized anti-CD6 antibody that reduces the secretion of multiple inflammatory cytokines. Authors concluded that the timely use of itolizumab can reduce the probability of death while its late prescription might not significantly reduce COVID-19 morbidity and mortality.

Key words: COVID-19, mathematical modeling, statistical analysis, itolizumab, interferon alpha 2B

1 INTRODUCTION

1.1 Importance

We develop a mathematical model for the dynamics of the immune response associated with COVID-19. Model results help to understand the effect of immunotherapies used in Cuban protocols on this infectious disease, and predict the best treatment strategies. We also present new clinical data for the use of itolizumab, a Cuban anti-inflammatory therapy. Statistical analysis of its efficacy in Cuban patients is in agreement with mathematical model predictions.

1.2 Preliminaries

COVID-19 is an acute respiratory disease caused by a highly pathogenic novel coronavirus SARS-CoV-2. The widely reported symptoms of COVID-19 are extremely variable, ranging from minimal symptoms to significant hypoxia with acute respiratory distress syndrome (ARDS) and multiorgan failure, which could be fatal [1].

COVID-19 is not a clear-cut disorder, but a gradually evolving pathology, characterized by a series of stages sustained by different molecular mechanisms. Earliest analyses of people with coronavirus in China suggested that it might not be the virus alone that damages the lungs and kills, but an overactive immune response might also contribute [2]. The disease can hence be divided into different phases including a respiratory and a proinflammatory stage [3].

Type I Interferons (IFNs) play a primary role in the inhibition of viral replication through the coordination of antiviral immune responses and modulation of inflammatory responses. The type I IFN response in SARS patients was observed to be deregulated in patients that experienced adverse outcomes and severe disease [4]. In addition, the viral infection can lead to an excessive immune reaction in some patients, which is a hyperinflammatory state, known as cytokine release syndrome or cytokine storm [1].

Even though the exact immune mechanisms of COVID-19-mediated pathogenesis are still under investigation [5], we propose a mathematical model to explain the role of the innate and adaptive immune response in the outcome of the disease. We also present new data and statistical analyses of the clinical use of itolizumab, a humanized anti-CD6 antibody that reduces the secretion of multiple inflammatory cytokines.

2 MATHEMATICAL MODEL PRESENTATION

The immune response induced by COVID-19 involves several cells and molecules that play different roles depending on the stage of viral infection. The first response against the virus is mediated by components of the innate immune response, where the antigen presenting cells (APCs) have an important role in processing virus antigens and secreting Type I IFN that directly acts in inhibiting virus replication inside infected cells. This process helps to control virus expansion, but the total or partial elimination of the virus depends on the magnitude of this response. The second response is mediated by components of the adaptive immune response, where CD8+ T cells play a crucial role. These cells arrive to the site of infection with a time delay after virus entry to the system, differentiating into cytotoxic T cells after antigen recognition and interleukin-6 (IL-6) signaling. Cytotoxic T cells are able to kill infected cells and finally eliminate the virus from the system. In patients with deficiency in types of immune response, the presence of a higher virus load and infected cells induce a persistent activation of APCs accompanied by a continuous secretion of type I IFN and IL-6. In this case of uncontrolled disease, type I IFN acts as a proinflammatory cytokine potentiating the continuous activation of APCs. Additionally, increased levels of IL-6 cause host cell damage which can lead to death.

We developed a mathematical model for the immunopathology associated with COVID-19. To the classical Virus+Target+Infected model, we added the dynamics of immune components such as type I IFN and IL-6 cytokines, and immune cells such as Dendritic, CD8+ and Cytotoxic CD8+ T cells. Model simulations reproduce the clinical observations for different patients, both good responders and immunodeficient, and provide an explanation for the effect of immunotherapies applied in different moments during virus infection.

2.1 Model Assumptions

We built the model based on relevant information from the immunopathology of COVID-19 disease, recently described in the literature. We centered our model on the processes concerning CD8+ T cell response, responsible for virus elimination; and both molecules, type I IFN and IL-6, for which there is a consensus about their main role during the immune response and posterior inflammatory damage (see Fig. 1).

To describe the dynamics of virus infection and the associated immune response, the model is based on the following assumptions:

1. Virus particles infect susceptible cells in a process that results in their replication [6].
2. IFN-type I inhibits the virus replication process in infected cells [7–9].
3. Dendritic cells (DCs) are the main source of type I IFN [10, 11].
4. High levels of type I IFN lead to a proinflammatory effect mediated by the induction of DCs activation [12].
5. IL-6 is generated by DCs in an infectious process [13].

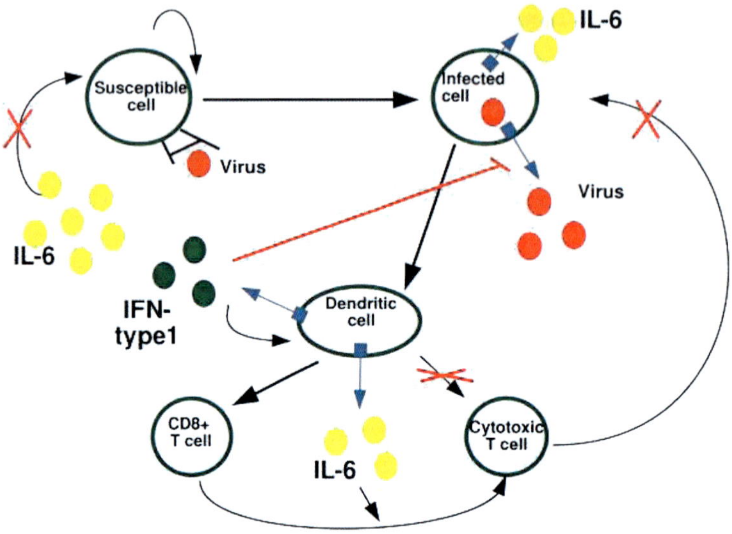

Figure 1: Immunopathology associated with COVID-19 disease, summarized in Model Assumptions. Arrows correspond to activation, creation, or secretion processes; arrows with red crosses indicate elimination processes; and the red line indicates inhibition process

6. Virus promotes IL-6 production by infected cells [14].
7. IL-6 induces the differentiation of CD8+ T cells into cytotoxic T cells [15].
8. High levels of IL-6 expression lead to profound inflammatory damage to susceptible cells [16].
9. Infected cells recruit DCs to the site of infection [17].
10. Cytotoxic CD8+ T cells kill infected epithelial cells [14, 18].
11. Disease severity is associated with a pronounced decrease in CD8+ T cells due to T cell exhaustion [19, 20].
12. Susceptible cells renovate in a homeostatic process [21].

Other processes have been described for COVID-19 disease, which we do not take into account in our model assumptions. For example, it has been reported that the virus can inhibit IFN-type I production by DCs, in a process depending on the viral load [14, 22]; increased levels of IL-6 can induce T cell exhaustion [23]; and the virus can directly infect T cells and induce cell death, but cannot replicate inside T cells [24]. There is not a consensus on the relevance of these mechanisms during COVID-19 disease. Thus, we will not include these processes in our model. Nevertheless, their effect can be taken into account by varying specific model parameter values in simulations without the need to include new terms in the model equations. For example, increasing the rate of T cell exhaustion or reducing the threshold of exhaustion helps to simulate a stronger induction of this process, mediated by both DCs and IL-6 produced by the same DCs.

The processes related to antibody-producing B cell dynamics and the consequent antibody response are not included in the model. We simplify our model considering only the effect of cytotoxic T cells during virus dynamics, described as the main cause of the elimination of virus-infected cells during infection [25]. This is a first approximation to study the effect of adaptive immune response in COVID-19.

Memory CD8+ T cell response is not included in the model. This type of response is relevant during reinfection or after vaccination. In the future, we will include the effect of Memory T cells in the dynamics of COVID-19 immunopathology. This will allow us to study the capacity of the generation of virus protection during a second infection, or after a preventive vaccination treatment.

2.2 Model Equations

Model assumptions are translated into a system of ordinary differential equations to describe the dynamics of susceptible cells (S), infected cells (I_c), virus particles (V), dendritic cells (D_c), type I IFN molecules (If_n), IL-6 molecules (IL), CD8+ T cells (T) and Cytotoxic (T_c) CD8+ T cells. Equations are given below (see variables and parameters definition in Tables 1, 2, and 3, respectively):

$$
\begin{aligned}
\frac{dS(t)}{dt} &= -k_i S(t)V(t) + kp_s S(t)\left(1 - \frac{S(t)+I_c(t)}{S_{max}}\right) - kd_s S(t)\frac{IL(t)}{IL(t)+n_s},\\
\frac{dI_c(t)}{dt} &= k_i S(t)V(t) - d_i I_c(t) - d_{tc} I_c(t)T_c(t),\\
\frac{dV(t)}{dt} &= k_v I_c(t)\left(1 - \frac{If_n(t)}{If_n(t)+k_{if}}\right) - d_v V(t),\\
\frac{dD_c(t)}{dt} &= k_{dc} I_c(t) + kp_{if}\frac{If_n(t)}{If_n(t)+kf_{dc}} D_c(t) - d_c D_c(t),\\
\frac{dIf_n(t)}{dt} &= k_f \frac{D_c(t)}{D_c(t)+n_{if}} - d_{ifn} If_n(t),\\
\frac{dIL(t)}{dt} &= k_{pdc}\frac{D_c(t)}{D_c(t)+n_{dc}} + k_{piv}\frac{IL(t)}{IL(t)+n_{ic}} - d_{il} IL(t),\\
\frac{dT(t)}{dt} &= H(t-t_c)\left[kp_T T(t)\frac{D_c(t)}{D_c(t)+n_{ac}} - kc_T T(t)\frac{IL(t)}{IL(t)+n_{IL}} - kd_T T(t)\right],\\
\frac{dT_c(t)}{dt} &= H(t-t_c)\left[kc_T T(t)\frac{IL(t)}{IL(t)+n_{IL}} - kc_{ex} T_(t)\frac{D_c(t)}{D_c(t)+n_{ex}}\right].
\end{aligned}
$$

Variables	**Nomenclature in equations**	**Dimension**
Susceptible cells	S	$cell/mL$
Infected cells	$I\nu$	$cell/mL$
Virus particles	V	$copies/mL$
Dendritic cells	Dc	$cells/mL$
IFN-type1 molecules	Ifn	pg/mL
IL-6 molecules	IL	pg/mL
CD8+ T cells	T, Tc	$cells/mL$

Table 1: Variables of the model, the nomenclature used in equations and their dimensions

The first three equations are similar to the classical Virus+Target+Infected model. The first equation assumes that the virus can infect susceptible cells through a process that leads to infected cells (second equation). Virus replicates inside the infected cells and is released at a rate k_v.

Model parameter	Symbol	Value	References	Classification
Rate of virus infection of susceptible cells	k_i	4×10^{-8} $[mL/copies.1/day]$	[26]	*Fitting results for COVID-19 patients*
Rate at which infected cells are cleared, as a consequence of cytopathic viral effects	d_i	1.0 $[1/day]$	[26]	*Fitting results for COVID-19 patients*
		0.014 $[1/day]$	[21]	
Rate of virus release from infected cells	k_v	3 $[copies/mL.1/day.1/cell]$	[26]	*Fitting results for COVID-19 patients*
Rate at which virus particles are cleared	d_v	2.4 $[1/day]$	[26]	*Previously estimated in humans for influenza and HIV (this process is not related to the immune system or viral particles per se)*
Dendritic cells recruitment rate by Infected cells	k_{dc}	0.22 $[1/day]$	[21]	*Taken from literature of previous mathematical model studies that estimate it*
Dendritic cells death rate	d_{dc}	0.3 $[1/day]$	[21]	*Taken from literature*
IFN-type1 production by Dendritic cells	$(*)k_f$	3.56 $[pg/mL/day]$	[21]	*Parameter estimated in vitro after monocytes and respiratory syncytial virus co-culture*
IFN-type1 production by Dendritic cells → cytokine production half-effect	n_{if}	0.54 $[10^9 cells/mL]$	[21]	*Parameter estimated in vitro after monocytes and respiratory syncytial virus co-culture*
Rate of IFN-type1 renal clearance	d_{ifn}	18 $[1/day]$	[21]	*Taken from literature*
IFN inhibition of viral production → cell related half-effect	k_{if}	4.7×10^{-4} $[pg/mL]$	[21]	*From measures of the mean inhibition of MERS-CoV replication of IFN-b*
IL-6 production by Dendritic cells	k_{pdc}	1872 $[pg/mL/day]$	[21]	*Estimated by data fitting in the literature*
IL-6 production by Dendritic cells → cytokine production half-effect	n_{dc}	4.47×10^5 $[cells/mL]$	[21]	*Estimated by data fitting in the literature*
IL-6 production by Infected cells	k_{piv}	11.89 $[pg/mL/day]$	[21]	*Estimated from in vitro culture of A549 cells infected with H5N1 and H7N9 virus*
IL-6 production by Infected cells → cytokine production half-effect	n_{ic}	0.7×10^9 $[cells/mL]$	[21]	*Estimated from in vitro culture of A549 cells infected with H5N1 and H7N9 virus*
Rate of IL-6 renal clearance	d_{il}	16.6 $[1/day]$	[21]	*Taken from literature*
Time of first infiltration of CD8+ T cell	t_c	5 $[days]$	[27]	*Taken from literature, from infected cell recruitment of CD8+ T cells*
		4.5 $[days]$	[21]	
Rate of CD8+ T cells proliferation	(**) kp_T	0.194 $[1/day]$	[26]	*Taken from literature*
		1 $[1/day]$	[21, 28]	
Rate of CD8+ T cells proliferation (antigen driven proliferation) → cell related half-effect	(**) n_{ac}	0.1 $[cells/mL]$	[21]	*Taken from literature*

Table 2: Parameter values used in model simulations. (*) Control parameters of the model varied in simulations around this reported value. (**) For T cell proliferation and exhaustion processes note that $kp_T < k_{ex}$, $n_{ac} < n_{ex}$, so that T cell proliferation prevails when antigen presentation levels are low, and T cell exhaustion when they are high [28, 29]. Note: more than one value are reported for some parameters; in those cases, we perform simulations using different values and we found no qualitative modifications in results. Continued

Model parameter	Symbol	Value	References	Classification
Cytotoxic CD8+ T cells differentiation rate by IL-6	kc_T	$4\ [1/day]$	[21]	*Taken from literature*
Cytotoxic CD8+ T cells differentiation rate by IL-6 → cell related half-effect	n_{il}	$3 \times 10^{-4}\ [pg/mL]$	[21]	*Taken from literature*
Half-life of T cells	kd_T	$0.1\ [1/day]$	[26, 27]	*Taken from literature*
		$0.4\ [1/day]$	[21]	
Rate of killing infected cells by the immune response	(*) d_{tc}	$0.42\ [mL/cells/day]$	[28]	*Baseline CTL killing rate*
Maximal rate of exhaustion (depending on the antigen load)	(**) k_{ex}	$2\ [1/day]$	[28]	*Taken from literature of T cell experiments*
Threshold of exhaustion mediated suppression of adaptive cells	(**) n_{ex}	$5\ [cells/mL]$	[28]	*Taken from literature of T cell experiments*
Rate of elimination of susceptible cells by IL-6	kd_S	$2\ [1/day]$	-	*Fixed in model simulations, at the same value of* k_{ex}
Rate of elimination of Susceptible cells by IL-6 → cell related half-effect	n_S	$5\ [cells/mL]$	-	*Fixed in model simulations, at the same value of* n_{ex}
Rate of Susceptible cells renovation	kp_s	$0.74\ [1/day]$	[21]	*Estimated from A549 cell proliferation, fitting to an exponential growth curve*
Maximal number of Epithelial (Susceptible+Infected) cells	S_{max}	$S(0)$	-	-
Rate of DCs estimulation by IFN-type1	kp_{if}	$0.5\ [1/day]$	-	*Fixed in model simulations, at a higher value in compare to* k_{dc}
Rate of DCs estimulation by IFN-type1 → cell related half-effect	$kfdc$	$10^{-2}\ [pg/mL]$	-	*Fixed in model simulations, inside the range of IFN-type1 concentration during immune response*
Initial concentration of Susceptible cells	$S(0)$	$1.6 \times 10^{8}\ [cells/mL]$	[21]	*Respiratory epithelial cells in human adult*
Initial concentration of Infected cells	$I(0)$	$0\ [cells/mL]$	-	-
Initial concentration of Viral particles	$V(0)$	$0.31\ [copies/mL]$	[26]	*Estimated using a regression model of COVID-19 patients data*
Initial concentration of Dendritic cells	$Dc(0)$	$0\ [cells/mL]$	-	-
Initial concentration of IFN-type1	$Ifn(0)$	$0\ [pg/mL]$	-	-
Initial concentration of IL-6 concentration	$IL(0)$	$0\ [pg/mL]$	-	-
Initial concentration of CD8+ T cells	(*) $T(0)$	$1.1 \times 10^{-4}\ [10^{9} cells/mL]$	[21]	*Steady state condition to guarantee the T cell homeostatic level (taken from literature)*
Initial concentration of cytotoxic CD8+ T cells	$Tc(0)$	$0\ [cells/mL]$	-	-

Table 3: Parameter values used in model simulations. (*) Control parameters of the model varied in simulations around this reported value. (**) For T cell proliferation and exhaustion processes note that $kp_T < k_{ex}$, $n_{ac} < n_{ex}$, so that T cell proliferation prevails when antigen presentation levels are low, and T cell exhaustion when they are high [28, 29]. Note: more than one value are reported for some parameters; in those cases, we perform simulations using different values and we found no qualitative modifications in results

This last process can be inhibited by type I IFN related signals, in a concentration-dependent manner. Infected cells and viral particles are eliminated from the system at a rate d_i (related with the half-life of these cells) and d_v (related with renal clearance), respectively. In the presence of Cytotoxic CD8+ T cells, infected cells are also eliminated at a rate d_{tc} of immune killing. The fourth equation describes the dynamics of dendritic cells, considering that infected cells recruit them to the site of infection with a rate k_{dc}, and are eliminated with a natural death rate d_{dc}. The fifth and sixth equations are related to the cytokine dynamics, taking into account the production of Type I IFN by dendritic cells, and IL-6 by dendritic and infected cells. The last terms in the equations correspond to renal clearance of molecules. The last two equations describe the delayed T cell related response. The time of first infiltration of CD8+ T cells is given by the parameter tc, where the Heaviside step function (H) is defined as: $H(t - tc) = 0$ if $t < t_c$, $H(t - tc) = 1$ if $t > t_c$. CD8+ T cells are activated after antigen recognition by dendritic cells and proliferate with a rate kp_T. These cells are eliminated with a natural death rate kd_T, or can also differentiate to Cytotoxic CD8+ T cells with a rate kc_T in an IL-6 dose-dependent process. Finally, the last term in the last equation represents the exhaustion process in cytotoxic cells that depends on the level of antigen presentation. Note that in the equations there are several terms that depend on the concentration level of the molecule or cell involved in a specific process (i.e., last term in the first equation). These terms are modeled as sigmoid functions, where a threshold parameter controls the concentration level at which the effect mediated by the indicated molecule or cell becomes relevant.

Model parameters are listed in Tables 2 and 3. Out of a total of 32 parameters, 12 are related to virus-mediated processes and 20 to the dynamics of the immune response. For virus-related parameters, we found 4 values estimated in the literature by fitting the data of COVID-19 patients. These model parameters that are specifically calibrated for SARS-CoV-2, include the rate of virus infection of susceptible cells (k_i), the rate at which infected cells are cleared as a consequence of cytopathic viral effects (d_i), the rate of virus release from infected cells (k_v), and the initial concentration of viral particles ($V(0)$). The other 8 parameters related to virus processes, which are fixed to values estimated in the literature from experiments using other kinds of virus. For immune response related parameters, 16 are fixed and taken from data reported in the literature and 4 are the result of studies for a range of biologically reasonable values and fixed in model simulations.

We used parameters controlling the type I IFN production rate by dendritic cells (k_f), the rate of killing infected cells by CD8+ cytotoxic T cells (d_{tc}) and the initial concentration of CD8+ T cells ($T(0)$) as control parameters. Variations of their values allow us to simulate different scenarios for the efficacy of innate and adaptive immune responses during COVID-19 disease, which lead to qualitatively different dynamical behaviors during model simulations.

2.3 Model Results

2.3.1 Simulating Different Scenarios for Immune Response Dynamics During COVID-19 Disease

We performed several simulations for a wide range of control parameter values. Model simulations reproduce qualitatively different dynamics, depending on the strength of the immune system response. Then, we present the results for two extreme situations, corresponding to cases where a strong immune response is developed during virus infection, and the opposite, where an immunodeficient response is triggered.

First, we simulate a situation in which the virus infection triggers a strong immune response mediated by type I IFN and CD8+ T cells (see Fig. 2A-B). This is obtained for high values of control parameters, in particular for the rate of type I IFN production by dendritic cells[1] (k_f) and the initial concentration of CD8+ T cells that recognize virus related antigens[2] ($T(0)$). In this

[1]This parameter value is modified with respect to the value reported after in vitro monocytes and respiratory syncytial virus co-culture [21].

[2]This parameter value is modified when compared to the value reported to guarantee the T cells homeostatic level in steady state conditions [21], considering that the majority (for a good response) or a minority (for an immunodeficient response) of cells are able to recognize virus-related antigens.

case, the developed type I IFN response is able to totally or partially inhibit virus replication. This response is followed by an effective cytotoxic T cell response that eliminates infected cells and consequently the remaining virus. The susceptible cells are protected in this scenario, due to the reduction obtained at peak viral load. The effective response to virus infection leads to a controlled inflammatory scenario after virus elimination, which ends up in a low/moderate damage to susceptible cells. This scenario can be interpreted as a mild infection, where patients have a low or medium level of lung tissue damage with a stable or even asymptomatic condition. Here, we reproduce the immune response dynamics for a good responder patient, usually a young and healthy person.

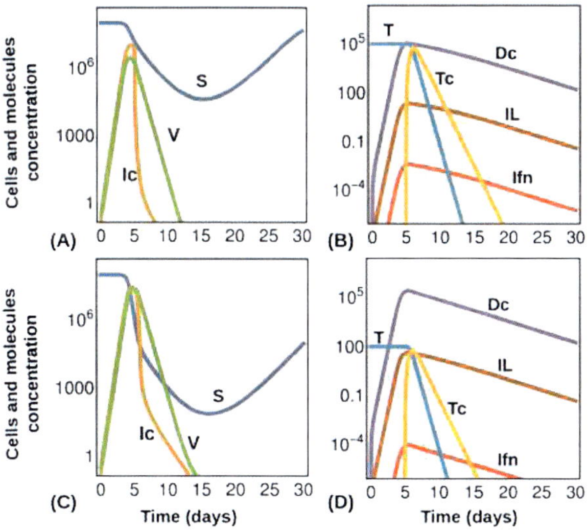

Figure 2: Dynamics of cells related to infection (panels at left column) and immune system response (panels at right column). Above, the response kinetic dynamics of a good responder to infection (panels A and B), with high secretion of Type I IFN and initial number of CD8+ T cells (control parameter values: $k_f = 3.56 \times 10^2$, $T(0) = 10^5$, $d_{tc} = 0.42$). Below (panels C and D), the dynamics obtained for infection in immunodeficient patients with lack of elevated levels of Type I IFN and CD8+ T cells (control parameter values: $k_f = 3.56, T(0) = 10^2, d_{tc} = 0.42$)

On the other extreme, we study the scenario where the immune response is deficient during virus infection, which is the worst situation for a patient (see Fig. 2C-D). This corresponds to the case when, during infection, the rate of type I IFN production (k_f) is low, as well as the initial concentration of CD8+ T cells ($T(0)$). In this scenario, the virus expanded infecting susceptible cells, which became infected cells with the ability to replicate the virus. The virus reached a higher peak in comparison with the scenario of a good response, as a consequence of a deficient type I IFN mediated inhibition and a posterior reduced cytotoxic CD8+ T cell response. During the virus clearance, IL-6 secreted by the elevated number of infected and dendritic cells accumulates in the system. This cytokine has an important role in the significant damage to susceptible cells that occurred during the posterior inflammatory process. This scenario can be interpreted as a severe infection, characteristic of patients in critical conditions. Even when it is mathematically possible at the end to recover a healthy cell population, by considering a model which includes a renovation process of susceptible cells, in real life, it is possible that the patients cannot survive this decrease in lung tissue cells. Here, we reproduce the dynamics obtained during an immunodeficient response, observed in elderly patients or individuals with comorbidities such as diabetes, cardiovascular disease, and hypertension.

2.3.2 Simulating the Effect of Cuban Immunotherapies to Treat COVID-19 in an Immunodeficiency Scenario

Understanding the impact of different immune mechanisms during COVID-19 infection is crucial to improve treatment strategies and control the damage provoked by the virus. Nowadays, there are still key open questions concerning this disease, related to: 1) improving treatment strategies to strengthen the antiviral immune response and controlling the inflammatory damage; and 2) to determine the best time window for the application of each treatment.

Cuban protocols to treat patients with COVID-19 include anti-inflammatory therapy such as Itolizumab, a new product that reduces the secretion of inflammatory cytokines as IL-6; and an anti-viral therapy using type I IFN injection. We used the developed model to study the impact of both treatments in modifying the immune response during COVID-19 and to predict the best moment for their application. Specifically, we simulate the treatment effects on immunodeficient patients that are the ones with a critical damage associated with virus infection.

To simulate the effect of type I IFN injection and IL-6 depletion therapies, we included new terms in the model equations for these cytokine dynamics, respectively. In particular, we added an external source of type I IFN that increases the amount of this cytokine in the system during a given period of time, and a new term that temporally increases the decay rate of IL-6 (see equation (9.1)). Three new parameters control the treatment simulations; dose (D), time of treatment initiation (t_i), and treatment duration (t_d). We simulate the effect of both therapies applied individually at different moments of the disease, and study the induced changes in susceptible cell damage as a measure of treatment efficacy.

$$\begin{aligned} \frac{dIf_n(t)}{dt} &= AIF(t) + k_f \frac{D_c(t)}{D_c(t) + n_{if}} - d_{ifn} If_n(t), \\ \frac{IL(t)}{dt} &= k_{pdc} \frac{D_c(t)}{D_c(t) + n_{dc}} + k_{piv} \frac{I_c(t)}{I_c(t) + n_{ic}} - d_{il} IL(t)\,(1 + AIL(t)). \end{aligned} \tag{9.1}$$

First, we simulate the effect of type I IFN injection. If this treatment starts during the building up of the immune response, it has a beneficial effect by blocking virus replication and consequently contributing to its control (see Fig. 3A-B). Treatment simulations predict a dose-dependent effect in reducing the virus load peak that causes a decrease in infected cell number. As a consequence of infection control, IL-6 is less secreted and consequently less accumulated in the system. This results in a prevention of susceptible cell damage, due to both virus and inflammation control, moving the system from a critical scenario without treatment, to a moderate one in the presence of therapy.

On the contrary, if type I IFN injection is applied later, beginning at the peak of the inflammatory reaction, the treatment has a proinflammatory effect that enhances the damage to susceptible cells (see Fig. 3C-D). In this scenario, the treatment has a less significant effect controlling virus replication due to the fact that the virus is cleared from the system. However, it has a relevant effect stimulating the activation of dendritic cells and therefore increasing the levels of IL-6 in the system, potentiating the inflammatory stage and the consequent damage to susceptible cells. Thus, in this case, the treatment will do more damage and reinforce the critical scenario obtained without treatment.

Finally, we simulate the injection of type I IFN starting early after virus infection, as Cuban protocols suggest as an effective strategy. In this case, the treatment is capable of eliminating the virus, even before it could damage susceptible cells (see Fig. 3E-F). Additionally, as a result of infection, an expanded cytotoxic CD8+ T cell population that eventually will generate memory cells remains in the system. This is the best treatment strategy predicted by the model, that prevents a critical development of the disease and provides protection against virus reinfection.

Next, we simulate the effect of an IL-6 depletion treatment, applied at different moments during COVID-19 progression. If the treatment is applied starting during the building up of the immune response, it blocks CD8+ T cells differentiation into cytotoxic cells (see Fig. 4A-B). This reduces the capacity of the immune system to eliminate the virus, increasing the infection of susceptible cells. Thus, in this case the treatment will trigger more damage to susceptible cells, even exacerbating the critical scenario obtained without treatment.

If IL-6 depletion is applied later, beginning at the peak of the inflammatory reaction, it can control the damage to susceptible cells by reducing IL-6 concentration (see Fig. 4C-D). In this scenario, the immune response mediated by CD8+ T cells was already developed and the virus is starting to be cleared from the system. Therefore, the damage to susceptible cells is mainly caused by the inflammation mediated by IL-6. Thus, in this case the treatment will improve the critical scenario obtained without treatment, moving the system to a moderate one.

Finally, if IL-6 depletion treatment is applied at a late stage of inflammation, beginning after the peak of T cell response and viral infection, it has no effect in controlling the damage to susceptible cells (see Fig. 4E-F). At this stage, there is already a significant level of damage that a temporally reduction of IL-6 concentration cannot reverse. Therefore, in this scenario, the treatment is totally ineffective.

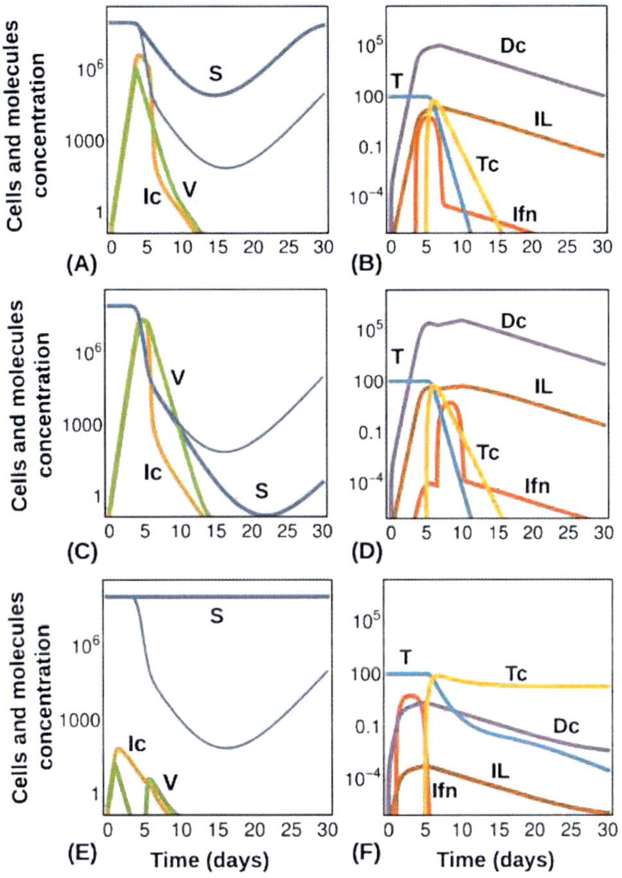

Figure 3: Simulation results for Type I IFN injection treatment in the immunodeficient patient. Panels show the dynamics obtained when the treatment starts: (Panels A-B) during the building up of the immune response (values of treatment control parameters: $D = 10^2$ pg/mL, $t_i = 3.5$ days, $t_d = 3.5$ days); (Panels C-D) at the peak of inflammatory reaction (values of treatment control parameters: $D = 10^2$ pg/mL, $t_i = 6.5$ days, $t_d = 3.5$ days); (Panels E-F) early after viral infection (values of treatment control parameters: $D = 10^2$ pg/mL, $t_i = 1.0$ day, $t_d = 4$ days). Dashed curve inserted in panels A, C, and E, corresponds to susceptible cell dynamics in the absence of treatment

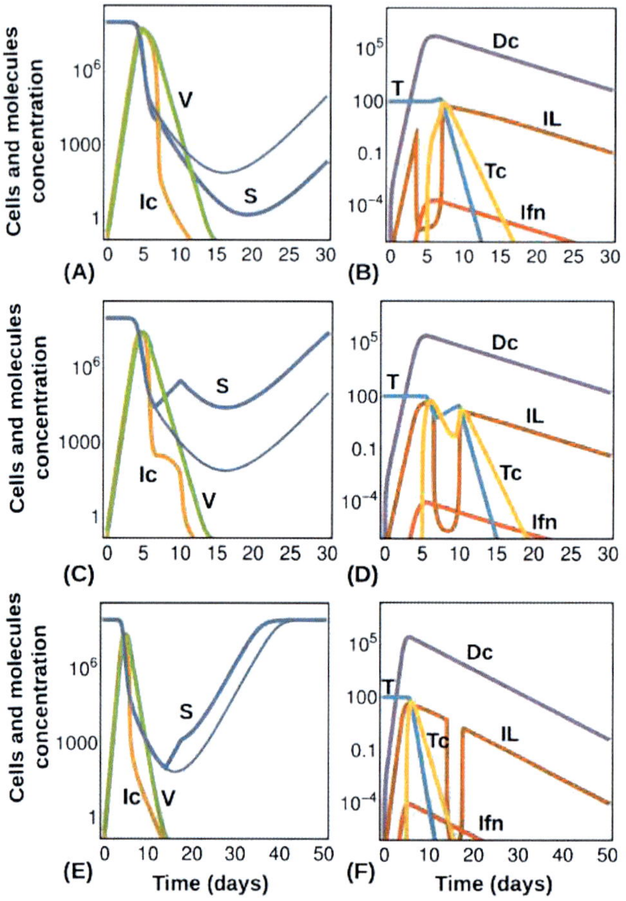

Figure 4: Simulation results for IL-6 depletion treatment in the immunodeficient patient. Panels show the dynamics obtained when the treatment starts: (Panels A-B) during the building up of the immune response (values of treatment control parameters: $D = 10^7$ pg/mL, $t_i = 3.5$ days, $t_d = 3.5$ days); (Panels C-D) at the peak of inflammatory reaction (values of treatment control parameters: $D = 10^7$ pg/mL, $t_i = 6.5$ days, $t_d = 3.5$ days); (Panels E-F) after the peak of T cell response and viral infection (values of treatment control parameters: $D = 10^7$ pg/mL, $t_i = 15.0$ day, $t_d = 3.5$ days). Dashed curve inserted in panels A,C, and E, corresponds to susceptible cell dynamics in the absence of treatment.

In summary, these results predict a good response to Type I IFN injection when the treatment is applied in COVID-19 patients that are still asymptomatic, at the beginning of virus infection; and, on the contrary, it is useless or even harmful when applied at a late stage in the presence of inflammation. On the other hand, IL-6 depletion therapy shows a time window of efficacy. This treatment is effective if applied at the beginning of inflammation, preventing the progression to critical stages of host cell damage. On the contrary, it could be harmful if applied early and has no effect at later stages.

3 ITOLIZUMAB ON COVID-19

3.1 Preliminary Evidences from the Clinical Practice

Itolizumab is a monoclonal antibody that recognizes CD6, which is a marker for T cell activation. The antibody acts in important aspects of the pathogenesis of COVID-19 by inhibiting the migration and overactivation of effector T cells. The fundamental effect of itolizumab is evidenced by the reduction of the secretion of multiple inflammatory cytokines (IL-6, IFN-gamma, TNF-alpha, and IL-17) and by the skewing towards a regulatory phenotype [30].

3.1.1 Itolizumab Reduces COVID-19 Lethality

In the first expanded access study, 68 SARS-CoV2 confirmed patients (30 men and 38 women) with moderate, severe, or critical disease, were treated with itolizumab in 10 Cuban hospitals from April 4 to May 13, 2020.

In the first 68 Cuban patients, the fatality rate at 14 days was 4% for patients in a moderate condition and 18% for patients in severe conditions. For critical patients, the lethality rate was 69%.

To assess the impact of itolizumab in comparison with untreated subjects, a control group ($n = 128$) was selected among the Cuban COVID-19 patients who received the rest of the drugs included in the national protocol (interferon alpha, lopinavir-ritonavir (kaletra) and chloroquine), but no immunomodulatory biologics according to the national database (June 2020). Control patients were paired with respect to a propensity score method with treated patients by age, sex, severity of the illness, and number of comorbidities. All severe and critically ill patients treated at the Intensive Care Unit (ICU) without immunomodulatory biologics were considered ($n = 62$). For moderately ill patients, controls with at least two comorbidities considered as factors of poor prognosis for COVID-19 (hypertension, cardiovascular disease, diabetes, cancer, chronic renal disease, obesity or chronic obstructive pulmonary disease (COPD)) were selected ($n = 66$). Both groups were homogeneous in terms of demographic factors and significant comorbidities, except for asthma and obesity, which had more incidence in the itolizumab group. Odds-ratios (OR) for death according to disease severity were estimated for controls vs itolizumab. Odds-ratio for disease worsening (risk of ICU admission) was estimated for moderately ill patients. Table 4 shows the baseline characteristics according to age, sex, and comorbidities in both groups.

Overall, 58,9% of patients were older than 65. One hundred thirteen patients (57.4%) had 2 or more associated diseases. The most prevalent concomitant conditions were hypertension (72.6 %), cardio-vascular disease (29.4 %), and diabetes mellitus (36.5 %).

Itolizumab reduced the probability of death of severe and moderate patients with 2 comorbidities in comparison to controls. The odds ratio for controls in severe conditions was 3.9 [95% CI 1.0; 14.3] as compared with patients treated with itolizumab. Moderate control patients at high risk of worsening had higher odds of ICU admission: 3.2 [95% CI 0.9; 11.4] or death, 6.9 [95% CI 0.9; 50] than itolizumab patients.

Time to death due to COVID-19 was analyzed by using a competitive risk model, such as the one proposed in [31] based on the hazard subdistribution. Accordingly, "discharge alive" was considered a competing event and patients were not censored at the time of discharge. Right censoring means that the unobserved time to death could be any time point larger than the observed, whereas patients who recover may in fact never die from COVID-19 [32]. Analysis was made with the SPSS 25 and the package cmprsk of R software. Time to recovery or death curves for itolizumab vs. control severe patients is shown in Fig. 5.

Patient characteristics		Control $N = 128$		Itulizumab $N = 69$		Total $N = 196$		
		Freq	%	Freq	%	Freq	%	χ^2 P-value
Age Group	0-18	0	0.0	0	0.0	0	0.0	0.564
	19-39	11	8.5	3	4.4	14	7.1	
	40-64	43	33.3	24	35.3	67	34.0	
	65 or more	75	58.1	41	60.3	116	58.9	
Sex	F	62	48.1	38	55.9	100	50.8	0.369
	M	67	51.9	30	44.1	97	49.2	
Number of comorbidities	≤ 1	60	46.5	24	35.3	84	42.6	0.172
	2 or more	69	53.5	44	64.7	113	57.4	
Hypertension		98	76.0	45	66.2	143	72.6	0.179
Diabetes Mellitus		50	38.8	22	32.4	72	36.5	0.437
Cardiovascular desease		35	27.1	23	33.8	58	29.4	0.411
Asthma		12	9.3	14	20.6	26	13.2	0.030
COPD		17	13.2	9	13.2	26	13.2	0.991
Cancer		15	11.6	3	4.4	18	9.1	0.121
Obesity		3	2.3	7	10.3	10	5.1	0.034
Chronic Renal Disease		18	14.0	9	13.2	27	13.7	0.889

Table 4: Baseline characteristics of patients treated with itolizumab vs. controls not receiving immunomodulatory drugs

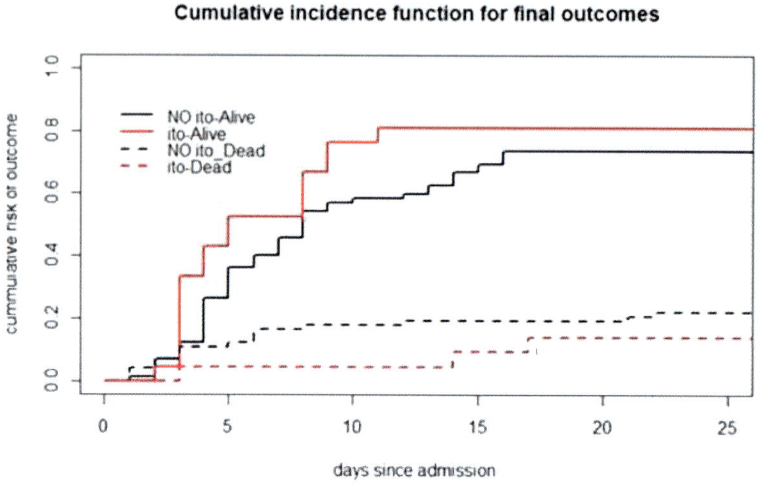

Figure 5: Competing risk curves of itolizumab vs control severe patients

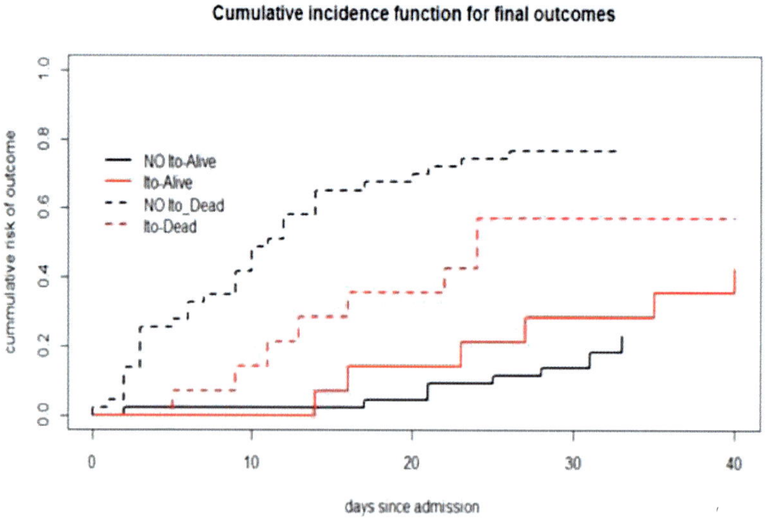

Figure 6: Competing risk curves of itolizumab vs control critical patients, interrumpting interferon alpha 2b upon worsening

In severe patients, the probability of recovery was much higher than the probability of a fatal outcome. The Kaplan-Meier estimate of recovery by day 14 were 80% and 60% with and without itolizumab, respectively.

In the first version of the national treatment protocol, interferon alpha 2b was not interrupted at the time of patient aggravation. The rationale behind this decision was to keep treatment with a well-known antiviral drug in severe and critical patients. However, since interferons can also have immunomodulatory and could further fuel the cytokine release syndrome [33, 34], the second version of the national protocol prescribed treatment interruption at the time of transition to severe or critical condition. In our series, the odds ratio for critical controls not receiving itolizumab was 1.8 [95% CI 0.4; 8.3]. An additional analysis was made for controls and itolizumab individuals who did not receive concurrent interferon. The odds of death of critical control patients lacking itolizumab was 6.2 [95% CI 0.9; 38.5]. The curve for time to recovery or death for itolizumab vs. control patients is shown in Fig. 6.

Overall, in critical patients, the probability of death is higher than the probability of recovery. However, itolizumab reduced the probability of death as compared with controls. The Kaplan-Meier estimate of death by day 14 was 20% with itolizumab and 60% without it.

3.1.2 Timely Prescription of Itolizumab Can Be Assisted by Biomarkers

Since the well-timed prescription of itolizumab was deemed to be crucial to reduce mortality, several biomarkers associated with inflammation were evaluated to identify patients most likely to progress to a severe form of the disease. The discriminative power of the neutrophil to lymphocyte ratio (NLR) and interleukin 6 (IL-6) on disease severity was evaluated by receiver operating curves (ROC) analyses.

NLR and IL-6 showed a very high sensitivity and specificity to predict disease severity. Fig. 7 shows ROC predictive curves of COVID-19 severity for NLR and IL-6.

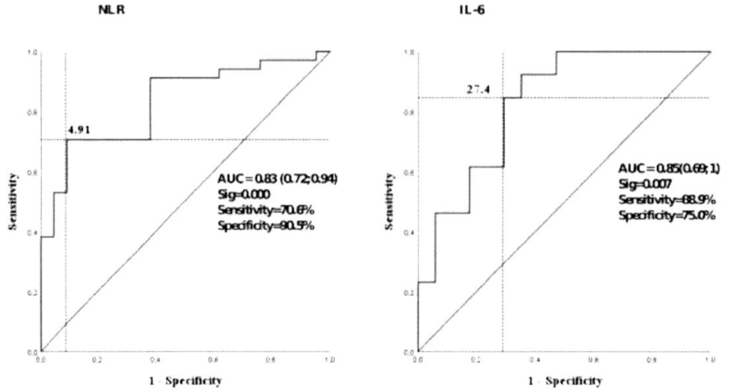

Figure 7: Neutrophil/Lymphocytes Ratio (NLR) and IL-6 as prognostic of the severity of the COVID-19 illness

NLR of 4.9 and IL-6 of 27.5 pg/ml distinguished nonsevere from severe patients with high sensitivity and specificity.

The discriminative power of the inflammatory markers (NLR and IL-6) on death due to COVID-19 was also evaluated by ROC analyses.

Fig. 8 shows ROC predictive curves of COVID-19 lethality for NLR and IL-6.

In patients treated with itolizumab, NLR thresholds of 8.22 and IL-6 of 52.8 pg/ml predicted death with high sensitivity and specificity.

According to these analyses, we concluded that in severe cases, itolizumab should be prescribed to patients showing a neutrophil to lymphocyte ratio (NLR) between 4.9 and 8.22 or an IL-6 concentration between 27.4 and 52.8 pg/ml. The use of itolizumab in patients with NLR above 8.22 or IL-6 higher than 52.8 will not significantly reduce the risk of death.

To validate our data, a competing risk model of the cumulative results (recovery or death) was adjusted to evaluate differences between subjects with higher or lower values of NLR, using the cutoff that predicted mortality (8.22). This analysis only included severe or critical patients treated with itolizumab. Time to recovery or death curves according NLR are shown in Fig. 9.

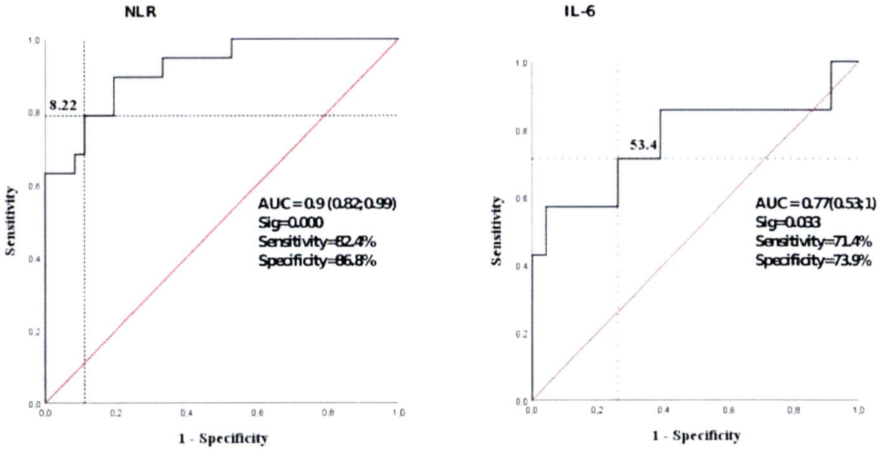

Figure 8: Neutrophil/Lymphocytes Ratio (NLR) and IL-6 as predictors of mortality of patients

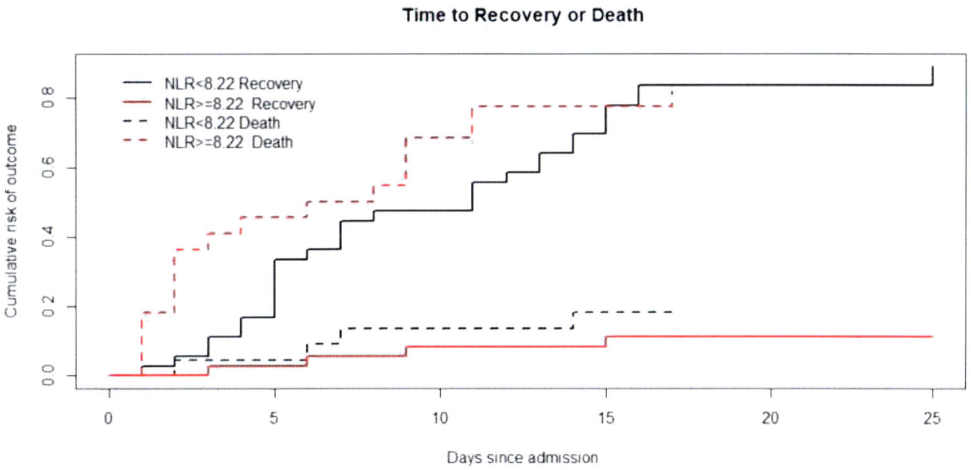

Figure 9: Competing risk curves of severe and critical itolizumab treated patients with NLR higher or lower than 8.22

Itolizumab patients with a NLR lower than 8.22, had a larger probability of recovery than of a fatal outcome. The probability of recovery was $\sim 70\%$ at day 14. However, itolizumab treated patients with a higher index of inflammation (NLR > 8.22) had a higher probability of death than recovery. The probability of recovery at day 14 was barely 15%.

3.1.3 Opportune Prescription of Itolizumab Considering Time from Symptoms Onset

In addition to the laboratory biomarkers associated with inflammation, we tried to determine which was the optimal time to use of itolizumab in relation to the symptoms onset. The discriminant power of the time between symptom initiation and itolizumab on death due to COVID-19 was evaluated by ROC analyses. Fig. 10 shows the ROC predictive curve of COVID-19 death considering the time between symptoms and the start of treatment with itolizumab.

We concluded that the effectiveness of treatment also depended on the time between symptom's onset and itolizumab administration. In our data set, the cut-off point associated with higher mortality was 7 days between the first symptoms and the inception of treatment with itolizumab. To confirm this finding, a competing risk model of cumulative effects (recuperation or death) was fit for itolizumab patients treated before or after day 7 (Fig. 11).

The recovery or fatality rate was evaluated at a later time point (30 days) since this analysis started at the time of the first symptoms (even before hospitalization) and not at the moment of hospital admission or itolizumab infusion.

After 30 days of symptom initiation, patients receiving itolizumab before day 7 had more than 75% chance of recovery, while their probability of death was less than 20%. On the contrary, subjects treated after day 7 had a higher probability of death around 50%.

4 CONCLUDING REMARKS

The developed mathematical model helps to understand the dynamics of the immune response during COVID-19 and its influence on the effectiveness of immunotherapies. In particular, we

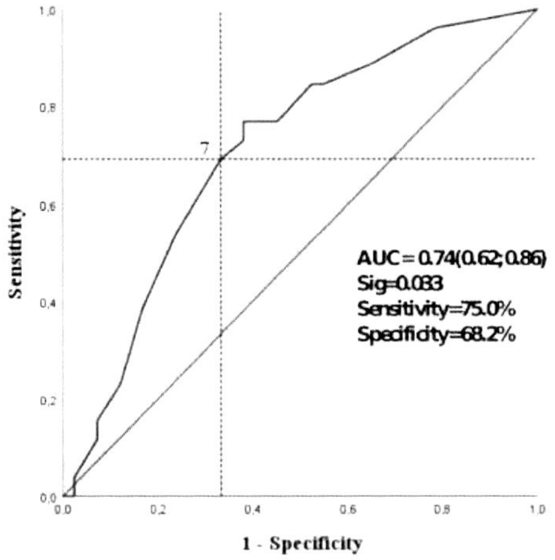

Figure 10: Time to symptoms and itolizumab administration as a predictor of patients' mortality. (AUC: area under the curve)

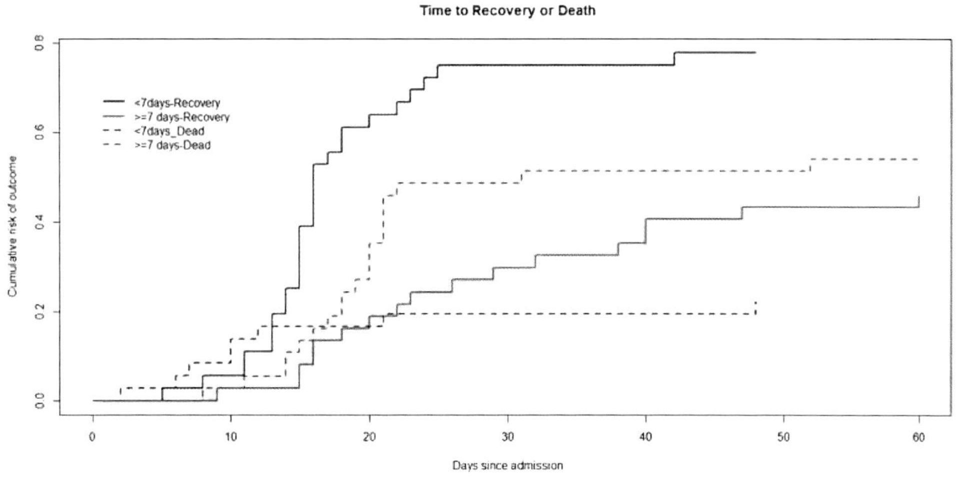

Figure 11: Competing risk curves of itolizumab treated patients before or after day 7

studied the best strategies for Cuban protocol application that includes interferon alpha 2B and itolizumab therapies. Model predictions of the best time windows for treatment application are in agreement with the results from statistical analysis of Cuban patient data. Additionally, the model allows to better understand the clinical impact of both treatments from an immunological point of view.

The main results can be summarized as follows:

1. Injection of Type I IFN is predicted to be effective if applied at early stages of virus infection, not at a late stage when the inflammation starts. Hence, the importance of patients receiving medical care since the first stages of infection, when this treatment is effective in controlling viral replication.

2. IL-6 depletion shows an intermediate time window of effectiveness: it needs to be applied at the beginning of inflammation, not before or after. Cuban protocols include a timely prescription of itolizumab, an antibody that reduces IL-6 concentrations, obtaining a decrease in the probability of death of severe and moderate patients at high risk of aggravation. The late prescription of itolizumab might not significantly reduce mortality.

3. Inflammatory biomarkers such as NLR and IL-6, and time from symptom onset, can be useful to recommend itolizumab administration.

5 CONSENT FOR PUBLICATION

Not applicable.

6 CONFLICT OF INTEREST

The authors declare no conflict of interest, financial or otherwise.

7 ACKNOWLEDGEMENTS

We wish to warmly acknowledge the support of the patients and the relatives who participated or gave the consent for enrollment in the clinical trials. The authors are also very grateful to all physicians, nurses and general staff that worked with the hospitalized COVID-19 patients.

References

[1] Atal S, Fatima Z. IL-6 Inhibitors in the Treatment of Serious COVID-19: A Promising Therapy? Pharmaceutical Medicine [Internet]. 2020 Jun 13 [cited 2021 Oct 3];34(4):223–31. Available from: https://doi.org/10.1007/s40290-020-00342-z

[2] Ledford H. How does COVID-19 kill? Uncertainty is hampering doctors' ability to choose treatments. Nature [Internet]. 2020 Apr [cited 2021 Oct 3];580(7803):311–2. Available from: https://doi.org/10.1038/d41586-020-01056-7

[3] Lippi G, Sanchis-Gomar F, Henry BM. COVID-19: unravelling the clinical progression of nature's virtually perfect biological weapon. Annals of Translational Medicine [Internet]. 2020 Jun [cited 2021 Oct 3];8(11):693. Available from: https://doi.org/10.21037/atm-20-3989

[4] Sariol A, Perlman S. Lessons for COVID-19 Immunity from Other Coronavirus Infections. Immunity [Internet]. 2020 Aug [cited 2021 Oct 3];53(2):248–63. Available from: https://doi.org/10.1016/j.immuni.2020.07.005

[5] Gubernatorova EO, Gorshkova EA, Polinova AI, Drutskaya MS. IL-6: Relevance for immunopathology of SARS-CoV-2. Cytokine & Growth Factor Reviews [Internet]. 2020

Jun [cited 2021 Oct 3];53:13–24. Available from: https://doi.org/10.1016/j.cytogfr.2020.05.009

[6] Hasan A, Al-Ozairi E, Al-Baqsumi Z, Ahmad R, Al-Mulla F. Cellular and Humoral Immune Responses in Covid-19 and Immunotherapeutic Approaches. ImmunoTargets and Therapy [Internet]. 2021 Mar [cited 2021 Oct 3];Volume 10:63-85. Available from: https://doi.org/10.2147/itt.s280706

[7] Crouse J, Kalinke U, Oxenius A. Regulation of antiviral T cell responses by type I interferons. Nature Reviews Immunology [Internet]. 2015 Mar 20 [cited 2021 Oct 3];15(4):231–42. Available from: https://doi.org/10.1038/nri3806

[8] Makris S, Paulsen M, Johansson C. Type I Interferons as Regulators of Lung Inflammation. Frontiers in Immunology [Internet]. 2017 Mar 10 [cited 2021 Oct 3];8. Available from: https://doi.org/10.3389/fimmu.2017.00259

[9] Seo YJ, Hahm B. Type I Interferon Modulates the Battle of Host Immune System Against Viruses. In: Advances in Applied Microbiology [Internet]. [place unknown]: Elsevier; 2010 [cited 2021 Oct 3]. p. 83–101. Available from: https://doi.org/10.1016/s0065-2164(10)73004-5

[10] Reizis B. Plasmacytoid Dendritic Cells: Development, Regulation, and Function. Immunity [Internet]. 2019 Jan [cited 2021 Oct 3];50(1):37–50. Available from: https://doi.org/10.1016/j.immuni.2018.12.027

[11] Cervantes-Barragan L, Lewis KL, Firner S, Thiel V, Hugues S, Reith W, Ludewig B, Reizis B. Plasmacytoid dendritic cells control T-cell response to chronic viral infection. Proceedings of the National Academy of Sciences [Internet]. 2012 Feb 6 [cited 2021 Oct 3];109(8):3012–7. Available from: https://doi.org/10.1073/pnas.1117359109

[12] King C, Sprent J. Dual Nature of Type I Interferons in SARS-CoV-2-Induced Inflammation. Trends in Immunology [Internet]. 2021 Apr [cited 2021 Oct 3];42(4):312–22. Available from: https://doi.org/10.1016/j.it.2021.02.003

[13] Tanaka T, Narazaki M, Kishimoto T. IL-6 in Inflammation, Immunity, and Disease. Cold Spring Harbor Perspectives in Biology [Internet]. 2014 Sep 4 [cited 2021 Oct 3];6(10):a016295. Available from: https://doi.org/10.1101/cshperspect.a016295

[14] Vabret N, Britton GJ, Gruber C, Hegde S, Kim J, Kuksin M, et al. Immunology of COVID-19: Current State of the Science. Immunity [Internet]. 2020 Jun [cited 2021 Oct 3];52(6):910–41. Available from: https://doi.org/10.1016/j.immuni.2020.05.002

[15] Li B, Jones LL, Geiger TL. IL-6 Promotes T Cell Proliferation and Expansion under Inflammatory Conditions in Association with Low-Level RORγt Expression. The Journal of Immunology [Internet]. 2018 Oct 12 [cited 2021 Oct 3];201(10):2934-46. Available from: https://doi.org/10.4049/jimmunol.1800016

[16] Arnaldez FI, O'Day SJ, Drake CG, Fox BA, Fu B, Urba WJ, Montesarchio V, Weber JS, Wei H, Wigginton JM, Ascierto PA. The Society for Immunotherapy of Cancer perspective on regulation of interleukin-6 signaling in COVID-19-related systemic inflammatory response. Journal for ImmunoTherapy of Cancer [Internet]. 2020 May [cited 2021 Oct 3];8(1):e000930. Available from: https://doi.org/10.1136/jitc-2020-000930

[17] Qian Z, Travanty EA, Oko L, Edeen K, Berglund A, Wang J, Ito Y, Holmes KV, Mason RJ. Innate Immune Response of Human Alveolar Type II Cells Infected with Severe Acute Respiratory Syndrome–Coronavirus. American Journal of Respiratory Cell and Molecular Biology [Internet]. 2013 Jun [cited 2021 Oct 3];48(6):742–8. Available from: https://doi.org/10.1165/rcmb.2012-0339oc

[18] Chen Z, John Wherry E. T cell responses in patients with COVID-19. Nature Reviews Immunology [Internet]. 2020 Jul 29 [cited 2021 Oct 3];20(9):529–36. Available from: https://doi.org/10.1038/s41577-020-0402-6

[19] Diao B, Wang C, Tan Y, Chen X, Liu Y, Ning L, Chen L, Li M, Liu Y, Wang G, Yuan Z, Feng Z, Zhang Y, Wu Y, Chen Y. Reduction and Functional Exhaustion of T Cells in Patients With Coronavirus Disease 2019 (COVID-19). Frontiers in Immunology [Internet]. 2020 May 1 [cited 2021 Oct 3];11. Available from: https://doi.org/10.3389/fimmu.2020.00827

[20] Zheng M, Gao Y, Wang G, Song G, Liu S, Sun D, Xu Y, Tian Z. Functional exhaustion of antiviral lymphocytes in COVID-19 patients. Cellular & Molecular Immunology [Internet]. 2020 Mar 19 [cited 2021 Oct 3];17(5):533–5. Available from: https://doi.org/10.1038/s41423-020-0402-2

[21] Jenner AL, Aogo RA, Alfonso S, Crowe V, Deng X, Smith AP, Morel PA, Davis CL, Smith AM, Craig M. COVID-19 virtual patient cohort suggests immune mechanisms driving disease outcomes. PLOS Pathogens [Internet]. 2021 Jul 14 [cited 2021 Oct 3];17(7):e1009753. Available from: https://doi.org/10.1371/journal.ppat.1009753

[22] Hadjadj J, Yatim N, Barnabei L, Corneau A, Boussier J, Smith N, et al. Impaired type I interferon activity and inflammatory responses in severe COVID-19 patients. Science [Internet]. 2020 Jul 13 [cited 2021 Oct 3];369(6504):718–24. Available from: https://doi.org/10.1126/science.abc6027

[23] Crisafulli S, Isgrò V, La Corte L, Atzeni F, Trifirò G. Potential Role of Anti-interleukin (IL)-6 Drugs in the Treatment of COVID-19: Rationale, Clinical Evidence and Risks. BioDrugs [Internet]. 2020 Jun 15 [cited 2021 Oct 3];34(4):415–22. Available from: https://doi.org/10.1007/s40259-020-00430-1

[24] Jamilloux Y, Henry T, Belot A, Viel S, Fauter M, El Jammal T, Walzer T, François B, Sève P. Should we stimulate or suppress immune responses in COVID-19? Cytokine and anti-cytokine interventions. Autoimmunity Reviews [Internet]. 2020 Jul [cited 2021 Oct 3];19(7):102567. Available from: https://doi.org/10.1016/j.autrev.2020.102567

[25] Kumar S, Nyodu R, Maurya VK, Saxena SK. Host Immune Response and Immunobiology of Human SARS-CoV-2 Infection. In: Medical Virology: From Pathogenesis to Disease Control [Internet]. Singapore: Springer Singapore; 2020 [cited 2021 Oct 3]. p. 43–53. Available from: https://doi.org/10.1007/978-981-15-4814-7_5

[26] Hernández-Vargas EA, Velasco-Hernández JX. In-host mathematical modelling of COVID-19 in humans. Annual Reviews in Control [Internet]. 2020 [cited 2021 Oct 3];50:448–56. Available from: https://doi.org/10.1016/j.arcontrol.2020.09.006

[27] Sahoo S, et al. Mechanistic modeling of the SARS-CoV-2 and immune system interplay unravels design principles for diverse clinicopathological outcomes. BioRxiv 2020.

[28] Conway JM, Perelson AS. Post-treatment control of HIV infection. Proceedings of the National Academy of Sciences [Internet]. 2015 Apr 13 [cited 2021 Oct 3];112(17):5467–72. Available from: https://doi.org/10.1073/pnas.1419162112

[29] Baral S, Raja R, Sen P, Dixit NM. Towards multiscale modeling of the CD8+ T cell response to viral infections. Wiley Interdisciplinary Reviews: Systems Biology and Medicine [Internet]. 2019 Feb 27 [cited 2021 Oct 3];11(4):e1446. Available from: https://doi.org/10.1002/wsbm.1446

[30] Loganathan S, Athalye SN, Joshi SR. Itolizumab, an anti-CD6 monoclonal antibody, as a potential treatment for COVID-19 complications. Expert Opinion on Biological Therapy

[Internet]. 2020 Jul 29 [cited 2021 Oct 3];20(9):1025–31. Available from: https://doi.org/10.1080/14712598.2020.1798399

[31] Fine JP, Gray RJ. A Proportional Hazards Model for the Subdistribution of a Competing Risk. Journal of the American Statistical Association [Internet]. 1999 Jun [cited 2021 Oct 3];94(446):496–509. Available from: https://doi.org/10.1080/01621459.1999.10474144

[32] Molenberghs G, Buyse M, Abrams S, Hens N, Beutels P, Faes C, Verbeke G, Van Damme P, Goossens H, Neyens T, Herzog S, Theeten H, Pepermans K, Abad AA, Van Keilegom I, Speybroeck N, Legrand C, De Buyser S, Hulstaert F. Infectious diseases epidemiology, quantitative methodology, and clinical research in the midst of the COVID-19 pandemic: Perspective from a European country. Contemporary Clinical Trials [Internet]. 2020 Dec [cited 2021 Oct 3];99:106189. Available from: https://doi.org/10.1016/j.cct.2020.106189

[33] Channappanavar R, Fehr AR, Vijay R, Mack M, Zhao J, Meyerholz DK, Perlman S. Dysregulated Type I Interferon and Inflammatory Monocyte-Macrophage Responses Cause Lethal Pneumonia in SARS-CoV-Infected Mice. Cell Host & Microbe [Internet]. 2016 Feb [cited 2021 Oct 3];19(2):181–93. Available from: https://doi.org/10.1016/j.chom.2016.01.007

[34] Channappanavar R, Fehr AR, Zheng J, Wohlford-Lenane C, Abrahante JE, Mack M, Sompallae R, McCray PB, Meyerholz DK, Perlman S. IFN-I response timing relative to virus replication determines MERS coronavirus infection outcomes. Journal of Clinical Investigation [Internet]. 2019 Jul 29 [cited 2021 Oct 3];129(9):3625–39. Available from: https://doi.org/10.1172/jci126363

CHAPTER 10

Vaccines Against SARS-CoV-2. Eradicating COVID-19

Barbara Dema[1], **Sthefany Pagliari**[1], **Arturo Reyes-Sandoval**[*12]

[*] **Corresponding author:** arturo.reyes@ndm.ox.ac.uk, Phone: +44 (0) 1865 287811

[1] The Jenner Institute, University of Oxford, Old Road campus Research Building, Roosevelt Drive, Oxford, OX3 7DQ, UK

[2] Instituto Politécnico Nacional, IPN. Av. Luis Enrique Erro s/n. Unidad Adolfo López Mateos, Mexico City, Mexico

Abstract. A year after the COVID-19 pandemic started, a global effort to develop vaccines and make them available to the public, has prompted a turning point in the history of vaccine development. The post-COVID era has accelerated the efforts to bring novel platform vaccine technologies such as nucleic acid or viral-vectored vaccines, which were proved to offer safety, efficacy, and speed in development and production, but have restricted records in the clinic. To date, five candidate vaccines have been approved for emergency use by different regulatory agencies across the world, after demonstrating their robust immunogenicity response and efficacy against SARS-COV-2 infection. We summarize and analyse the progression of those vaccines with major research development and results in peer-reviewed journals.

Key words: COVID-19, SARS-CoV-2, vaccines, viral vectors, adenovirus, RNA vaccines, DNA vaccines, pandemic.

1 INTRODUCTION

1.1 Importance

Despite advances in many directions, from epidemiologic control to specific treatments, prevention based on immunization is the cornerstone of the strategy to cope with the pandemic. This chapter highlights its importance and exposes the uncertainties and challenges still remaining after more than one year of worldwide efforts towards safe and effective vaccines.

1.2 Preliminaries

Severe Acute Respiratory Syndrome coronavirus 2 (SARS-Cov2) is the newly discovered virus responsible for coronavirus disease 2019 (COVID-19). The COVID-19 outbreak reported in late 2019, emerged in the city of Wuhan (Hubei, China) and spread fast all over the world, making it a new public health concern [1, 2]. On 11 March 2020, the World Health Organization (WHO) officially had to consider the global COVID-19 outbreak as a pandemic due to the high number of cases continuing to disseminate at a remarkable pace in many worldwide territories.

Since the beginning of the COVID-19 pandemic, many effective measures have been taken in place to prevent the disease transmission, but most of these measures are not sustainable and have caused major disruptions to the economy as well as social and psychological issues. The ability of the virus to propagate in either symptomatic or asymptomatic patients made the control of the disease is a real challenge for the authorities, and vaccination is the most important tool to protect against COVID-19 [3, 4].

The development of a new vaccine usually takes at least 10-15 years and needs to be evaluated for safety, immunogenicity, and efficacy in humans before it is licensed for use. An initial preclinical phase is conducted to identify a suitable target antigen. Both *in vitro* and *in vivo* evaluations will be performed to assess the ability of the new candidate to induce an effective immune response. The clinical phase intends to establish the safety and efficacy of a new vaccine in humans prior to its being licensed by regulatory agencies and getting into the clinic.

During a global health emergency, the development of a new vaccine must be accelerated to prevent and control the disease without compromising on safety. The COVID-19 vaccine has shown how fast a new candidate development can be achieved when sufficient resources are made available. With the recent COVID-19 pandemic, a new era in vaccinology using nucleic acid or viral vector technology has contributed to setting a fast-track development.

In this chapter, we highlight the different strategies that were introduced to develop a new COVID-19 vaccine since the start of the race for an effective and safe vaccine. We describe the current vaccines developed under different platforms and analyse the vaccines approved for emergency use based on results in peer-reviewed journals.

2 VACCINE DEVELOPMENT PROCESS

The development of a new vaccine is a result of a long process which involves several stages from laboratory research to regulatory submission for clinical trials. Regulatory agencies classify the process of the development of a new vaccine into preclinical (*in vitro* and *in vivo* animal tests) and clinical (clinical trials in humans) stages.

The preclinical phase is a requirement to take a new vaccine candidate from the laboratory to humans. The first step is exploratory and consists of the generation of the antigen that might induce an immune response and help to prevent the disease. A new antigen can be characterized according to the delivery platform used, such as protein, genetic material or viral. Later, it will be assessed in *in vitro* and *in vivo* assays to test the correct expression and immunogenicity. Studies in animal models give an idea of the immune response that might be expected in humans, which may suggest a safe starting dose and a better route of administration. In some cases, the protection of the new vaccine can also be evaluated by performing challenge studies using vaccinated animals to infect with the target pathogen.

After the decision to move forward the new vaccine candidate into human trials, the developers must submit the preclinical trial results in the form of an Investigational New Drug application (IND) to the regulatory agencies. The sponsor (developer) describes the proposed study and identifies an established manufacturer able to provide information to demonstrate compliance with the principles of Good Manufacturing Practices (GMP). GMPs ensures that the vaccine will be consistently produced and controlled with the quality standards appropriate to their purpose and required by marketing authorization.

In the United States, the U.S. Food and Drug Administration (FDA) and FDA's Center for Biologics Evaluation and Research (CBER) are responsible for ensuring rigorous scientific and regulatory processes. They pursue the development of vaccines guaranteeing the safety, quality, and effectiveness of vaccines [5]. The authorization of development, scientific evaluation, approval, and monitoring of COVID-19 vaccines in the European Union (EU) is under European Medicines Agency (EMA) and other independent regulators in EU and European Economic Area (EEA) countries. At an international level, the World Health Organization (WHO) makes recommendations and assistance in the evaluation of a clinical trials (development and regulatory review) and many countries adopt such standards set out by the WHO [6, 7].

When the vaccine is ready to start studies in humans and the regulatory review has been accepted, the standard vaccine development typically undergoes a long process of clinical evaluation which depends on the nature of a particular vaccine and its intended use may impact specific data needs. However, usually, the stages will sequentially go through three clinical phases of development.

The investigational products will be studied in human for the first time under phase I, phase II, and phase III clinical trials and are governed by good clinical practice (GCP).

Phase I: Moreover nominated as human pharmacology studies, the vaccine is given to a small number of healthy volunteers (20-100) or patients (depending on the therapeutic area) to find a proper way to administer the vaccine before moving into a larger study. In this phase, the study will primarily check the safety, reactogenicity (possible side effects), and often the adequate dose, route of administration, and schedule of immunisation are determined [5, 8]. Phase I takes 1 week to several months and once it achieves satisfactory results with no safety concerns, phase II continues the safety assessment.

Phase II: The therapeutic exploratory studies intend to evaluate the immunogenicity of the vaccine, provide preliminary estimates on the rates of common adverse events, and identify the optimal dose (number of doses are needed, schedule of immunizations and method of delivery) helping to establish therapeutic doses for large-scale Phase III studies. Several hundreds of volunteers with varying health statuses and from different demographic groups are involved and closely monitored. A control group or placebo group, consisting of people who may not receive a target vaccine, but another vaccine related to a different disease is included in randomized and well-controlled designs. The group vaccinated with placebo will be compared to the group receiving the vaccine under study [5, 8].

Phase III: Clinical efficacy and safety studies are essential for the registration and approval of the new vaccine and are designed to evaluate and show how an efficacious the vaccine is against infection or alternative treatment. The percentage reduction in incidence among the vaccinated volunteers were compared to the incidence in the placebo group. A large-scale clinical trial with thousands of volunteers is made to provide additional safety data among the rare adverse events. At the end of this phase, the developer of a vaccine can submit the results to the regulatory authorities as part of a marketing authorisation application. These Phase III studies are randomized and double blind.

A phase IV trial is considered a post-marketing surveillance and it is not mandatory but may be performed after a vaccine is released to continue monitoring the safety and to study long-term effects in the population. Once the vaccine has been developed, the national regulators will decide whether to introduce a vaccine in their countries.

2.1 Fast-Track Procedures for COVID-19 Vaccine

The process to develop a new vaccine is a high-cost study involving many steps that can take many years to achieve and have the vaccine available for commercial use. This long period involves not just the time to get the results from each clinical trial conducted, but also the period to get funding, the time to recruit volunteers to take part in the study, negotiation to manufacturers and the review of the efficacy and safety evidence required, including regulatory review and approval in the country. However, during a public health emergency such as the urgent need for COVID-19 vaccine, development may be atypical, and a fast-tracked process is essential.

The EMA put in place rapid review procedures related to COVID-19 and exceptionally started evaluating data while the development was still ongoing. It delivered assessments of high-quality applications from sponsors in the shortest possible timeframes rather than waiting for all data to be made available along with the formal applications [9]. The COVID-19 vaccines have been developed following the same legal requirements for quality, safety, and efficacy as for all other vaccines but some steps during the process have to be conducted in parallel with the clinical trials. For example, new COVID-19 vaccines using a platform with previous experience in humans were conducted phase I at the same time as preclinical studies, and some aspects of manufacture and control were based on the vaccine platform, which in some instances reduced the need for product-specific data [10].

Typically, the manufacturing of the new vaccine starts after approval by the regulators, but to guarantee the distribution of COVID-19 vaccine would occur quickly after the approval, the process has been anticipated long before the results came in, even though it entails a financial risk for companies to start producing the vaccine.

The decision of whether to approve vaccines for national use is made by local authorities based on the WHO recommendations. In the EU, when the evidence for any COVID-19 vaccine shows that the benefits of vaccination are greater than any known potential risks, marketing authorisation can be granted.

3 MAJOR COVID-19 VACCINE APPROACHES

There are currently around 267 new vaccines in different preclinical (184 vaccines) or clinical (83 vaccines) stages of the development process. The WHO keeps a draft landscape document listing all novel coronavirus SARS-Cov2 vaccines, which is updated regularly and can be found online at `https://www.who.int/publications/m/item/draft-landscape-of-covid-19-candidate-vaccines`. The types of vaccines can be classified depending on the platform used to deliver the antigen:

1. original virus attenuated or inactivated;
2. other viruses, replicative or non-replicative;
3. genetic material, DNA or RNA;
4. proteins delivered in subunits.

3.1 Original Virus as Vaccine Platform

The SAR-CoV-2 virus itself is used as a vaccine, but the infectious capabilities and therefore the pathogenicity, are modified by either attenuation or inactivation mechanisms. Inactivation of the virus may be achieved through methods like ultraviolet or gamma irradiation, high pressure, visible ultrashort pulsed laser, formalin or other chemical compounds, and low-energy electron irradiation. Attenuation of a virus involves the modification of the virus genetic signature by adapting the virus to unfavourable conditions such as growth in nonhuman cells or by rationally modifying it with either codon deoptimization, mutagenesis or recombination. Even though attenuated and traditional inactivated vaccines are being extremely valued, high-titer preparation of these vaccines in cell culture under the conditions of biosafety level-3 has its challenges because they are live viruses. A great advantage of the whole virus vaccine is that they preserve the immunogenicity of all antigens of the virus and not only stimulate humoral immunity, but also stimulate cellular immune responses in a similar way to live viruses. In fact, apart from the ability of viral particles of cross-presentation to CD4 and CD8 T cells via MHC class II and MHC class I molecules, respectively, they contain PAMPs (Pathogen-associated molecular patterns), which are constitutive components of the virus or bacteria such as nucleic acids, polysaccharides, Lipopolysaccharides, Lipid A, monophosphoryl lipid A, bacterial peptidoglycans, etc. PAMPs are used by the innate immune compartment through Toll like receptor 7 to induce T cell-mediated responses as well as the production of cytokines which induce potent cellular immune responses [11].

Eighteen inactivated vaccines are described to be in different phases of development, eight of them in clinical stage [12]. However, just three live-attenuated vaccines have been listed and are still in preclinical stages. Inactivated vaccines, unlike attenuated vaccines, are more advantageous because they do not cause disease, which has been a safety concern over the years. In fact, the main difficulty of attenuated vaccines is the possible reversion of the pathogen to its virulent form as happened with the oral poliovirus vaccine [13].

Due to the devastating consequences of the SAR-CoV-2 pandemic, the urge to get scientific results led to publishing the results of preclinical assays in mouse, rat, and nonhuman primate (NHP) models on bioRxiv, a free online archive for unpublished preprints in the life sciences that additionally lacks peer-review, edition or typeset before being posted online. We will base our review on the vaccines developed with scientific results in scientific peer-reviewed journals.

Sinovac developed the first inactivated vaccine supported by a peer-reviewed scientific journal (Science) published in May 2020 [14]. The laboratory based in Beijing (China) chose a Chinese strain (GenBank accession number MT407650) to develop a purified inactivated SARS-CoV-2 virus vaccine identified as PiCoVacc. The isolate was obtained from bronchoalveolar fluid of hospitalized patients, which showed 99.8 to 100 sequence identity with other isolates from China, Italy, United Kingdom, Switzerland, and Spain. The virus was propagated by passaging ten times in Vero cells demonstrating excellent genetic stability. Then PiCoVacc was inactivated with β-propiolactone. Immunogenicity of the vaccine was tested in BALB/c mice and Wistar rats. After a Prime-Boost immunization strategy using Alum as an adjuvant, they observed that PiCoVacc induces an antibody immune response that peaks after 6 weeks and covers the spike, receptor binding domain (RBD), and N-viral proteins. The maximum neutralising titers peaked at week 7 by using the microneutralization (MN50) assay [14]. NHP species (Rhesus macaque) develop a COVID-19-like disease caused by SARS-CoV-2 infection [15], providing a great insight into the pathogenic mechanism and facilitating the development of vaccines and therapeutics against SARS-CoV-2.

When PicoVacc was administered three times intramuscularly to rhesus macaques, the S-specific antibody and neutralizing antibody titers obtained three weeks after immunisation were similar to those of sera from the recovered COVID-19 patients. To evaluate the protective efficacy, the macaques were intratracheally inoculated with a different SARS-CoV-2 strain (MT407649). Vaccinated macaques were largely protected with a $6\mu g$-dose, observing undetectable viral loads in different pulmonary specimens [14]. Considering the described "Cytokine Storm" induced by excessive T cell responses which exacerbates COVID-19 pathogenicity [16], Sinovac evaluated the safety profile of PicoVacc in macaques. Haematological, biochemical, and histopathological evaluation showed no notable changes in the vaccinated groups compared to the sham and placebo groups [14].

Sinovac's vaccine candidate (now named as CoronaVac) entered phase 1/2 clinical trials in April-May 2020 to evaluate safety, tolerance, and immunogenicity in elderly (> 60 years old) and adults (18-59 years old) (NTC04383574, NCT04352608). Although the results have not been published yet, the company press release (`http://www.sinovac.com/?optionid=754`) informed that the vaccine induces neutralising antibodies 14 days after vaccination with a 0, 14-day schedule and the neutralizing antibody seroconversion rate is above 90%. No severe adverse events were reported in either phase I (143 volunteers) or phase 2 (600 volunteers) trials. The Phase 1/2 clinical trial among adolescents and children (3-17 years old) is expected to begin soon (NCT04551547), since it was approved by the Ethics committee in September. Considering those early results, the Phase III clinical trial started in July 2020 sponsored by Instituto Butantan in Brazil, and seeks to test the efficacy and safety, aiming to support the licensure of CoronaVac (NCT04456595). This case-driven, randomised, double-blinded, two-dose, placebo-controlled phase III clinical trial is multicentred (Brazil, Turkey, Indonesia, and Chile) and it will be developed in two stages: the first stage with 1,300 healthcare adult workers (18-59 years old) and a second stage with 12,000 adults of general population. The estimated completion date is for October 2021, but preliminary and promising successful results obtained from Brazil and Turkey cohorts were press-released on February 2021: by December 2020, a total of 12,396 health workers were enrolled, with 253 positive cases collected in the observation period. After 14 days following the two-dose vaccination in a 0, 14-day schedule, the efficacy rate against the disease was 50.65% for all cases, 83.70% for cases requiring medical treatment and 100% for hospitalised, severe and fatal cases.

The Beijing Institute of Biological Products Limited company developed a SARS-CoV-2 inactivated vaccine candidate which was published in August 2020 by Cell [17]. They used the strain 19nCov-CDC-Tan-HBO2 (W2020(COVID-19-BJ-P7)01) isolated from Vero cells which were directly infected via the throat swabs of patients to prevent possible mutations during viral culture and isolation. The genetic stability was confirmed after 10 generations (sequence homology more than 99.95%) and the inactivation with β-propiolactone showed elimination of the viral infectivity, good stability, and replicability of the process. The vaccine BBIBP-CorV was produced following a new strategy based on a novel carrier-in-basket reactor. The immunogenicity studies in Balb/c mice showed that the three-dose (D0/D7/D14) intraperitoneal adjuvanted (aluminium hydroxide) administration induces the highest Neutralising antibody titers (microtitration method) with 100% of seroconversion rate which was also confirmed in rabbits and guinea pig models. Efficacy studies in NHP (macaques), demonstrated that a prime-boost regimen, intramuscular injection with BBIBP-CorV (low dose $2\mu g$) could efficiently block infection of SARS-CoV-2 and COVID-19 disease. Safety studies proved no clinical signs of distress nor histopathologic changes after euthanasia in guinea pigs and rats [17]. No evidence of antibody-dependent enhancement (ADE) was observed in rhesus macaques. The phase 1/2 clinical trial of BBIBP-CorV was recently published in Lancet [18]. The randomised, double-blind, placebo-controlled trial aimed to test safety and immunogenicity in healthy adults and aged people (18-80 years old). Two-dose immunization was safe and well tolerated in both age groups. A robust humoral immune response was observed in 100% of vaccine recipients, although delayed in the group aged 60 years and older (day 42 compared to days 14-28 in younger adults) as well as a reduced magnitude of neutralising antibodies [18]. A two-dose immunisation with $4\mu g$ of vaccine on days 0 and 21 or days 0 and 28 achieved higher neutralising antibody titers than the single $8\mu g$ or $4\mu g$ dose on days 0 and 14. A phase III clinical trial to evaluate the efficacy, immunogenicity, and safety of the BBIBP-CorV vaccine started in July 2020 in the United Arab Emirates (ChiCTR2000034780) and in August 2020 in other countries such as Jordan, Egypt, Bahrain (NCT04510207) as well as Morocco (ChiCTR2000039000) and Peru (NCT04612972). The studies were expected to be completed by the end of the year 2021, however, in December Chinese regulators granted a conditional approval to be used broadly with an efficacy rate of 79% based on an interim analysis of Phase 3 trials. The United Arab Emirates and Bahrain gave full approval to the BBIBP-CorV vaccine with an efficacy rate of 86% in December 2020 (`https://www.nytimes.com/interactive/2020/health/sinopharm-covid-19-vaccine.html`). These interim results have not been scientifically published by the time this review has been written.

3.2 Other Viruses as Vaccine Platform

Recombinant-vectored vaccines are a powerful technology for delivering heterologous antigens. The antigen against which immunity is sought comes from a foreign transgene inserted into a competent viral vector without replacing any vector genes. The vector genome carries out all viral amplification and transmission functions and the transgene does not contribute to any process benefiting vector reproduction [19]. This technology was developed forty years ago using the vaccinia virus vector expressing the hepatitis B surface antigen (HBsAg) [20]. Since then, viral vectors have been successfully introduced in many veterinary species [21], but only one has been licensed for human vaccination (rVSV-ZEBOV for Ebola Virus) [22]. Several viruses have been used as vectors for vaccine development: poxviruses, adenoviruses, herpesviruses, arenaviruses, retroviruses, paramyxoviruses, and flaviviruses among others [23]. One of the main advantages of viral vectors is their ability to evoke a robust adaptive immune response in the absence of an adjuvant. In fact, viral vectors express diverse PAMPS, which activate innate immunity and, at the same time, their capacity to infect cells and express encoded antigens which are shed into the extracellular milieu or directed to host intracellular processing pathways ensuring highly efficient induction of both humoral and cytotoxic (CD8+) T cell responses [24]. To ensure safety for human use, targeted gene deletion is a widely used strategy to reduce or eliminate the replicative capacity without loss of potency. Replicant competent vectors are biological active and produce virus progeny in the vaccinated host but may be attenuated to pathogenicity either because of mutations in the vector, because of the chimeric nature of the vaccine itself, because the vector is used in a heterologous host or due to a combination of all these factors. A replication-deficient virus vector is so severely attenuated that it cannot undergo a complete replication cycle in infected cells [25]. The main disadvantage of viral vectors is that the transgene specific immune response may be dampened by preexisting or *de novo* adaptive immune responses to antigenic targets within the vector itself. Strategies such as the use of higher doses or heterologous prime-boost regimens have been used to overcome this situation [24].

Eighteen vaccines have been described to be in the clinical phases of vaccine development, twelve of them non-replicating viral vectors and five replicating ones. Additionally, another 41 (19 replicant-competent and 22 non-replicant) are in preclinical development [12]. Adenovirus vectored vaccines are currently the furthest along in clinical testing. Adenoviruses are non-enveloped, icosahedral, double-stranded DNA viruses that can broadly infect vertebrates including humans and NHP. Human adenoviruse serotype 5-based vectors (Ad5) have been broadly studied in many laboratory and clinical trials over the last decades, demonstrating its potent antigen-specific immune responses in both preclinical and clinical studies [26]. This is the case of the recombinant non-replicative Ad5-nCoV vaccine candidate (Convidecia^{TM}) developed by the Chinese company Cansino Biologics, which expresses the spike protein of the SARS-CoV-2 virus. No preclinical study has been published, but phase 1 [27], phase 2 [28] and a currently opened phase 3 clinical trial (NCT04526990, NCT04540419) have been performed to test the immunogenicity, safety, tolerability and efficacy of the vaccine. Phase 1 and Phase 2 clinical trials have shown that a single dose of 5×10^{10} viral particles is safe, tolerable and elicits seroconversion at day 28 post vaccination of neutralising antibodies in almost 50% of the participants and S-specific binding antibodies in 97% of them. Positive specific T-cell responses measured by IFNγ-ELISPOT, were found in 88% of the participants. An interim analysis of the phase III clinical trials was reported by CanSinoBIO on its press-released website (`http://www.cansinotech.com/html/1///179/180/651.html`), shows an overall efficacy of 65.28% at preventing all symptomatic COVID-19 diseases, 28 days after single dose vaccination. However, Ad5-nCoV has an efficacy of 90.07% at preventing severe disease 28 days after a single vaccination. On February 2021, CanSino Biologics applied to the National Medical Products administration (NMPA) in China to get a conditional marketing authorization.

The limitations of these studies are the short-term report (28 days after vaccination), the higher reactogenicity in the high dose ($1.5 \times 10^{11} vp$) with severe self-limiting and transient adverse events and the presence of preexisting immunity to the Ad5 vector which gets more prominent with age, thus hampering the immune responses to vaccination. Indeed, 40-60% of Americans carry detectable levels of neutralising antibodies against Ad5 wild-type viruses and in China around 74% and even higher in Africa and other Asian countries [29]. The development of novel recombinant human adenoviruses with low seroprevalence among healthy individuals that circumvent anti-Ad5 immunity and are also highly immunogenic has been of great importance in recent years [26]. This is the case of the recombinant non-replicant Ad26-CoV2.S vaccine candidate developed by Janssen Vaccines (Johnson and Johnson) company in the US. The viral vector carries the wild-type leader sequence with full-length spike and mutation of the furin cleavage site and proline-stabilizing mutations (S.PP) [30]. Preclinical evaluation of this vaccine was done in NHP (rhesus macaques) [31] and Syrian golden hamsters [32]. Large animal models offer an important advantage due to the ability to use the natural routes of challenge and therefore obtain more relevant correlates of immune mediated protection [33]. Mercado *et al.* have shown that a single immunization with the Ad26-CoV2.S vaccine induced robust neutralising antibody responses and provided complete protection against SARS-CoV-2 challenge in five out of 6 macaques (one macaque had low levels of virus in nasal swabs). In addition, they demonstrated that serum titers of neutralizing antibodies may be a potential biomarker of vaccine protection since the titers correlate with protection in both bronchoalveolar lavage (BAL) and nasal swabs after challenge. However, a big caveat is that this model is clinically mild and it does not represent the severe clinical disease with respiratory failure and mortality that affects humans. Hamsters, on the contrary, as a result of their homology to the human ACE2 receptor [34], shows a severe clinical picture after intranasal SARS-CoV-2 infection, with high levels of virus replication in different tissues, extensive pneumonia, weight loss and mortality. Indeed, the Ad26 vaccine elicited binding and neutralising antibody responses which were correlated with protection against clinical disease as well as reduced virus replication in the upper and lower respiratory tract [32]. A randomised, double-blind, Placebo-controlled Phase 1/2 clinical trial of Ad26.CoV2.S started in June 2020 in different states of US, with more than 1000 volunteers (NCT04436276). Although no results have been reported yet, Johnson & Johnson announced through its press release website (`https://www.janssen.com/johnson-johnson-initiates-pivotal-global-phase-3-clinical-trial-janssens-covid-19-vaccine-candidate`) that had launched in September 2020 a large, pivotal, multicountry Phase 3 ENSAMBLE clinical trial (NCT04505722) with the enrolment of up to 60,000 volunteers. This was supported by the positive interim results demonstrating the safety profile and immunogenicity after a single vaccination on the Phase 1/2 clinical study. The latest news released on January 29th, 2021 by Johnson & Johnson, show that the coprimary endpoint of 28 days following a single-dose vaccination demonstrated 72% efficacy in the US and 66% efficacy overall at preventing moderate to severe COVID-19. The vaccine candidate was 85% effective in preventing severe disease across all regions studied and complete protection against COVID-19 related Hospitalization and Death (Johnson & Johnson Announces Single-Shot Janssen COVID-19 Vaccine Candidate Met Primary Endpoints in Interim Analysis of its Phase 3 ENSEMBLE Trial | Janssen). In February 2021, the company submitted a conditional Marketing Authorization Application (cMAA) to the European Medicines Agency (EMA).

The Gamaleya Research Institute (Russia) has developed a heterologous recombinant adenoviral vaccine to overcome the preexisting immunity against human adenoviruses [35]. The vaccine Gam-COVID-Vac is based on a heterologous prime-boost vaccination with first rAd26 and secondly with rAd5, both coding the spike glycoprotein or S. This approach was tested in a non-randomised phase 1/2 clinical trial. They demonstrated that, despite the formation of neutralising antibodies against recombinant adenoviruses, the S specific immune response was not affected [35]. The vaccine is highly immunogenic, inducing strong humoral and cellular immune responses in 100% of participants with an antibody titers higher than that of convalescent plasma. Although preclinical data are not published yet, they assured robust humoral and cellular immune responses in NHP, providing protection from SARS-CoV-2 infection as well as complete protection in a lethal model of immunosuppressed hamsters. A randomised, double-blind, placebo-controlled phase 3 clinical trial started in august 2020 to assess the efficacy, immunogenicity, and safety of the Gam-COVID-Vac vaccine (NCT04530396, NCT04564716). It aims to include 40,000 volunteers aged at least 18 years. The interim results of the phase 3 Gam-COVID-Vac trial showed that the vaccine is 91.6% efficacious against COVID-19 after 21 days of the first dose (day of receiving the second dose). Although the study was not designed to assess the efficacy of a single-dose regimen, it allowed them to observe a possible partial protective effect of a single dose [36].

The level of neutralizing antibodies to simian adenoviruses is very low in human population and a number of different replicant-deficit vaccine vectors such as ChAd3, ChAd63, or ChAdOx1

[29, 37], have been previously used as a vaccine platform in different clinical trials. The University of Oxford (partnered with AstraZeneca) developed the ChAdOx1 nCov-19 (AZD1222) vaccine encoding the codon-optimized full-length spike protein of SARS-CoV-2 based on the previously demonstrated Middle East Respiratory syndrome coronavirus (MERS-CoV). ChAdOx1 is derived from the isolate Y25 whose seroprevalence in the human population was found to be 0% in the UK and 9% in Gambia [38]. Preclinical studies in mice (inbred Balb/c and outbred CD1), pigs [39] and NHP (rhesus macaques) [40] have shown that a single dose induces antibody responses but are significantly enhanced after a homologous boost. The SARS-CoV-2 neutralising antibody titers in pigs after a single immunisation appear broadly comparable to those in sera from human following asymptomatic infection, whereas titers in prime-boost pigs were more comparable to serum from recovered COVID-19 patients [41]. Vaccination with one or two doses of ChAdOx1 nCov-19 prevents or strongly reduces virus replication in the lower respiratory tract after inoculation of rhesus macaques with SARS-CoV-2. However, no reduction was detected in viral shedding from the nose in either the prime-only or prime-boost regimen [40]. An immune-enhanced disease related to SARS coronavirus immunization has been associated with a T_H2 response in mice [42] and diffuse alveolar damage and cellular infiltrates in NHP [43]. However, vaccination with ChAdOx1 nCov-19 promotes a T_H1 response (IFNγ, IL-2) in mice and NHP, and no markers of disease enhancement were detected in pulmonary tissues of NHPs, such as influx of cells or diffuse alveolar damage [40]. A phase 1/2, single-blind, randomised controlled clinical trial started in April 2020 with 1077 participants in different centres all over the UK (NCT04568031) [44]. It was demonstrated that a single dose of ChAdOx1 nCov-19 elicited an increase in Spike-specific antibodies by day 28 and neutralising antibodies in all participants after a booster dose. The correlation of neutralisation assays with IgG quantitation might indicate that a standardised ELISA would be sufficient to predict protection. A strong cellular immunity after vaccination resulted in marked increases in Spike -specific IFNγ producer's effector T cell responses as early as day 7, peaking at day 14 and maintained up to day 56. A Phase 3 clinical trial has started since July 2020 in US, Brazil, South Africa, India, and the UK to evaluate safety, efficacy, and immunogenicity of

ChAdOx1 nCov-19 (ISRCTN89951424, NCT04516746, NCT04540393, CTRI/2020/08/027170). First preliminary completion date was expected to be in December 2020, which was strongly impatiently awaited. The interim report [45] and *a posteriori* full primary analysis [46] with data obtained from different studies (UK, Brazil, and South Africa) showed a significant vaccine efficacy of 70.4% after two doses and protection of 64.1% after at least one standard dose against symptomatic disease. Interestingly, an efficacy of 90% was seen in those who received a low dose as prime in the UK study, which a more exploratory subgroup analysis demonstrated to be restricted to participants aged 18-55 years and with greater intervals (>8 weeks) between doses. Indeed, a more extended analysis showed that the vaccine efficacy after a second dose was higher in those with a longer prime-boost interval, reaching 81.3% with a dosing interval of 12 weeks or more compared to 55.1% in those with an interval of less than 6 weeks [46]. Another important question revealed in this study, although just analysed in UK population, was that ChAdOx1 nCoV-19 might have a substantial effect on transmission by reducing the number of infected individuals in the population. The UK Medicines and Healthcare products Regulatory Agency (MHRA) authorised for emergency supply the AstraZeneca COVID-19 vaccine (AZD1222) on the 30th December of 2020 followed by the emergency use authorization in INDIA, Argentina, Dominican Republic, El Salvador, Mexico and Morocco, on January 06th 2021 for active immunisation of adults. The European Union granted a conditional marketing authorization for active immunisation in individuals 18 years of age and older on the 29th January of 2021 (https://www.astrazeneca.com/media-centre/press-releases.html).

The vaccines that have a more advance run in the clinical trials are administered intramuscularly. However, mucosal immunization through the nasopharyngeal route can elicit local immune responses, including secretory IgA antibodies that confer protection at or near the site of inoculation of respiratory pathogens [47]. In fact, some recent preclinical studies in different animal models show the differences in immunogenicity and efficacy of intranasal versus intramuscular vaccine immunisations. The Beijing Institute of Biotechnology tested the vaccine Ad5-nCov (Cansino Biologics) in mice and ferrets observed for the first time that a single inoculation leads to complete protection of the upper and lower respiratory tracts. Interestingly, the neutralising antibody titers were higher in the high-dose intranasal groups than in the intramuscular groups, but the splenic cellular response was higher in the intramuscular groups in a dose-dependent way [48]. A group at the Washington University School of Medicine in Saint Louis, Missouri, led by Dr. Diamond, developed a chimpanzee adenovirus-vectored vaccine encoding the stabilized spike protein (ChAd-SARS-CoV-2S) and found that a single intranasal immunisation confers sterilising immunity in mice expressing the human ACE2. In fact, they hypothesized that the greater protection observed compared to the intramuscular administration was based on the mucosal immune response generated. High levels of anti-SARS-CoV-2 IgA were detected in serum and lung and B cells secreting IgA in spleen only in mice vaccinated via the intranasal route [49]. Of all viral vectored vaccines that have entered clinical trials, just the one developed by Casino Biologics (Ad5-nCov) has started a Phase 1 clinical trial to evaluate the safety and immunogenicity of mucosal vaccination (NCT04552366), although the type of administration, whether it is intranasal or other, is not detailed. Safety profiles of mucosal immunization are yet to be stablished in humans for many of the formulation's approaches [50], but the obvious benefits of directly stimulating the mucosal immune response are clear and could be the next step to follow.

Other viral vectors have been used to deliver SARS-CoV-2 antigens and they have also entered into early clinical trials. This is the case of non-replicating viral vectors such as Modified Vaccinia Virus Ankara (MVA) developed by the University of Munich (NCT04569383) or replicating competent viral vectors such as the Measles-vector based developed by the Institut Pasteur (NCT04497298) or the recombinant vesicular Stomatitis Virus by the Israel Institute for Biological research (NCT04608305). However, not much information about them has been published yet.

3.3 Genetic Material as Vaccine Platform

Vaccines based on nucleic acids (DNA, RNA) have gained great popularity due to their cost-effectiveness, ease of design and production, and, in the case of DNA, stability. From vaccine administration to antigen expression, DNA vaccines and RNA vaccines are processed through different pathways. Once encountered the cell to be transfected, the DNA must cross the cytoplasmic and nuclear membranes, be transcribed into mRNA, and move back to the cytoplasm and initiate translation. However, additionally, the stability and translation of mRNA inside the cell is crucial for the antigen to be expressed [51].

DNA vaccines are usually produced from purified bacterial plasmid preparations. DNA sequences contain the antigen gene to which the immune response is expected and is flanked by an eukaryotic promoter/enhancer and a transcription/polyadenylation sequence to induce gene expression in the host cell. Some of these plasmids also contain an antibiotic resistance gene to be used for selection during the production process [52]. Clinical trials using DNA vaccines evoked efficient induction of cellular and humoral immune responses, but the level of these responses most often was not sufficient to elicit significant clinical benefits. To overcome the poor immunogenicity, several strategies have been described for either optimization of DNA vaccines or approaches to improve their delivery to antigen presenting cells (APC) [53]. These strategies include the use of activated dendritic cell promoters such as Fascin-1 [54]; codon optimisation of antigen to enhance strongly the expression [55]; introduction of epitope-specific changes in the antigen to increase the affinity of MHC/peptide complexes to T cell receptors [56, 57]; coadministration with adjuvants which promotes the so-called danger signal (co-stimulators and pro-inflammatory mediators) [58] or intrinsic adjuvancy of plasmid DNA with encoding transcription factors to stimulate APC such as IRF [59] or NF-κB [60]; deletion of prokaryotic sequences of the plasmid after its propagation in bacteria yielding minicircle DNA [61]; bi-cistronic genes to enable expression of several genes [62]; DNA sequences which mediate nuclear translocation such as the simian virus (SV)40 enhancer region [63]; nano-carriers to shield the DNA vaccine from degradation by DNases and other vaccines [64]. Finally, the administration routes of DNA vaccines determine the immune response generated due to the number of APCs successfully transfected. Systemic administration such as intravenous aims to reach APCs located in secondary lymphoid organs. The skin constitutes an interesting target due to the high frequency of cutaneous DCs and many transfection strategies have been used to test their suitability in the clinic such as needle-free biolistic transfection, microneedles, electroporation [53]. Despite all efforts, just a limited number of DNA vaccines have been licensed for veterinary use, since safety concerns for use in the clinic have been raised regarding the probability of stable integration of transfected DNA into the genome of somatic or even germ cells, causing dysregulated gene expression and mutations [52]. However, many authors have demonstrated otherwise [65, 66].

RNA based vaccines confer several advantages over DNA based vaccines such as nonintegrating, natural degradation, but concerns with stability have been extensively raised. Two forms of RNA vaccines have been developed: conventional and self-amplifying. Conventional vaccines include just the simplest version of an open reading frame (ORF) for the target antigen, flanked by untranslated regions (UTRs) and with a terminal Poly (A) tail. Self-amplifying RNA vaccines consist of an engineered viral genome (usually alphavirus) containing genes encoding the RNA replication machinery, whereas the structural protein sequences are replaced by the gene of interest. While conventional RNA vaccines drive transient antigen expression, self-amplifying vaccines result in higher antigen expression which persist for several days *in vivo* although delayed in time [67]. Stability and translation of mRNA is crucial for a successful RNA vaccine as well as the administration route and the formulation which determine the kinetics and magnitude of antigen expression, and the potency of the immune response. Most of the vaccines need to be transported and stored in an uninterrupted cold-chain process, requirements which are not met in poor rural areas of tropical countries. Optimizations in formulations to develop more thermostable mRNA vaccines has been lately studied, such as dried mRNA [68], lyophilized [69], or protamine-encapsulated [70]. mRNA vaccines have the advantage of being produced in cell-free systems that can eliminate the concern of bacterial contamination and lack the potential for chromosomal integration and long-lasting expression [67]. Lipid nanoparticles (LNP) when loaded with nucleoside modified conventional mRNA, have been used to examine the influence of the route of administration on the kinetics of antigen expression [71]. In fact, intramuscular and intradermal injections offered the best levels and duration of effect [72]. LNPs are a popular delivery vehicle which have been proved to induce potent cellular and humoral immune responses when self-amplifying mRNA is encapsulated [73]. Interestingly, recently a study has shown that modified mRNA encapsulated into LNPs has an adjuvant effect and induces a potent T follicular helper response and a large number of germinal centre B cells with long living and high affinity neutralizing antibodies [74]. Dendritic cells are crucial to the effectiveness of RNA-based vaccines. More specifically, RNA sensors such as Toll-like receptors (TLRs) and RIG-I-Like receptors, located in different DCs compartments, after activation, can increase antigen presentation, promote cytokine secretion and stimulate B cell responses [67].

DNA and RNA based vaccines provide an advantage over other platforms since they do not require bioreactor culture techniques to scale up during the manufacturing process, allowing the development process to be faster for a pandemic. In fact, there are seventeen vaccines in clinical development (3 RNA based vaccines and 15 DNA based vaccines), and 38 in preclinical development (15 DNA based vaccines and 23 RNA based vaccines).

Moderna (Cambridge, Massachusetts) in collaboration with the National Institute of Allergy and Infectious diseases (NIAID) developed an mRNA vaccine based on a prefusion stabilised protein vaccine strategy, effective for enveloped viruses such as the respiratory syncytial virus (RSV) [75]. S proteins undergo marked structural rearrangement to fuse virus and host cell membranes, enabling delivery of the viral genome into the target cell. When prefusion proteins are stabilised, the neutralisation-sensitive epitopes are preserved making them highly immunogenic. To produce the prefusion-stabilised SARS-CoV-2 S protein, two proline mutations were substituted into the S protein residues 986 and 987. The mRNA was purified by oligo-dT affinity purification and encapsulated in a lipid nanoparticle, composed of four lipids, through a modified ethanol-drop nanoprecipitation process at a ratio of 2.5:1 (lipid:mRNA) [76]. Interestingly, five days after for the release of the genomic sequence of SARS-CoV-2 isolates, the good manufacturing practice (GMP) production of the mRNA-LNP (mRNA-1273) was initiated in parallel with the preclinical evaluation. This allowed a first-in-human phase I clinical trial just 66 days after and a phase II trial 74 days later. Corbett *et al.* [76] demonstrated in mice models that $1\mu g$ of mRNA-1273 is enough to induce a robust pseudovirus-neutralising activity, CD8 T cell responses, and balanced T_H1 and T_H2 responses (important to avoid vaccine-associated enhanced respiratory disease linked to T_H2 biased immune response). Protective immunity was assessed with the mouse-adapted SARS-CoV-2, which contains the substitution Q498Y/P499T in the receptor-binding domain enabling the virus to bind to the mouse angiotensin-converting enzyme 2 (ACE2) receptor and infect and replicate in the upper and lower respiratory tract. Viral replication in the lungs was undetectable for more than three months following prime-boost regimen. It is worth to mention that the level of pseudovirus-neutralising activity induced by $1\mu g$ mRNA-1273 in mice was of a similar magnitude to that induced by $100\mu g$ mRNA-1273 in humans [77]. A two-immunisation regimen of NHP with the mRNA-1273 vaccine showed protection against upper and lower airway viral replication even with a high dose challenge of SARS-CoV-2 ($8 \times 10^5 PFU$), which has important implications not only in preventing disease but also in the transmission of the virus [78]. A phase 1, dose escalation, open-label clinical trial was conducted to determine the safety, reactogenicity, and immunogenicity of mRNA-1273 (NCT04283461). Preliminary results demonstrated no-trial-limiting safety concerns and a rapid and robust immunogenicity profile with high neutralising antibody responses elicited in a dose-dependent manner. Seroconversion was quick for binding antibodies (2 weeks after the first vaccination), but pseudovirus neutralising activity was low before the second vaccination, supporting the need of a two-dose vaccination schedule [77]. A phase 1 dose-scalation clinical trial study involving older adults (>56 years old) was performed later, showing mild or moderate adverse events and the $100\mu g$ dose one inducing higher binding and neutralising antibody titers [79]. Widge *et al.* have revealed that three months after booster vaccinations, the levels of binding and neutralising antibodies remain high in all participants [80]. A phase 3 randomised, observer-blinded, placebo-controlled trial was performed across the US, enrolled 30,420 volunteers (NCT04470427) whose primary results indicated that the mRNA-1273 vaccine showed a 94.1% efficacy at preventing COVID-19 illness, including severe disease [81]. On December 2020, the Food and Drug Administration (FDA) authorized the emergency use of mRNA-1273 Moderna's vaccine against COVID-19 in individuals 18 years of age or older (`https://investors.modernatx.com/news-releases`).

BioNTech, a German company, together with Pfizer, an American company, launched a coordinated program to develop two lipid nanoparticle-formulated, nucleoside-modified mRNA vaccine candidates which were lately evaluated in phase 1 clinical trials. One of these candidates was BNT162b1, which encoded the SARS-CoV-2 receptor-binding domain (RBD) trimerized by the addition of a T4 fibritin fold on domain to increase its immunogenicity through multivalent display. The second candidate was BNT162b2, which encoded the full-length spike protein of SARS-CoV-2 modified by two proline mutations to lock the prefusion conformation and to mimic the intact virus to elicit virus neutralising antibodies [82]. Immunisation with either two vaccines in mice induced high antibody titers that inhibit pseudovirus entry and strong T_{FH} and T_{H1}-type CD4+ T cell response. However, BNT162b2 appears to be more efficient at eliciting antigen-specific cytotoxic IFNγ CD8+ T cells. Both candidates protected 2-4 -year-old macaques from challenge with infectious SARS-CoV-2, but BNT162b2 provided greater evidence of protection of the lower respiratory tract since no detectable SARS-CoV-2 RNA in the bronchoalveolar lavage samples was detected starting 3 days after challenge [82]. A placebo-controlled, observer-blinded, dose escalation, phase 1 trial conducted in the United states was performed to evaluate the safety and immunogenicity of BNT162b1 and BNT162b2 in healthy adults 18-55 years and 65-85 years old [83] (NCT04368728). The results obtained in this study guided them to move forward the vaccine BNT162b2 ($30\mu g$ dose) into a phase 2-3 clinical trial based on different outcomes: milder systemic reactogenicity particularly in older adults; although the immune responses elicited by both vaccines were similar, 7 and 14 days after the second dose, the 50% and 90% neutralising antibody titers in older adults elicited by BNT162b2 exceeded those of the convalescent sera. A multinational randomised observer-blinded efficacy trial of the two-dose regimen of BNT162b2 underwent with 43,548 participants 16 years old and older (NCT04368728). The results showed that at least 7 days after the second dose of BNT162b2 ($30\mu g$) was 95% effective against COVID-19 [84]. Although the study was not designed to assess the efficacy of a single-dose regimen, in the interval between the first and second dose, an efficacy of 52% was observed, reaching full efficacy against the disease after the second dose, highlighting the need of two doses for full efficacy. In December 2020, the US food and Drug Administration (FDA) and European Medicines Agency (EMA) authorised emergency use to prevent COVID-19 for use in individuals 16 years of age and older. Interestingly, Pfizer BioNTech launched in February 2021 a Phase 2/3 trial to evaluate the safety and efficacy in pregnant women vaccinated during their 24-34 weeks of gestation (NCT04754594), as informed on their press-release website (`https://investors.biontech.de/news-releases/news-release-details/pfizer-and-biontech-commence-global-clinical-trial-evaluate`).

A big concern worldwide is the emergence of new variants which have been associated with increased transmission, higher viral load, and extensive mutations in the spike protein: ΔH69/V70, ΔY144, N501Y, A570D, D614G, P681H, T716I, S982A and D1118H. One of these mutations, N501Y, was of particular concern because it is located in the receptor binding site, which makes the mutation to bind more tightly to its cellular receptor, ACE-2 [85]. This is the case of the B.1.1.7 variant and B.1.351, first identified in UK and the Republic of South Africa, respectively. A recent study, although still not peer-reviewed, showed that the variants B.1.1.7 and B.1.351 are resistant to convalescent serum (3 or 11-fold, respectively) and vaccine serum (2 or 6.5-fold, respectively), which might threaten the protective efficacy of current vaccines [86]. However, Moderna's vaccine seems to retain neutralizing activity against these emerging variants as communicated by a website press-release. And in the meantime, an additional variant-specific vaccine candidate (mRNA-1273.351), against variant B.1.351 has completed he manufacturing process and a phase 1 clinical trial to determine his boosting immunity capacity is about to start (`https://investors.modernatx.com/news-releases`). Pfizer has shown that BNT162b2-immune serum neutralised SARS-CoV-2 (USA/WA-1/2020 background strain) with an introduced N501Y mutation as efficiently as SARS-CoV-2 without mutation [87, 88]. Additionally, it has been reported that the titers of a 50% neutralization assay of immunised sera from individuals with $30\mu g$ BNT162b2 against the SARS-CoV-2 lineage B1.1.7 spike-pseudotyped VSV, although statistically reduced, was not indicating a biologically significant change in neutralisation activity. Although further experiments are recommended, it seems that the UK variant will unlikely escape the BNT162b2-mediated protection [89].

Inovio Pharmaceuticals is a US company specialised in DNA medicine to treat several infectious or noninfectious diseases. DNA plasmids with a target antigen are delivered directly into the body's cells through the electroporation device CELLECTRA® which has been shown to be well-tolerated in healthy adults [90]. Inovio generated an optimised DNA sequence of the SAR-CoV-2 spike glycoprotein and cloned into the expression vector pGX0001. This plasmid was considered the vaccine candidate INO-4800 after confirming the successful expression of the spike protein at both the RNA and protein level in different *in vitro* studies. Humoral and T cell responses were observed in mouse and guinea pig's preclinical studies after intramuscular and dermal injections, respectively. Importantly, anti-SARS-CoV-2 binding antibodies were found in lung washes of INO-4800 immunised mice and guinea pigs, which have the potential to protect against infection of these tissues and prevent lower respiratory disease associated with severe cases of COVID-19 [91]. A phase 1 open-label multi-centre, dose escalation, clinical trial (NCT0433610) was performed to evaluate the safety, tolerability, and immunogenicity of INO-4800 in a two-dose regimen (weeks 0 and 4), administered intradermally followed by electroporation using the CELLECTRA® 2000 device. INO-4800 was well tolerated with a successful safety profile across the two-dose groups with just product-related grade 1 adverse events and without an increase of adverse events post the second dose. Cellular and humoral responses were observed after the second dose of INO-4800. Thirty-six out of 38 participants seroconverted by generating binding, and/or neutralizing antibodies with titers among the range of convalescent sera. T cell response was dominated by T CD8+ co-producing IFN-γ and TNF-α, without the increase of IL-4 [92]. A phase 2/3 randomized, placebo-controlled, multicentre clinical trial has been registered to start soon to evaluate the safety, immunogenicity, and efficacy of INO-4800 followed by electroporation using CELLECTRA® 2000 device, in individuals of 18 years of age and older (NCT04642638).

3.4 Protein/Peptides Delivered as Subunit Vaccines

They are denominated subunit vaccines and involve the manufacturing *in vitro* of key recombinant proteins or peptides. In the last decades, recombinant protein technology has become efficient, relatively inexpensive, and therefore relatively widely available. Since they lack any of the infectious components, subunit vaccines are considered a safer approach compared to vaccines derived from live viruses. There are available many systems to produce recombinant protein including microbial systems such as *Escherichia coli* and yeast, as well as insect cells or mammalian cells. *E.coli* expression systems do not provide posttranslational modifications (PMT), such as glycosylation, which affect protein characteristics such as solubility, stability, or even correct folding. PMTs therefore affect the nature of the immune response and consequently, the functionality of the vaccine. Due to the complexity of SARS-CoV-2, it is difficult to properly produce these antigens in *E.coli*, and other systems have been chosen. Yeast has been the protein production system selected by several currently licensed hepatitis B vaccines [93] since the inclusion of PMT facilitates proper folding and the secretion of recombinant proteins extracellularly makes the purification simpler. Most of the COVID-19 recombinant protein vaccine candidates are expressed in mammalian expression systems, which constitute the majority of recombinant biologics [94]. Although they are more expensive, mammalian systems are appreciated for their ability to express glycoproteins with their native structures and PMT. COVID-19 subunit vaccines, like the ones from Novavax, Sanofi, and Adimmune, are produced in insect cells through a baculovirus expression vector [95]. Insect cells express recombinant proteins that are usually well-folded, soluble, and often contain the desired PMTs, however, the N-glycosylation is not equivalent to that of higher eukaryotes.

The SARS-CoV-2 spike glycoprotein has been discovered to be the one that triggers the most potent neutralizing antibody response, which epitopes are within the N-terminal domain (NTD) and in the receptor binding domain (RBD) [96] where the most potent ones could block ACE-2 binding site [97]. The NTD region has eight potential sites of glycosylation, making it more vulnerable to different patterns of glycosylation affecting the ability of triggering neutralizing antibodies. However, no glycosylation sites have been found within or proximal to the RBD domain [98].

Subunit vaccines elicit only a weak immune response which is potentiated when formulated in combination with adjuvants. Adjuvants are immunostimulants that trigger specific cell receptors and induce an innate immune response at the site of injection and in the draining lymph nodes. Aluminium hydroxide (alum) is one of the most used in vaccine development worldwide. Alum enhances the phagocytosis of the antigen and activates the proinflammatory NLRP3 pathway, inducing a strong humoral immune response in combination with the secretion of T_H2-biased cytokines [99]. T_H2 biased immune responses might induce vaccine-related eosinophilic lung disease and eosinophil-associated T_H2 immunopotentiation, which is of great concern in COVID-19 disease aiming to polarize the T-cell response towards type 1 immunity [100]. MF59® is an oil-in-water emulsion developed by Novartis and contains squalene oil and two surfactants, tween-80 and Span-85 emulsified in a citric acid buffer. MF59 impacts the apoptosis-associated speck-like protein containing a caspase recruitment domain and stimulates IL-4 and Stat-6 signalling [101]. CpG adjuvants are synthetic DNA fragments containing unmethylated CpG sequences. They are potent stimulators through toll-like receptor 9 (TLR9), inducing the activation and maturation of plasmacytoid dendritic cells and enhancing the differentiation of B cells into antibody-secreting plasma cells [102]. AS03 is a squalene-based oil-in-water emulsion containing alpha-tocopherol produced by GSK. AS03 can induce proinflammatory cytokines and chemokines but independently of type-1 interferon. This pro-inflammatory response is associated with improvement recruitment, activation, and maturation of antigen-presenting cells at the injection site [103]. Matrix M (Novavax) consists of nanosized particles of different saponin fractions (Fraction-A and Fraction-C) stabilised with cholesterol and phospholipids [104]. Matrix-M has been proved to enhance T_H1 and T_H2 immune responses, inducing high levels of neutralising antibodies and enhancing immune cell trafficking [105].

There are 26 candidate subunit vaccines that have entered in clinical development phases, of which just two (Novavax and Clover Biopharmaceuticals) have started phase 3 clinical trials. Still, around 68 protein subunit candidate vaccines have been registered in preclinical development.

Novavax developed the subunit vaccine NVX-CoV2373, consisting in the full-length SARS-CoV-2 spike glycoprotein with two mutations: a furin cleavage site (RRAR$\rightarrow$QQAQ) to be protease resistant and two proline substitutions (K986P, V987P) to stabilize the structure in different environmental stress conditions [106]. In mice, the candidate NVX-CoV2373 adjuvanted with Matrix-M induces, in a dose-dependent manner, high titers of antibodies which are neutralising and block hACE2 receptor binding. Additionally, prime-boost regimen with adjuvant significantly protected from SARS-CoV-2 virus in mice previously transduced with adenovirus encoding human ACE2 receptor, which makes them permissive to infection. The administration of Matrix-M with NVX-CoV2373 led to an antigen-specific CD4+ T cell development, which was balanced between T_H1 and T_H2 phenotypes, in most animals, or with a predominance of T_H1 phenotype. The immunogenicity studies performed in NHP (olive baboons) of the adjuvanted vaccine were consistent with the results obtained in mice, supporting the role of Matrix M in promoting the generation of neutralising antibodies and dose sparing. Furthermore, baboons receiving the vaccine had eight-fold higher binding and receptor inhibiting antibodies compared to COVID-19 convalescent serum [106]. In a parallel study, cynomolgus macaques immunized with NVX-CoV2373 and Matrix M adjuvant, induced anti-S antibody that was able to neutralize and block the binding of hACE2 receptor. They also demonstrated that after intranasal and intratracheal challenge with SARS-CoV-2, immunised macaques were protected against upper and lower respiratory tract infections and pulmonary disease [107]. A randomised, placebo-controlled phase $1/2$ clinical trial (NCT04368988) to test safety and immunogenicity in healthy adults they have shown that the two-dose regimen of $5\mu g$ and $25\mu g$ of NVX-CoV2373 plus Matrix M had acceptable safety findings and induced high immune responses, with levels of neutralising antibodies of a magnitude seen in convalescent sera [108]. At the end of January 2021, Novavax announced on its press release website that the preliminary results of the UK Phase 3 clinical trial (NCT04611802) had an estimated vaccine efficacy of

89.3% (https://ir.novavax.com/news-releases/news-release-details/novavax-covid-19-vaccine-demonstrates-893-efficacy-uk-phase-3), however no published results have been found for the writing of this review.

Clover Biopharmaceuticals partnered with GlaxoSmithKline developed a subunit vaccine candidate based on the Trimer Tag technology. cDNA encoding the ectodomain of wild-type SARS-CoV-2 Spile (S) protein was subcloned into the pTRIMER mammalian expression vector to allow in-frame fusion to trimer tag, which is capable of self-trimerization via disulphide bonds [109]. Then S-Trimer is expressed on a high level as a disulphide bond-linked trimer secreted protein and partially cleaved at S1/S2 boundary by furin protease [110]. In studies with rodents and NHP, immunization with S-Trimer adjuvanted with either AS03 or CpG1018 plus alum, induces robust high levels of neutralising antibodies and cell-mediated immune responses. Interestingly, they observed that the adjuvant AS03 induced a greater humoral immune response by producing higher levels of neutralising antibodies than CpG 1018 plus alum. Whereas CpG 1018 plus alum appeared to induce a cellular immune response with a more strongly Th1-biased in rodents. However, S-Trimer adjuvanted with either AS03 or CpG 1018 plus alum can induce protective immunity against SARS-CoV-2 in NHP, with no signs of disease enhancement [111]. A phase 1 clinical trial was started in June 2020 (NCT04405908) to evaluate the safety and immunogenicity of a two-dose S-Trimer (SCB-2019) vaccine adjuvanted with either S03 or CpG/Alum [112]. This randomized, double-blind placebo-controlled trial was conducted in Australia with participants in two age groups: 18-57 years and 55-75 years. Vaccination was well tolerated with mild injection-site pain in formulations containing AS03 adjuvant compared to the CpG/Alum adjuvant. SCB-2019 with fixed doses of either AS03 or CpG/Alum adjuvants induced higher titer and high seroconversion rates on day 36 after the second dose of binding and neutralising antibodies in both younger and older adults. However, when adjuvanted with CpG/Alum, the immune responses were lower than with AS03 and in dose-dependent way. Both adjuvanted SCB-2019 formulations elicited T_H1 biased CD4+ T cell responses [112]. Based on these results, $9\mu g$ SCb-2019 adjuvanted with AS03 and $30\mu g$ SCb-2019 adjuvanted with CpG/Alum are the preferred candidates to be taken into the phase 2/3 clinical trial (NCT04672395) which is still waiting to open recruitment.

4 CONCLUDING REMARKS

An optimal COVID-19 vaccine is expected to induce high titers of neutralizing antibodies, elicit a robust and long-lasting memory T_H1 cell-mediated immune response, but low T_H2 cell-biased responses to avoid any enhanced respiratory disease, and provide cross-protection among the different new emergent SARS-CoV-2 variants. In just one year, more than two hundred candidate vaccines have been enlisted by the WHO, five of them have been authorised for emergency use in different countries around the world. The quick and efficient response is essential to control and, as a long-term goal, reduces dramatically the impact of the pandemic. However, many uncertain and unknown parameters make the COVID-19 vaccine not yet ideal to be able to eradicate SARS-CoV-2.

The new emergent variants are a matter of concern for the community because they may reduce the efficacy and probably a multitarget vaccine or other strategy might be required to be developed. The correlates of protection are still not elucidated and although neutralizing antibodies seem to play an important role in reducing infection, other immunologic components might be essential, such as IFNγ T-cell response. In addition, it is difficult to compare results from different vaccines since not standardized assays for neutralisation and challenge studies have been developed. Careful longitudinal studies will be needed to determine the duration of any protection immunity and establish immunisation programmes which in turn require further exploration. For instance, many of the vaccines tested are administered intramuscularly or a few intradermally, and considering the lung disease acquired with SARS-CoV-2 infection, it is still unclear whether a possible mucosal vaccination through the nasal cavity might induce a strong immune response in the respiratory tract and, in turn, reduce oral dissemination.

In general, COVID-19 has become a turning point in the history of the development of vaccines and although it has demonstrated an intense and global effort for a pandemic control strategy, there are still challenges to face.

5 CONSENT FOR PUBLICATION

Not applicable.

6 CONFLICT OF INTEREST

The authors declare no conflict of interest, financial or otherwise.

7 ACKNOWLEDGEMENTS

We want to express our gratitude to all the staff at the Oxford University Jenner Institute dedicated to COVID-19 vaccine research.

References

[1] Huang C, Wang Y, Li X, Ren L, Zhao J, Hu Y, et al. Clinical features of patients infected with 2019 novel coronavirus in Wuhan, China. The Lancet [Internet]. 2020 Feb [cited 2021 Sep 29];395(10223):497–506. Available from: https://doi.org/10.1016/s0140-6736(20)30183-5

[2] Zhu N, Zhang D, Wang W, Li X, Yang B, Song J, Zhao X, Huang B, Shi W, Lu R, Niu P, Zhan F, Ma X, Wang D, Xu W, Wu G, Gao GF, Tan W. A Novel Coronavirus from Patients with Pneumonia in China, 2019. New England Journal of Medicine [Internet]. 2020 Feb 20 [cited 2021 Sep 29];382(8):727–33. Available from: https://doi.org/10.1056/nejmoa2001017

[3] Wilder-Smith A, Freedman DO. Isolation, quarantine, social distancing and community containment: pivotal role for old-style public health measures in the novel coronavirus (2019-nCoV) outbreak. Journal of Travel Medicine [Internet]. 2020 Feb 13 [cited 2021 Sep 29];27(2). Available from: https://doi.org/10.1093/jtm/taaa020

[4] Brooks SK, Webster RK, Smith LE, Woodland L, Wessely S, Greenberg N, Rubin GJ. The Psychological Impact of Quarantine and How to Reduce It: Rapid Review of the Evidence. SSRN Electronic Journal [Internet]. 2020 [cited 2021 Sep 29]. Available from: https://doi.org/10.2139/ssrn.3532534

[5] FDA. Available from: https://www.fda.gov/vaccines-blood-biologics/development-approval-process-cber/vaccine-development-101 2021.

[6] Baay MF, Richie TL, Neels P, Cavaleri M, Chilengi R, Diemert D, Hoffman SL, Johnson R, Kirkpatrick BD, Knezevic I, Laurens M, McShane H, Njuguna P, Older Aguilar A, Pollard AJ, Riddle M, Sauerwein R, Southern J, Tribble D, Wildfire A. Human challenge trials in vaccine development, Rockville, MD, USA, September 28–30, 2017. Biologicals [Internet]. 2019 Sep [cited 2021 Sep 29];61:85–94. Available from: https://doi.org/10.1016/j.biologicals.2018.02.002

[7] WHO. Expert Committe on Biological Standardization. Annex 9, Guidelines on clinical evaluation of vaccines: regulatory expectations. Replacement of Annex 1. WHO Technical Reports Series2017. p. 503–75.

[8] EMA. Clinical trials in human medicines 2021. Available from: https://www.ema.europa.eu/en/human-regulatory/research-development/clinical-trials-human-medicines.

[9] EMA. Fast-track procedures for treatments and vaccines for COVID-19 2021. Available from: https://www.ema.europa.eu/en/news/covid-19-how-ema-fast-tracks-development-support-approval-medicines-vaccines.

[10] FDA, CBER. Nonbinding Recommendations Development and Licensure of Vaccines to Prevent COVID-19. Guidance for Industry. 2020.

[11] Sabbaghi A, Miri SM, Keshavarz M, Zargar M, Ghaemi A. Inactivation methods for whole influenza vaccine production. Reviews in Medical Virology [Internet]. 2019 Jul 23 [cited 2021 Sep 29];29(6). Available from: https://doi.org/10.1002/rmv.2074

[12] Organization WH. Draft landscape of COVID-19 candidate vaccines WHO Publications

Overview 19 October 2020 Available from: https://www.who.int/publications/m/item/draft-landscape-of-covid-19-candidate-vaccines.

[13] Famulare M, Chang S, Iber J, Zhao K, Adeniji JA, Bukbuk D, Baba M, Behrend M, Burns CC, Oberste MS. Sabin Vaccine Reversion in the Field: a Comprehensive Analysis of Sabin-Like Poliovirus Isolates in Nigeria. Journal of Virology [Internet]. 2015 Oct 14 [cited 2021 Sep 29];90(1):317–31. Available from: https://doi.org/10.1128/jvi.01532-15

[14] Gao Q, Bao L, Mao H, Wang L, Xu K, Yang M, et al. Development of an inactivated vaccine candidate for SARS-CoV-2. Science [Internet]. 2020 May 6 [cited 2021 Sep 29];369(6499):77–81. Available from: https://doi.org/10.1126/science.abc1932

[15] Yu P, Qi F, Xu Y, Li F, Liu P, Liu J, et al. Age-related rhesus macaque models of COVID-19. Animal Models and Experimental Medicine [Internet]. 2020 Mar [cited 2021 Sep 30];3(1):93–7. Available from: https://doi.org/10.1002/ame2.12108

[16] Zheng HY, Zhang M, Yang CX, Zhang N, Wang XC, Yang XP, Dong XQ, Zheng YT. Elevated exhaustion levels and reduced functional diversity of T cells in peripheral blood may predict severe progression in COVID-19 patients. Cellular & Molecular Immunology [Internet]. 2020 Mar 17 [cited 2021 Sep 30];17(5):541–3. Available from: https://doi.org/10.1038/s41423-020-0401-3

[17] Wang H, Zhang Y, Huang B, Deng W, Quan Y, Wang W, et al. Development of an Inactivated Vaccine Candidate, BBIBP-CorV, with Potent Protection against SARS-CoV-2. Cell [Internet]. 2020 Aug [cited 2021 Sep 30];182(3):713–21. Available from: https://doi.org/10.1016/j.cell.2020.06.008

[18] Xia S, Zhang Y, Wang Y, Wang H, Yang Y, Gao GF, et al. Safety and immunogenicity of an inactivated SARS-CoV-2 vaccine, BBIBP-CorV: a randomised, double-blind,

placebo-controlled, phase 1/2 trial. The Lancet Infectious Diseases [Internet]. 2021 Jan [cited 2021 Sep 30];21(1):39–51. Available from: https://doi.org/10.1016/s1473-3099(20)30831-8

[19] Bull JJ, Nuismer SL, Antia R. Recombinant vector vaccine evolution. PLOS Computational Biology [Internet]. 2019 Jul 19 [cited 2021 Sep 30];15(7):e1006857. Available from: https://doi.org/10.1371/journal.pcbi.1006857

[20] Smith GL, Mackett M, Moss B. Infectious vaccinia virus recombinants that express hepatitis B virus surface antigen. Nature [Internet]. 1983 Apr [cited 2021 Sep 30];302(5908):490–5. Available from: https://doi.org/10.1038/302490a0

[21] Pastoret PP, Brochier B. The development and use of a vaccinia-rabies recombinant oral vaccine for the control of wildlife rabies; a link between Jenner and Pasteur. Epidemiology and Infection [Internet]. 1996 Jun [cited 2021 Sep 30];116(3):235–40. Available from: https://doi.org/10.1017/s0950268800052535

[22] First FDA-approved vaccine for the prevention of Ebola virus disease, marking a critical milestone in public health preparedness and response. Case Medical Research [Internet]. 2019 Dec 19 [cited 2021 Sep 30]. Available from: https://doi.org/10.31525/cmr-24aaf8a

[23] Draper SJ, Heeney JL. Viruses as vaccine vectors for infectious diseases and cancer. Nature Reviews Microbiology [Internet]. 2009 Dec 7 [cited 2021 Sep 30];8(1):62–73. Available from: https://doi.org/10.1038/nrmicro2240

[24] Ewer KJ, Lambe T, Rollier CS, Spencer AJ, Hill AV, Dorrell L. Viral vectors as vaccine platforms: from immunogenicity to impact. Current Opinion in Immunology [Internet]. 2016 Aug [cited 2021 Sep 30];41:47–54. Available from: https://doi.org/10.1016/j.coi.2016.05.014

[25] Condit RC, Williamson AL, Sheets R, Seligman SJ, Monath TP, Excler JL, Gurwith M, Bok K, Robertson JS, Kim D, Michael Hendry R, Singh V, Mac LM, Chen RT. Unique safety issues associated with virus-vectored vaccines: Potential for and theoretical consequences of recombination with wild type virus strains. Vaccine [Internet]. 2016 Dec [cited 2021 Sep 30];34(51):6610–6. Available from: `https://doi.org/10.1016/j.vaccine.2016.04.060`

[26] Abbink P, Lemckert AA, Ewald BA, Lynch DM, Denholtz M, Smits S, Holterman L, Damen I, Vogels R, Thorner AR, O'Brien KL, Carville A, Mansfield KG, Goudsmit J, Havenga MJ, Barouch DH. Comparative Seroprevalence and Immunogenicity of Six Rare Serotype Recombinant Adenovirus Vaccine Vectors from Subgroups B and D. Journal of Virology [Internet]. 2007 Feb 28 [cited 2021 Sep 30];81(9):4654–63. Available from: `https://doi.org/10.1128/jvi.02696-06`

[27] Zhu FC, Li YH, Guan XH, Hou LH, Wang WJ, Li JX, et al. Safety, tolerability, and immunogenicity of a recombinant adenovirus type-5 vectored COVID-19 vaccine: a dose-escalation, open-label, non-randomised, first-in-human trial. The Lancet [Internet]. 2020 Jun [cited 2021 Sep 30];395(10240):1845–54. Available from: `https://doi.org/10.1016/s0140-6736(20)31208-3`

[28] Zhu FC, Guan XH, Li YH, Huang JY, Jiang T, Hou LH, et al. Immunogenicity and safety of a recombinant adenovirus type-5-vectored COVID-19 vaccine in healthy adults aged 18 years or older: a randomised, double-blind, placebo-controlled, phase 2 trial. The Lancet [Internet]. 2020 Aug [cited 2021 Sep 30];396(10249):479–88. Available from: `https://doi.org/10.1016/s0140-6736(20)31605-6`

[29] Guo J, Mondal M, Zhou D. Development of novel vaccine vectors: Chimpanzee adenoviral vectors. Human Vaccines & Immunotherapeutics [Internet]. 2018 Jan 23

[cited 2021 Sep 30];14(7):1679–85. Available from: https://doi.org/10.1080/21645515.2017.1419108

[30] Bos R, Rutten L, van der Lubbe JE, Bakkers MJ, Hardenberg G, Wegmann F, et al. Ad26 vector-based COVID-19 vaccine encoding a prefusion-stabilized SARS-CoV-2 Spike immunogen induces potent humoral and cellular immune responses. npj Vaccines [Internet]. 2020 Sep 28 [cited 2021 Sep 30];5(1). Available from: https://doi.org/10.1038/s41541-020-00243-x

[31] Mercado NB, Zahn R, Wegmann F, Loos C, Chandrashekar A, Yu J, et al. Single-shot Ad26 vaccine protects against SARS-CoV-2 in rhesus macaques. Nature [Internet]. 2020 Jul 30 [cited 2021 Sep 30];586(7830):583–8. Available from: https://doi.org/10.1038/s41586-020-2607-z

[32] Tostanoski LH, Wegmann F, Martinot AJ, Loos C, McMahan K, Mercado NB, et al. Ad26 vaccine protects against SARS-CoV-2 severe clinical disease in hamsters. Nature Medicine [Internet]. 2020 Sep 3 [cited 2021 Sep 30];26(11):1694–700. Available from: https://doi.org/10.1038/s41591-020-1070-6

[33] Kiros TG, Levast B, Auray G, Strom S, van Kessel J, Gerdts V. The Importance of Animal Models in the Development of Vaccines. In: Innovation in Vaccinology [Internet]. Dordrecht: Springer Netherlands; 2012 [cited 2021 Sep 30]. p. 251–64. Available from: https://doi.org/10.1007/978-94-007-4543-8_11

[34] Chan JF, Zhang AJ, Yuan S, Poon VK, Chan CC, Lee AC, et al. Simulation of the Clinical and Pathological Manifestations of Coronavirus Disease 2019 (COVID-19) in a Golden Syrian Hamster Model: Implications for Disease Pathogenesis and Transmissibility. Clinical Infectious Diseases [Internet]. 2020 Mar 26 [cited 2021 Sep 30]. Available from: https://doi.org/10.1093/cid/ciaa325

[35] Logunov DY, Dolzhikova IV, Zubkova OV, Tukhvatullin AI, Shcheblyakov DV, Dzharullaeva AS, et al. Safety and immunogenicity of an rAd26 and rAd5 vector-based heterologous prime-boost COVID-19 vaccine in two formulations: two open, non-randomised phase 1/2 studies from Russia. The Lancet [Internet]. 2020 Sep [cited 2021 Sep 30];396(10255):887–97. Available from: https://doi.org/10.1016/s0140-6736(20)31866-3

[36] Logunov DY, Dolzhikova IV, Shcheblyakov DV, Tukhvatulin AI, Zubkova OV, Dzharullaeva AS, et al. Safety and efficacy of an rAd26 and rAd5 vector-based heterologous prime-boost COVID-19 vaccine: an interim analysis of a randomised controlled phase 3 trial in Russia. The Lancet [Internet]. 2021 Feb [cited 2021 Sep 30];397(10275):671–81. Available from: https://doi.org/10.1016/s0140-6736(21)00234-8

[37] Gilbert SC, Warimwe GM. Rapid development of vaccines against emerging pathogens: The replication-deficient simian adenovirus platform technology. Vaccine [Internet]. 2017 Aug [cited 2021 Sep 30];35(35):4461–4. Available from: https://doi.org/10.1016/j.vaccine.2017.04.085

[38] Dicks MD, Spencer AJ, Edwards NJ, Wadell G, Bojang K, Gilbert SC, Hill AV, Cottingham MG. A Novel Chimpanzee Adenovirus Vector with Low Human Seroprevalence: Improved Systems for Vector Derivation and Comparative Immunogenicity. PLoS ONE [Internet]. 2012 Jul 13 [cited 2021 Sep 30];7(7):e40385. Available from: https://doi.org/10.1371/journal.pone.0040385

[39] Graham SP, McLean RK, Spencer AJ, Belij-Rammerstorfer S, Wright D, Ulaszewska M, et al. Evaluation of the immunogenicity of prime-boost vaccination with the replication-deficient viral vectored COVID-19 vaccine candidate ChAdOx1 nCoV-19. npj Vaccines [Internet]. 2020 Jul 27 [cited 2021 Sep 30];5(1). Available from: https://doi.org/10.1038/s41541-020-00221-3

[40] van Doremalen N, Lambe T, Spencer A, Belij-Rammerstorfer S, Purushotham JN, Port JR, et al. ChAdOx1 nCoV-19 vaccine prevents SARS-CoV-2 pneumonia in rhesus macaques. Nature [Internet]. 2020 Jul 30 [cited 2021 Sep 30];586(7830):578–82. Available from: `https://doi.org/10.1038/s41586-020-2608-y`

[41] Choe PG, Kang CK, Suh HJ, Jung J, Kang E, Lee SY, Song KH, Kim HB, Kim NJ, Park WB, Kim ES, Oh MD. Antibody Responses to SARS-CoV-2 at 8 Weeks Postinfection in Asymptomatic Patients. Emerging Infectious Diseases [Internet]. 2020 Oct [cited 2021 Sep 30];26(10). Available from: `https://doi.org/10.3201/eid2610.20211`

[42] Tseng CT, Sbrana E, Iwata-Yoshikawa N, Newman PC, Garron T, Atmar RL, Peters CJ, Couch RB. Immunization with SARS Coronavirus Vaccines Leads to Pulmonary Immunopathology on Challenge with the SARS Virus. PLoS ONE [Internet]. 2012 Apr 20 [cited 2021 Sep 30];7(4):e35421. Available from: `https://doi.org/10.1371/journal.pone.0035421`

[43] Liu L, Wei Q, Lin Q, Fang J, Wang H, Kwok H, Tang H, Nishiura K, Peng J, Tan Z, Wu T, Cheung KW, Chan KH, Alvarez X, Qin C, Lackner A, Perlman S, Yuen KY, Chen Z. Anti-spike IgG causes severe acute lung injury by skewing macrophage responses during acute SARS-CoV infection. JCI Insight [Internet]. 2019 Feb 21 [cited 2021 Sep 30];4(4). Available from: `https://doi.org/10.1172/jci.insight.123158`

[44] Folegatti PM, Ewer KJ, Aley PK, Angus B, Becker S, Belij-Rammerstorfer S, et al. Safety and immunogenicity of the ChAdOx1 nCoV-19 vaccine against SARS-CoV-2: a preliminary report of a phase 1/2, single-blind, randomised controlled trial. The Lancet [Internet]. 2020 Aug [cited 2021 Sep 30];396(10249):467–78. Available from: `https://doi.org/10.1016/s0140-6736(20)31604-4`

[45] Voysey M, Clemens SA, Madhi SA, Weckx LY, Folegatti PM, Aley PK, et al. Safety and efficacy of the ChAdOx1 nCoV-19 vaccine (AZD1222) against SARS-CoV-2: an interim

analysis of four randomised controlled trials in Brazil, South Africa, and the UK. The Lancet [Internet]. 2021 Jan [cited 2021 Sep 30];397(10269):99–111. Available from: https://doi.org/10.1016/s0140-6736(20)32661-1

[46] Voysey M, Costa Clemens SA, Madhi SA, Weckx LY, Folegatti PM, Aley PK, et al. Single-dose administration and the influence of the timing of the booster dose on immunogenicity and efficacy of ChAdOx1 nCoV-19 (AZD1222) vaccine: a pooled analysis of four randomised trials. The Lancet [Internet]. 2021 Mar [cited 2021 Sep 30];397(10277):881–91. Available from: https://doi.org/10.1016/s0140-6736(21)00432-3

[47] Neutra MR, Kozlowski PA. Mucosal vaccines: the promise and the challenge. Nature Reviews Immunology [Internet]. 2006 Feb [cited 2021 Sep 30];6(2):148–58. Available from: https://doi.org/10.1038/nri1777

[48] Wu S, Zhong G, Zhang J, Shuai L, Zhang Z, Wen Z, et al. A single dose of an adenovirus-vectored vaccine provides protection against SARS-CoV-2 challenge. Nature Communications [Internet]. 2020 Aug 14 [cited 2021 Sep 30];11(1). Available from: https://doi.org/10.1038/s41467-020-17972-1

[49] Hassan AO, Kafai NM, Dmitriev IP, Fox JM, Smith BK, Harvey IB, et al. A Single-Dose Intranasal ChAd Vaccine Protects Upper and Lower Respiratory Tracts against SARS-CoV-2. Cell [Internet]. 2020 Oct [cited 2021 Sep 30];183(1):169–84. Available from: https://doi.org/10.1016/j.cell.2020.08.026

[50] Yusuf H, Kett V. Current prospects and future challenges for nasal vaccine delivery. Human Vaccines & Immunotherapeutics [Internet]. 2016 Dec 9 [cited 2021 Sep 30];13(1):34–45. Available from: https://doi.org/10.1080/21645515.2016.1239668

[51] Brisse M, Vrba SM, Kirk N, Liang Y, Ly H. Emerging Concepts and Technologies in Vaccine

Development. Frontiers in Immunology [Internet]. 2020 Sep 30 [cited 2021 Sep 30];11. Available from: https://doi.org/10.3389/fimmu.2020.583077

[52] Myhr AI. DNA Vaccines: Regulatory Considerations and Safety Aspects. Current Issues in Molecular Biology [Internet]. 2017 [cited 2021 Sep 30]:79–88. Available from: https://doi.org/10.21775/cimb.022.079

[53] Hobernik D, Bros M. DNA Vaccines–How Far From Clinical Use? International Journal of Molecular Sciences [Internet]. 2018 Nov 15 [cited 2021 Sep 30];19(11):3605. Available from: https://doi.org/10.3390/ijms19113605

[54] Sudowe S, Ludwig-Portugall I, Montermann E, Ross R, Reske-Kunz AB. Transcriptional targeting of dendritic cells in gene gun-mediated DNA immunization favors the induction of type 1 immune responses. Molecular Therapy [Internet]. 2003 Oct [cited 2021 Sep 30];8(4):567–75. Available from: https://doi.org/10.1016/s1525-0016(03)00242-9

[55] Lopes A, Vanvarenberg K, Préat V, Vandermeulen G. Codon-Optimized P1A-Encoding DNA Vaccine: Toward a Therapeutic Vaccination against P815 Mastocytoma. Molecular Therapy - Nucleic Acids [Internet]. 2017 Sep [cited 2021 Sep 30];8:404–15. Available from: https://doi.org/10.1016/j.omtn.2017.07.011

[56] Hoppes R, Oostvogels R, Luimstra JJ, Wals K, Toebes M, Bies L, Ekkebus R, Rijal P, Celie PH, Huang JH, Emmelot ME, Spaapen RM, Lokhorst H, Schumacher TN, Mutis T, Rodenko B, Ovaa H. Altered Peptide Ligands Revisited: Vaccine Design through Chemically Modified HLA-A2–Restricted T Cell Epitopes. The Journal of Immunology [Internet]. 2014 Oct 13 [cited 2021 Sep 30];193(10):4803–13. Available from: https://doi.org/10.4049/jimmunol.1400800

[57] Pielak RM, O'Donoghue GP, Lin JJ, Alfieri KN, Fay NC, Low-Nam ST, Groves JT.

Early T cell receptor signals globally modulate ligand: receptor affinities during antigen discrimination. Proceedings of the National Academy of Sciences [Internet]. 2017 Oct 30 [cited 2021 Sep 30];114(46):12190–5. Available from: https://doi.org/10.1073/pnas.1613140114

[58] Joffre O, Nolte MA, Spörri R, Sousa CR. Inflammatory signals in dendritic cell activation and the induction of adaptive immunity. Immunological Reviews [Internet]. 2009 Jan [cited 2021 Sep 30];227(1):234–47. Available from: https://doi.org/10.1111/j.1600-065x.2008.00718.x

[59] Sasaki S, Amara RR, Yeow WS, Pitha PM, Robinson HL. Regulation of DNA-Raised Immune Responses by Cotransfected Interferon Regulatory Factors. Journal of Virology [Internet]. 2002 Jul 1 [cited 2021 Sep 30];76(13):6652–9. Available from: https://doi.org/10.1128/jvi.76.13.6652-6659.2002

[60] Shedlock D, Tingey C, Mahadevan L, Hutnick N, Reuschel E, Kudchodkar S, Flingai S, Yan J, Kim J, Ugen K, Weiner D, Muthumani K. Co-Administration of Molecular Adjuvants Expressing NF-Kappa B Subunit p65/RelA or Type-1 Transactivator T-bet Enhance Antigen Specific DNA Vaccine-Induced Immunity. Vaccines [Internet]. 2014 Mar 25 [cited 2021 Sep 30];2(2):196–215. Available from: https://doi.org/10.3390/vaccines2020196

[61] Stenler S, Blomberg P, Smith CE. Safety and efficacy of DNA vaccines. Human Vaccines & Immunotherapeutics [Internet]. 2014 Feb 19 [cited 2021 Sep 30];10(5):1306–8. Available from: https://doi.org/10.4161/hv.28077

[62] Vargas JE, Salton G, Sodré de Castro Laino A, Pires TD, Bonamino M, Lenz G, Delgado-Cañedo A. pLR: A lentiviral backbone series to stable transduction of bicistronic genes and exchange of promoters. Plasmid [Internet]. 2012 Nov [cited 2021 Sep 30];68(3):179–85. Available from: https://doi.org/10.1016/j.plasmid.2012.06.001

[63] Kanazawa T, Yamazaki M, Fukuda T, Takashima Y, Okada H. Versatile Nuclear Localization Signal-Based Oligopeptide as a Gene Vector. Biological & Pharmaceutical Bulletin [Internet]. 2015 [cited 2021 Sep 30];38(4):559–65. Available from: https://doi.org/10.1248/bpb.b14-00706

[64] Cai P, Zhang X, Wang M, Wu YL, Chen X. Combinatorial Nano-Bio Interfaces. ACS Nano [Internet]. 2018 Jun 8 [cited 2021 Sep 30];12(6):5078–84. Available from: https://doi.org/10.1021/acsnano.8b03285

[65] Wolff JA, Ludtke JJ, Acsadi G, Williams P, Jani A. Long-term persistence of plasmid DNA and foreign gone expression in mouse muscle. Human Molecular Genetics [Internet]. 1992 [cited 2021 Sep 30];1(6):363–9. Available from: https://doi.org/10.1093/hmg/1.6.363

[66] Manam S, Ledwith BJ, Barnum AB, Troilo PJ, Pauley CJ, Harper LB, Griffiths II TG, Niu Z, Denisova L, Follmer TT, Pacchione SJ, Wang Z, Beare CM, Bagdon WJ, Nichols WW. Plasmid DNA Vaccines: Tissue Distribution and Effects of DNA Sequence, Adjuvants and Delivery Method on Integration into Host DNA. Intervirology [Internet]. 2000 [cited 2021 Sep 30];43(4-6):273–81. Available from: https://doi.org/10.1159/000053994

[67] Zhang C, Maruggi G, Shan H, Li J. Advances in mRNA Vaccines for Infectious Diseases. Frontiers in Immunology [Internet]. 2019 Mar 27 [cited 2021 Sep 30];10. Available from: https://doi.org/10.3389/fimmu.2019.00594

[68] Jones KL, Drane D, Gowans EJ. Long-term storage of DNA-free RNA for use in vaccine studies. BioTechniques [Internet]. 2007 Nov [cited 2021 Sep 30];43(5):675–81. Available from: https://doi.org/10.2144/000112593

[69] Alberer M, Gnad-Vogt U, Hong HS, Mehr KT, Backert L, Finak G, Gottardo R, Bica MA, Garofano A, Koch SD, Fotin-Mleczek M, Hoerr I, Clemens R, von Sonnenburg F.

Safety and immunogenicity of a mRNA rabies vaccine in healthy adults: an open-label, non-randomised, prospective, first-in-human phase 1 clinical trial. The Lancet [Internet]. 2017 Sep [cited 2021 Oct 1];390(10101):1511–20. Available from: https://doi.org/10.1016/s0140-6736(17)31665-3

[70] Stitz L, Vogel A, Schnee M, Voss D, Rauch S, Mutzke T, Ketterer T, Kramps T, Petsch B. A thermostable messenger RNA based vaccine against rabies. PLOS Neglected Tropical Diseases [Internet]. 2017 Dec 7 [cited 2021 Oct 1];11(12):e0006108. Available from: https://doi.org/10.1371/journal.pntd.0006108

[71] Pardi N, Tuyishime S, Muramatsu H, Kariko K, Mui BL, Tam YK, Madden TD, Hope MJ, Weissman D. Expression kinetics of nucleoside-modified mRNA delivered in lipid nanoparticles to mice by various routes. Journal of Controlled Release [Internet]. 2015 Nov [cited 2021 Oct 1];217:345–51. Available from: https://doi.org/10.1016/j.jconrel.2015.08.007

[72] Lindgren G, Ols S, Liang F, Thompson EA, Lin A, Hellgren F, Bahl K, John S, Yuzhakov O, Hassett KJ, Brito LA, Salter H, Ciaramella G, Loré K. Induction of Robust B Cell Responses after Influenza mRNA Vaccination Is Accompanied by Circulating Hemagglutinin-Specific ICOS+ PD-1+ CXCR3+ T Follicular Helper Cells. Frontiers in Immunology [Internet]. 2017 Nov 13 [cited 2021 Oct 1];8. Available from: https://doi.org/10.3389/fimmu.2017.01539

[73] Oberli MA, Reichmuth AM, Dorkin JR, Mitchell MJ, Fenton OS, Jaklenec A, Anderson DG, Langer R, Blankschtein D. Lipid Nanoparticle Assisted mRNA Delivery for Potent Cancer Immunotherapy. Nano Letters [Internet]. 2016 Dec 5 [cited 2021 Oct 1];17(3):1326–35. Available from: https://doi.org/10.1021/acs.nanolett.6b03329

[74] Pardi N, Hogan MJ, Naradikian MS, Parkhouse K, Cain DW, Jones L, et al. Nucleoside-modified mRNA vaccines induce potent T follicular helper and germinal center

B cell responses. Journal of Experimental Medicine [Internet]. 2018 May 8 [cited 2021 Oct 1];215(6):1571–88. Available from: https://doi.org/10.1084/jem.20171450

[75] McLellan JS, Chen M, Joyce MG, Sastry M, Stewart-Jones GB, Yang Y, et al. Structure-Based Design of a Fusion Glycoprotein Vaccine for Respiratory Syncytial Virus. Science [Internet]. 2013 Oct 31 [cited 2021 Oct 1];342(6158):592–8. Available from: https://doi.org/10.1126/science.1243283

[76] Corbett KS, Edwards DK, Leist SR, Abiona OM, Boyoglu-Barnum S, Gillespie RA, et al. SARS-CoV-2 mRNA vaccine design enabled by prototype pathogen preparedness. Nature [Internet]. 2020 Aug 5 [cited 2021 Oct 1];586(7830):567–71. Available from: https://doi.org/10.1038/s41586-020-2622-0

[77] Jackson LA, Anderson EJ, Rouphael NG, Roberts PC, Makhene M, Coler RN, et al. An mRNA Vaccine against SARS-CoV-2 – Preliminary Report. New England Journal of Medicine [Internet]. 2020 Nov 12 [cited 2021 Oct 1];383(20):1920–31. Available from: https://doi.org/10.1056/nejmoa2022483

[78] Corbett KS, Flynn B, Foulds KE, Francica JR, Boyoglu-Barnum S, Werner AP, et al. Evaluation of the mRNA-1273 Vaccine against SARS-CoV-2 in Nonhuman Primates. New England Journal of Medicine [Internet]. 2020 Oct 15 [cited 2021 Oct 1];383(16):1544–55. Available from: https://doi.org/10.1056/nejmoa2024671

[79] Anderson EJ, Rouphael NG, Widge AT, Jackson LA, Roberts PC, Makhene M, et al. Safety and Immunogenicity of SARS-CoV-2 mRNA-1273 Vaccine in Older Adults. New England Journal of Medicine [Internet]. 2020 Dec 17 [cited 2021 Oct 1];383(25):2427–38. Available from: https://doi.org/10.1056/nejmoa2028436

[80] Widge AT, Rouphael NG, Jackson LA, Anderson EJ, Roberts PC, Makhene M, et al. Durability of Responses after SARS-CoV-2 mRNA-1273 Vaccination. New England Journal

of Medicine [Internet]. 2021 Jan 7 [cited 2021 Oct 1];384(1):80–2. Available from: https://doi.org/10.1056/nejmc2032195

[81] Baden LR, El Sahly HM, Essink B, Kotloff K, Frey S, Novak R, et al. Efficacy and Safety of the mRNA-1273 SARS-CoV-2 Vaccine. New England Journal of Medicine [Internet]. 2020 Dec 30 [cited 2021 Oct 1]. Available from: https://doi.org/10.1056/nejmoa2035389

[82] Vogel AB, Kanevsky I, Che Y, Swanson KA, Muik A, Vormehr M, et al. BNT162b vaccines protect rhesus macaques from SARS-CoV-2. Nature [Internet]. 2021 Feb 1 [cited 2021 Oct 1];592(7853):283–9. Available from: https://doi.org/10.1038/s41586-021-03275-y

[83] Walsh EE, Frenck RW, Falsey AR, Kitchin N, Absalon J, Gurtman A, et al. Safety and Immunogenicity of Two RNA-Based Covid-19 Vaccine Candidates. New England Journal of Medicine [Internet]. 2020 Dec 17 [cited 2021 Oct 1];383(25):2439–50. Available from: https://doi.org/10.1056/nejmoa2027906

[84] Polack FP, Thomas SJ, Kitchin N, Absalon J, Gurtman A, Lockhart S et al. Safety and efficacy of the bnt162b2 mrna covid-19 vaccine. New England Journal of Medicine [Internet]. 2020 Dec 31 [cited 2021 Oct 1];383(27):2603–15. Available from: https://doi.org/10.1056/nejmoa2034577

[85] Starr TN, Greaney AJ, Hilton SK, Ellis D, Crawford KH, Dingens AS, Navarro MJ, Bowen JE, Tortorici MA, Walls AC, King NP, Veesler D, Bloom JD. Deep Mutational Scanning of SARS-CoV-2 Receptor Binding Domain Reveals Constraints on Folding and ACE2 Binding. Cell [Internet]. 2020 Sep [cited 2021 Oct 1];182(5):1295–310. Available from: https://doi.org/10.1016/j.cell.2020.08.012

[86] Wang P, Liu L, Iketani S, Luo Y, Guo Y, Wang M, et al. Increased Resistance of SARS-CoV-2 Variants B.1.351 and B.1.1.7 to Antibody Neutralization. bioRxiv. 2021.

[87] Xie X, Liu Y, Liu J, Zhang X, Zou J, Fontes-Garfias CR, Xia H, Swanson KA, Cutler M, Cooper D, Menachery VD, Weaver SC, Dormitzer PR, Shi PY. Neutralization of SARS-CoV-2 spike 69/70 deletion, E484K and N501Y variants by BNT162b2 vaccine-elicited sera. Nature Medicine [Internet]. 2021 Feb 8 [cited 2021 Oct 1];27(4):620–1. Available from: https://doi.org/10.1038/s41591-021-01270-4

[88] Shi PY, Xie X, Zou J, Fontes-Garfias C, Xia H, Swanson K, et al. Neutralization of N501Y mutant SARS-CoV-2 by BNT162b2 vaccine-elicited sera. Res Sq. 2021.

[89] Muik A, Wallisch AK, Sänger B, Swanson KA, Mühl J, Chen W, Cai H, Maurus D, Sarkar R, Türeci Ö, Dormitzer PR, Şahin U. Neutralization of SARS-CoV-2 lineage B.1.1.7 pseudovirus by BNT162b2 vaccine-elicited human sera. Science [Internet]. 2021 Mar 12 [cited 2021 Oct 1];371(6534):1152–3. Available from: https://doi.org/10.1126/science.abg6105

[90] Diehl MC, Lee JC, Daniels SE, Tebas P, Khan AS, Giffear M, Sardesai NY, Bagarazzi ML. Tolerability of intramuscular and intradermal delivery by CELLECTRA®adaptive constant current electroporation device in healthy volunteers. Human Vaccines & Immunotherapeutics [Internet]. 2013 Oct 4 [cited 2021 Oct 1];9(10):2246–52. Available from: https://doi.org/10.4161/hv.24702

[91] Smith TR, Patel A, Ramos S, Elwood D, Zhu X, Yan J, et al. Immunogenicity of a DNA vaccine candidate for COVID-19. Nature Communications [Internet]. 2020 May 20 [cited 2021 Oct 1];11(1). Available from: https://doi.org/10.1038/s41467-020-16505-0

[92] Tebas P, Yang S, Boyer JD, Reuschel EL, Patel A, Christensen-Quick A, et al. Safety and

immunogenicity of INO-4800 DNA vaccine against SARS-CoV-2: A preliminary report of an open-label, Phase 1 clinical trial. EClinicalMedicine [Internet]. 2020 Dec [cited 2021 Oct 1]:100689. Available from: https://doi.org/10.1016/j.eclinm.2020.100689

[93] Valenzuela P, Medina A, Rutter WJ, Ammerer G, Hall BD. Synthesis and assembly of hepatitis B virus surface antigen particles in yeast. Nature [Internet]. 1982 Jul [cited 2021 Oct 1];298(5872):347–50. Available from: https://doi.org/10.1038/298347a0

[94] Tripathi NK, Shrivastava A. Recent Developments in Bioprocessing of Recombinant Proteins: Expression Hosts and Process Development. Frontiers in Bioengineering and Biotechnology [Internet]. 2019 Dec 20 [cited 2021 Oct 1];7. Available from: https://doi.org/10.3389/fbioe.2019.00420

[95] Smith GE, Summers MD, Fraser MJ. Production of human beta interferon in insect cells infected with a baculovirus expression vector. Molecular and Cellular Biology [Internet]. 1983 Dec [cited 2021 Oct 1];3(12):2156–65. Available from: https://doi.org/10.1128/mcb.3.12.2156

[96] Wrapp D, Wang N, Corbett KS, Goldsmith JA, Hsieh CL, Abiona O, Graham BS, McLellan JS. Cryo-EM structure of the 2019-nCoV spike in the prefusion conformation. Science [Internet]. 2020 Feb 19 [cited 2021 Oct 1];367(6483):1260–3. Available from: https://doi.org/10.1126/science.abb2507

[97] Liu L, Wang P, Nair MS, Yu J, Rapp M, Wang Q, et al. Potent neutralizing antibodies against multiple epitopes on SARS-CoV-2 spike. Nature [Internet]. 2020 Jul 22 [cited 2021 Oct 1];584(7821):450–6. Available from: https://doi.org/10.1038/s41586-020-2571-7

[98] Walls AC, Park YJ, Tortorici MA, Wall A, McGuire AT, Veesler D. Structure, Function, and Antigenicity of the SARS-CoV-2 Spike Glycoprotein. Cell [Internet]. 2020 Apr

[cited 2021 Oct 1];181(2):281–92. Available from: https://doi.org/10.1016/j.cell.2020.02.058

[99] He P, Zou Y, Hu Z. Advances in aluminum hydroxide-based adjuvant research and its mechanism. Human Vaccines & Immunotherapeutics [Internet]. 2015 Feb [cited 2021 Oct 1];11(2):477–88. Available from: https://doi.org/10.1080/21645515.2014.1004026

[100] Simon HU, Karaulov AV, Bachmann MF. Strategies to Prevent SARS-CoV-2-Mediated Eosinophilic Disease in Association with COVID-19 Vaccination and Infection. International Archives of Allergy and Immunology [Internet]. 2020 [cited 2021 Oct 1];181(8):624–8. Available from: https://doi.org/10.1159/000509368

[101] Ko EJ, Kang SM. Immunology and efficacy of MF59-adjuvanted vaccines. Human Vaccines & Immunotherapeutics [Internet]. 2018 Aug 29 [cited 2021 Oct 1];14(12):3041–5. Available from: https://doi.org/10.1080/21645515.2018.1495301

[102] Oberemok VV, Laikova KV, Yurchenko KA, Marochkin NA, Fomochkina II, Kubyshkin AV. SARS-CoV-2 will constantly sweep its tracks: a vaccine containing CpG motifs in 'lasso' for the multi-faced virus. Inflammation Research [Internet]. 2020 Jul 12 [cited 2021 Oct 1];69(9):801–12. Available from: https://doi.org/10.1007/s00011-020-01377-3

[103] Garçon N, Vaughn DW, Didierlaurent AM. Development and evaluation of AS03, an Adjuvant System containing α-tocopherol and squalene in an oil-in-water emulsion. Expert Review of Vaccines [Internet]. 2012 Jan [cited 2021 Oct 1];11(3):349–66. Available from: https://doi.org/10.1586/erv.11.192

[104] Magnusson SE, Altenburg AF, Bengtsson KL, Bosman F, de Vries RD, Rimmelzwaan GF, Stertman L. Matrix-M^{TM} adjuvant enhances immunogenicity of both protein- and modified

vaccinia virus Ankara-based influenza vaccines in mice. Immunologic Research [Internet]. 2018 Mar 28 [cited 2021 Oct 1];66(2):224–33. Available from: https://doi.org/10.1007/s12026-018-8991-x

[105] Magnusson SE, Reimer JM, Karlsson KH, Lilja L, Bengtsson KL, Stertman L. Immune enhancing properties of the novel Matrix-M^{TM} adjuvant leads to potentiated immune responses to an influenza vaccine in mice. Vaccine [Internet]. 2013 Mar [cited 2021 Oct 1];31(13):1725–33. Available from: https://doi.org/10.1016/j.vaccine.2013.01.039

[106] Tian JH, Patel N, Haupt R, Zhou H, Weston S, Hammond H, et al. SARS-CoV-2 spike glycoprotein vaccine candidate NVX-CoV2373 immunogenicity in baboons and protection in mice. Nature Communications [Internet]. 2021 Jan 14 [cited 2021 Oct 1];12(1). Available from: https://doi.org/10.1038/s41467-020-20653-8

[107] Guebre-Xabier M, Patel N, Tian JH, Zhou B, Maciejewski S, Lam K, Portnoff AD, Massare MJ, Frieman MB, Piedra PA, Ellingsworth L, Glenn G, Smith G. NVX-CoV2373 vaccine protects cynomolgus macaque upper and lower airways against SARS-CoV-2 challenge. Vaccine [Internet]. 2020 Nov [cited 2021 Oct 1];38(50):7892–6. Available from: https://doi.org/10.1016/j.vaccine.2020.10.064

[108] Keech C, Albert G, Cho I, Robertson A, Reed P, Neal S, et al. Phase 1-2 Trial of a SARS-CoV-2 Recombinant Spike Protein Nanoparticle Vaccine. New England Journal of Medicine [Internet]. 2020 Dec 10 [cited 2021 Oct 1];383(24):2320–32. Available from: https://doi.org/10.1056/nejmoa2026920

[109] Liu H, Su D, Zhang J, Ge S, Li Y, Wang F, Gravel M, Roulston A, Song Q, Xu W, Liang JG, Shore G, Wang X, Liang P. Improvement of Pharmacokinetic Profile of TRAIL via Trimer-Tag Enhances its Antitumor Activity in vivo. Scientific Reports [Internet]. 2017 Aug

21 [cited 2021 Oct 1];7(1). Available from: https://doi.org/10.1038/s41598-017-09518-1

[110] Ma J, Su D, Sun Y, Huang X, Liang Y, Fang L, Ma Y, Li W, Liang P, Zheng S. Cryo-electron Microscopy Structure of S-Trimer, a Subunit Vaccine Candidate for COVID-19. Journal of Virology [Internet]. 2021 May 10 [cited 2021 Oct 1];95(11). Available from: https://doi.org/10.1128/jvi.00194-21

[111] Liang JG, Su D, Song TZ, Zeng Y, Huang W, Wu J, et al. S-Trimer, a COVID-19 subunit vaccine candidate, induces protective immunity in nonhuman primates. Nature Communications [Internet]. 2021 Mar 1 [cited 2021 Oct 1];12(1). Available from: https://doi.org/10.1038/s41467-021-21634-1

[112] Richmond P, Hatchuel L, Dong M, Ma B, Hu B, Smolenov I, Li P, Liang P, Han HH, Liang J, Clemens R. Safety and immunogenicity of S-Trimer (SCB-2019), a protein subunit vaccine candidate for COVID-19 in healthy adults: a phase 1, randomised, double-blind, placebo-controlled trial. The Lancet [Internet]. 2021 Feb [cited 2021 Oct 1];397(10275):682–94. Available from: https://doi.org/10.1016/s0140-6736(21)00241-5

APPENDIX

Appendix: COVID-19 in charts

In this appendix we present some charts which represent in some sense the evolution of the pandemic COVID-19. These graphics were retrieved on September 7, 2021 from the web page Our World in Data[1]. The raw data on confirmed cases and deaths for all countries is sourced from the COVID-19 Data Repository by the Center for Systems Science and Engineering (CSSE) at Johns Hopkins University[2].

The first and second group of figures show the time series of the number of daily new confirmed COVID-19 cases and deaths, respectively (their rolling 7-day average). Please note that the number of confirmed cases is lower than the number of actual cases, because of limited testing, and the number of confirmed deaths may not be an accurate count of the real number of actual deaths from COVID-19, due to limited testing and challenges in the attribution of the cause of death. Note also that these factors have been changing with time as new information about COVID-19 were available.

[1][Hannah Ritchie, Edouard Mathieu, Lucas Rodés-Guirao, Cameron Appel, Charlie Giattino, Esteban Ortiz-Ospina, Joe Hasell, Bobbie Macdonald, Diana Beltekian and Max Roser (2020) - "Coronavirus Pandemic (COVID-19)". Published online at OurWorldInData.org. Retrieved from: `https://ourworldindata.org/coronavirus` [Online Resource]].

[2][Dong E, Du H, Gardner L. An interactive web-based dashboard to track COVID-19 in real time. Lancet Inf Dis. 20(5):533–534. doi: 10.1016/S1473-3099(20)30120-1], `https://github.com/CSSEGISandData/COVID-19`.

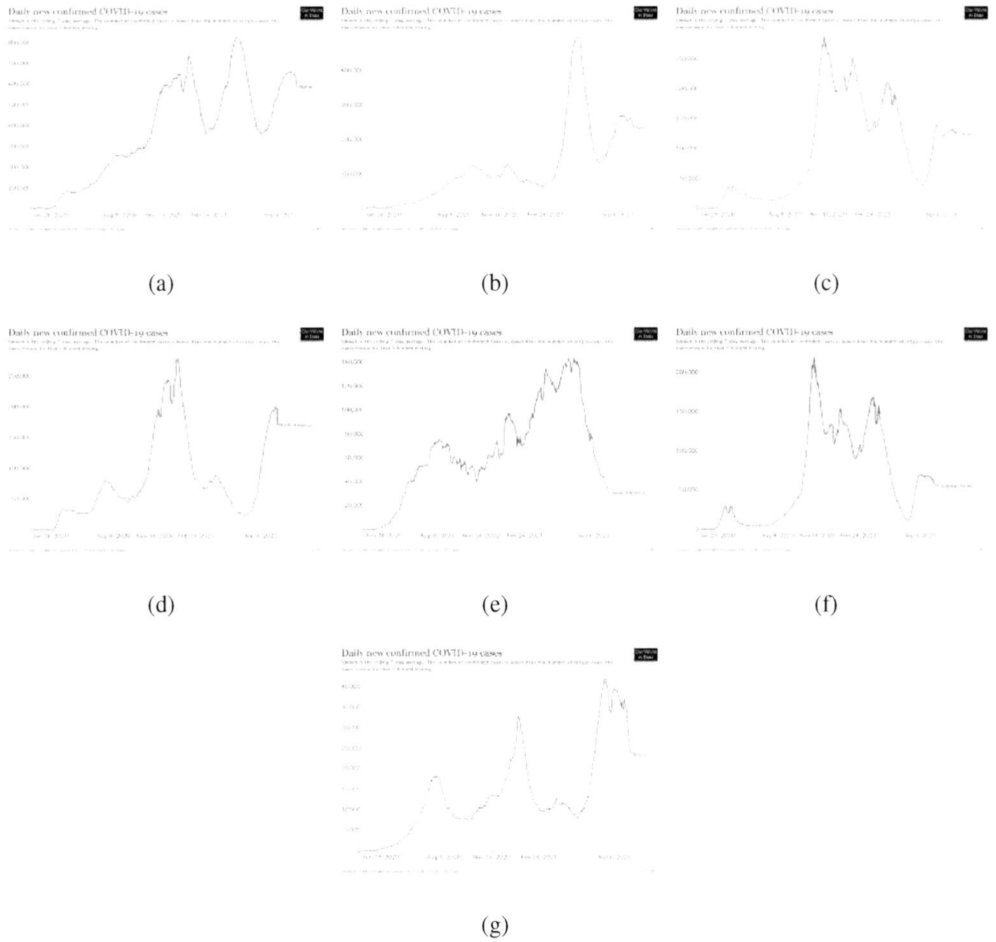

Figure 1: Daily new confirmed COVID-19 cases for different regions. (a) World, (b) Asia, (c) Europe, (d) North America, (e) South America, (f) European Union, (g) Africa

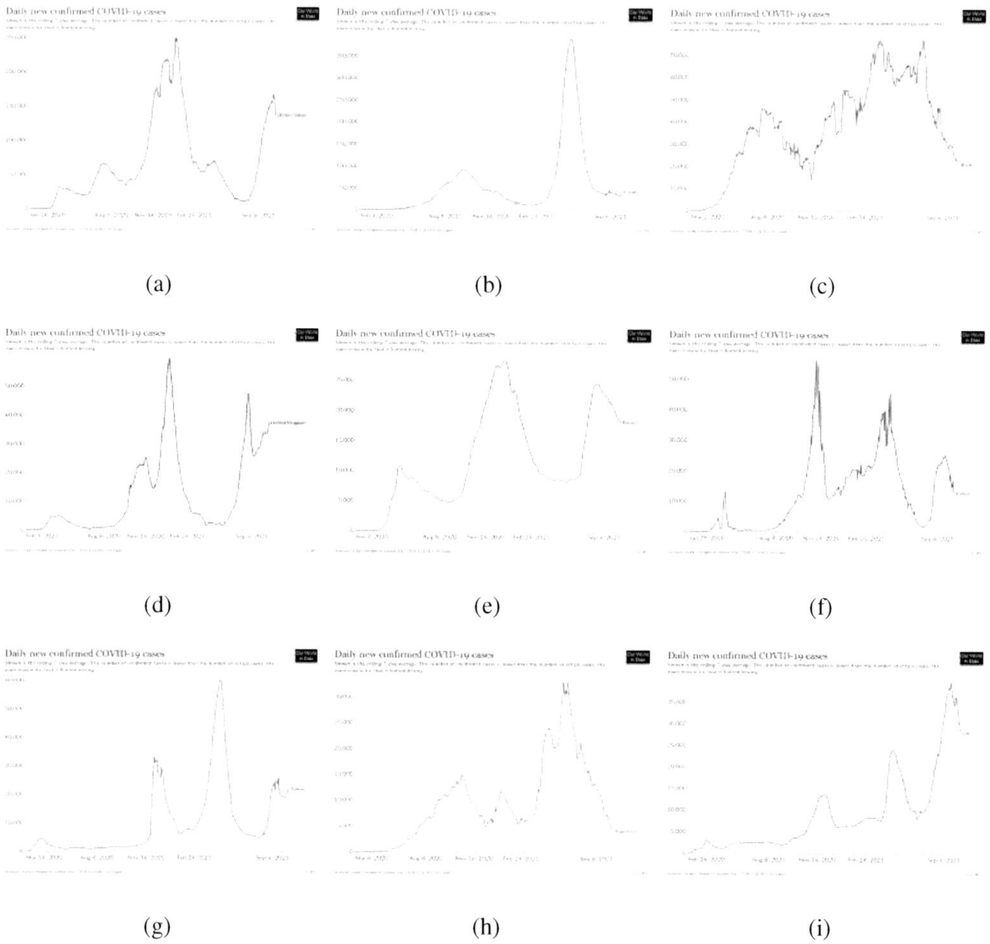

Figure 2: Daily new confirmed COVID-19 cases for different countries. (a) United States, (b) India, (c) Brazil, (d) United Kingdom, (e) Russia, (f) France, (g) Turkey, (h) Argentina, (i) Iran

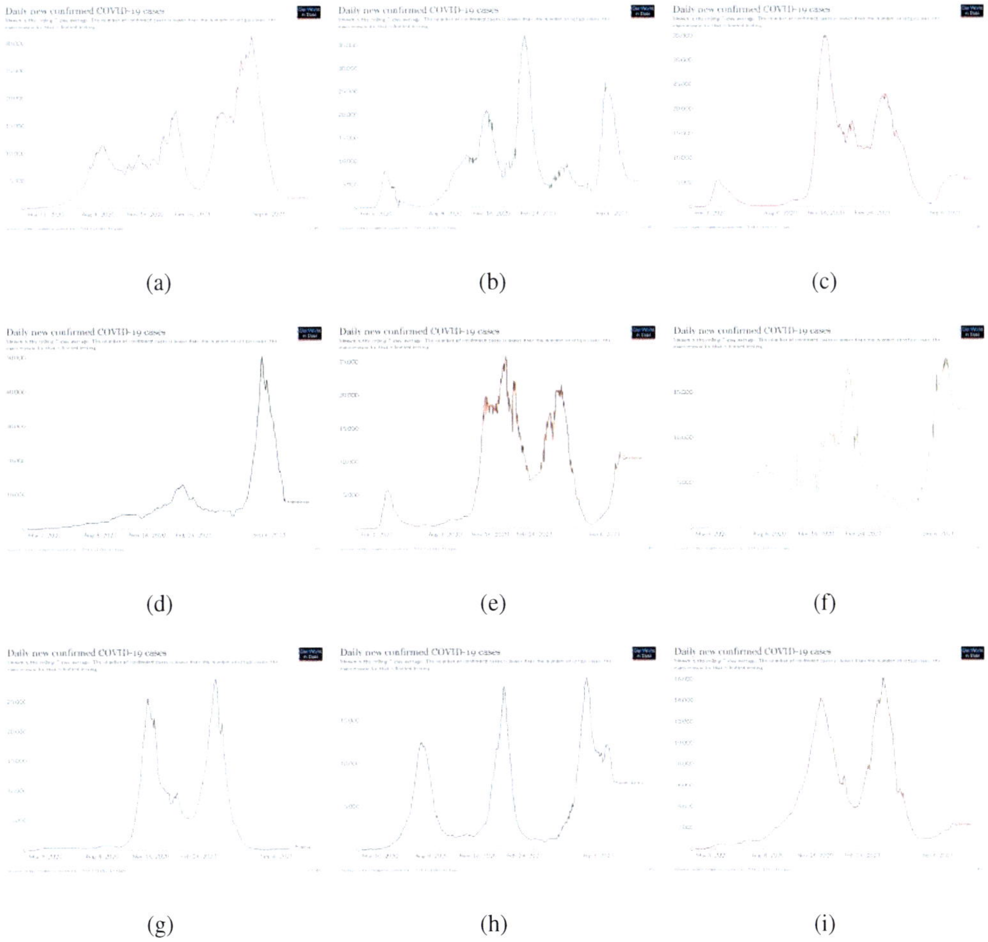

Figure 3: Daily new confirmed COVID-19 cases for different countries. (a) Colombia, (b) Spain, (c) Italy, (d) Indonesia, (e) Germany, (f) Mexico, (g) Poland, (h) South Africa, (i) Ukraine

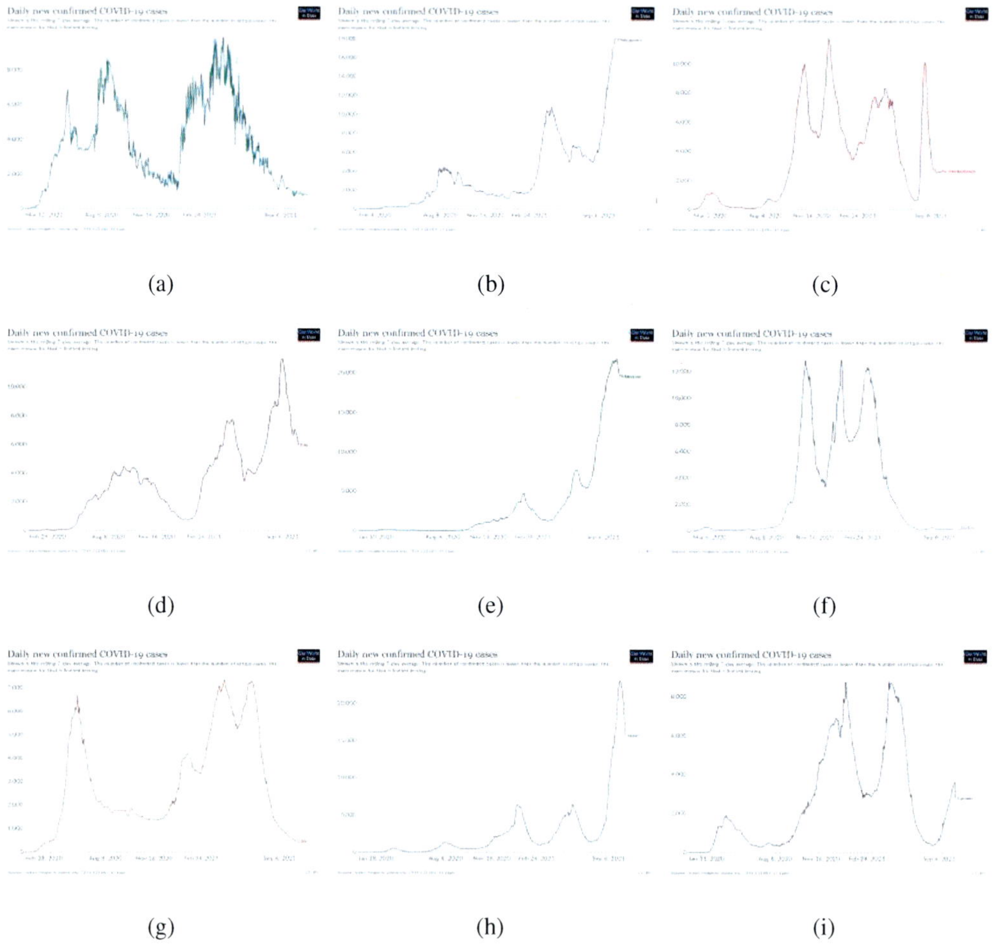

Figure 4: Daily new confirmed COVID-19 cases for different countries. (a) Peru, (b) Philippines, (c) Netherlands, (d) Iraq, (e) Malaysia, (f) Czechia, (g) Chile, (h) Japan, (i) Canada

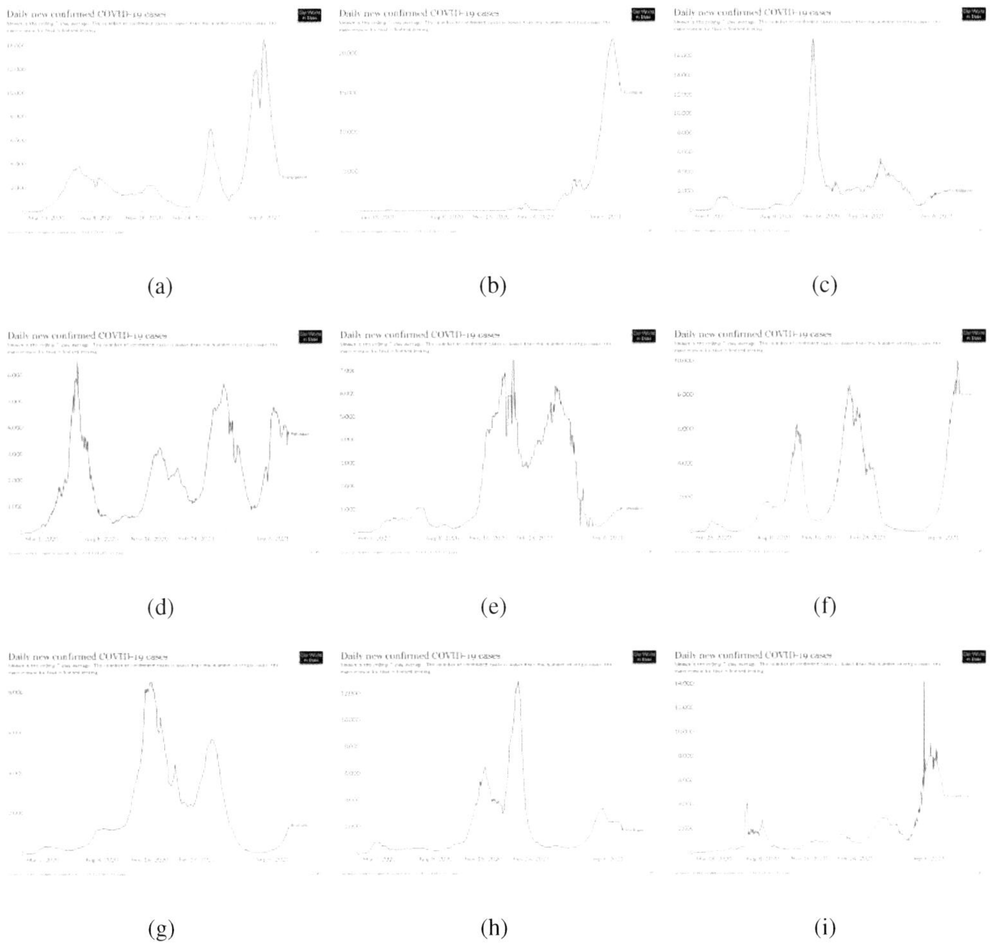

Figure 5: Daily new confirmed COVID-19 cases for different countries. (a) Bangladesh, (b) Thailand, (c) Belgium, (d) Pakistan, (e) Sweden, (f) Israel, (g) Romania, (h) Portugal, (i) Kazakhstan

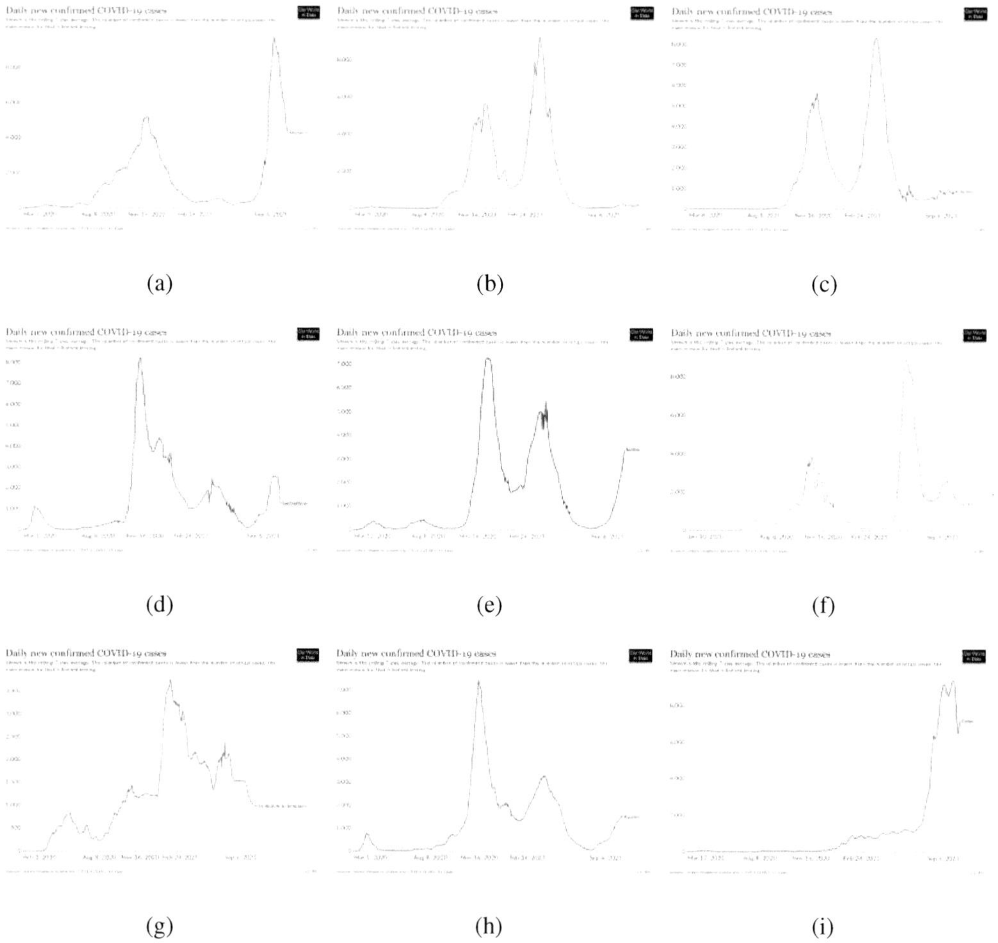

Figure 6: Daily new confirmed COVID-19 cases for different countries. (a) Morocco, (b) Hungary, (c) Jordan, (d) Switzerland, (e) Serbia, (f) Nepal, (g) United Arab Emirates, (h) Austria, (i) Cuba

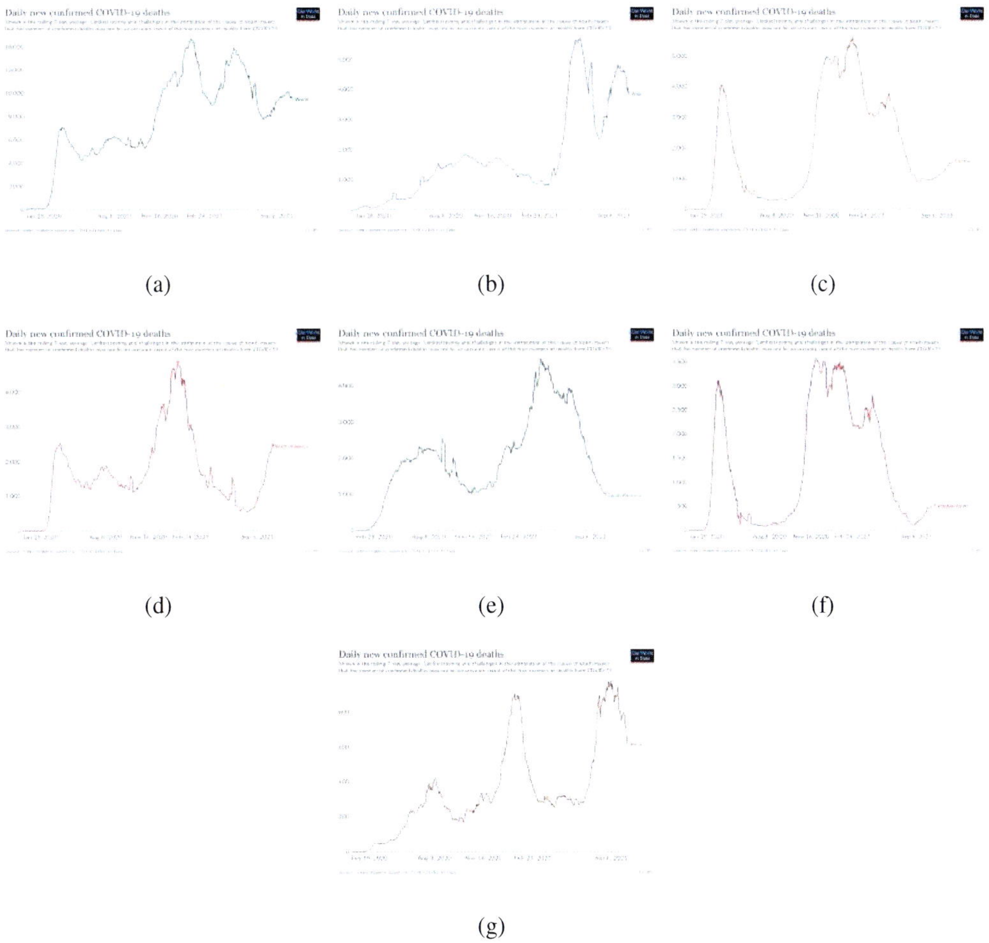

Figure 7: Daily new confirmed COVID-19 deaths for different regions. (a) World, (b) Asia, (c) Europe, (d) North America, (e) South America, (f) European Union, (g) Africa

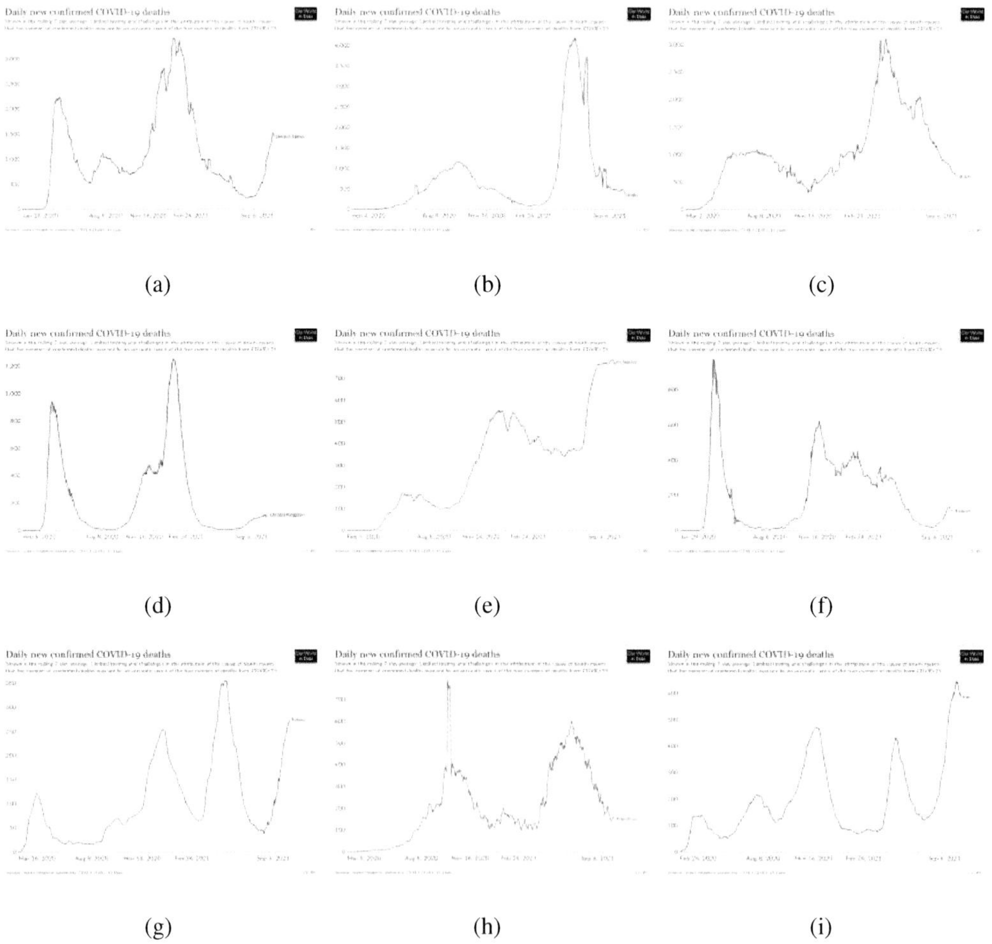

Figure 8: Daily new confirmed COVID-19 deaths for different countries. (a) United States, (b) India, (c) Brazil, (d) United Kingdom, (e) Russia, (f) France, (g) Turkey, (h) Argentina, (i) Iran

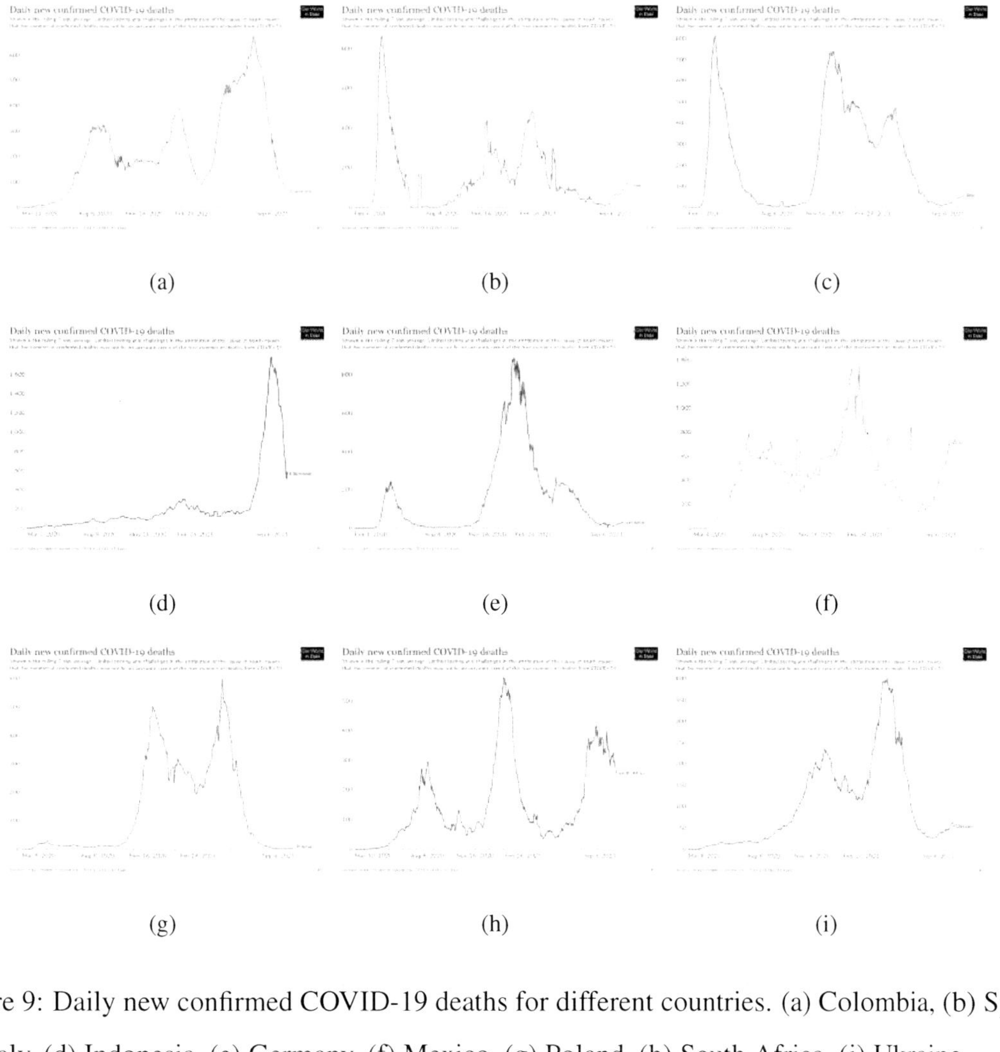

Figure 9: Daily new confirmed COVID-19 deaths for different countries. (a) Colombia, (b) Spain, (c) Italy, (d) Indonesia, (e) Germany, (f) Mexico, (g) Poland, (h) South Africa, (i) Ukraine

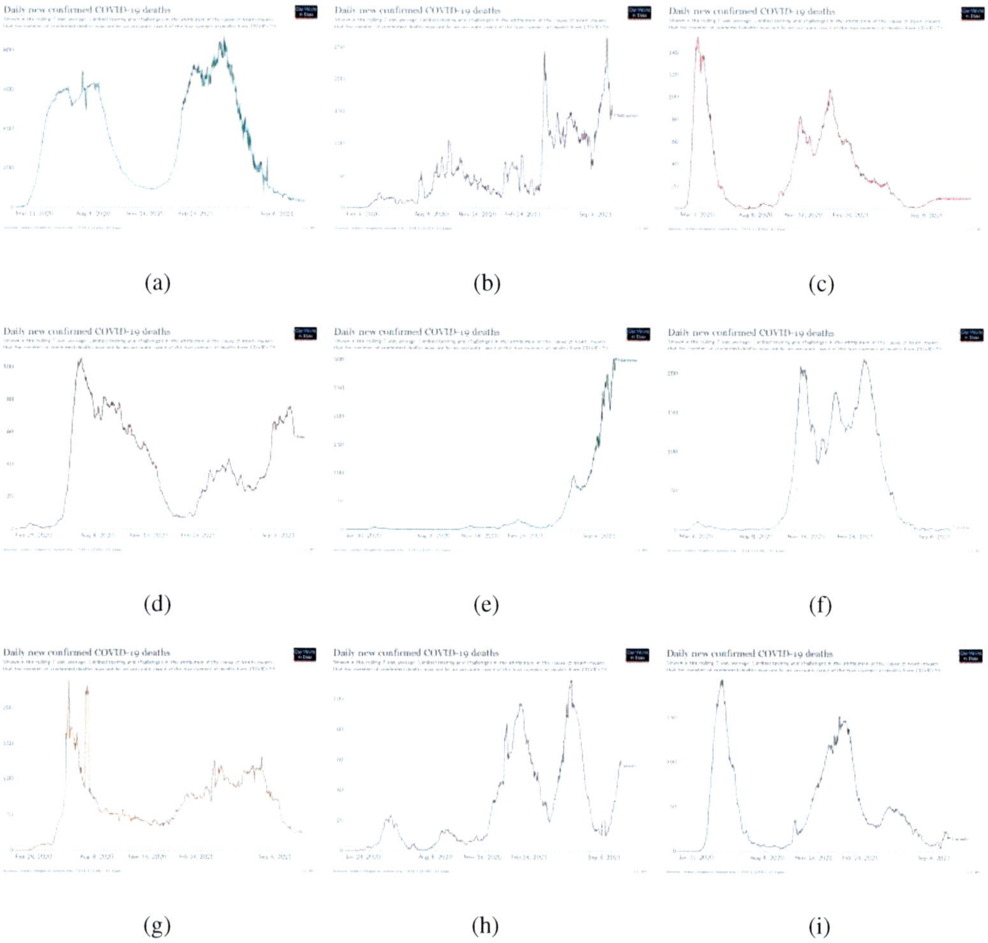

Figure 10: Daily new confirmed COVID-19 deaths for different countries. (a) Peru, (b) Philippines, (c) Netherlands, (d) Iraq, (e) Malaysia, (f) Czechia, (g) Chile, (h) Japan, (i) Canada

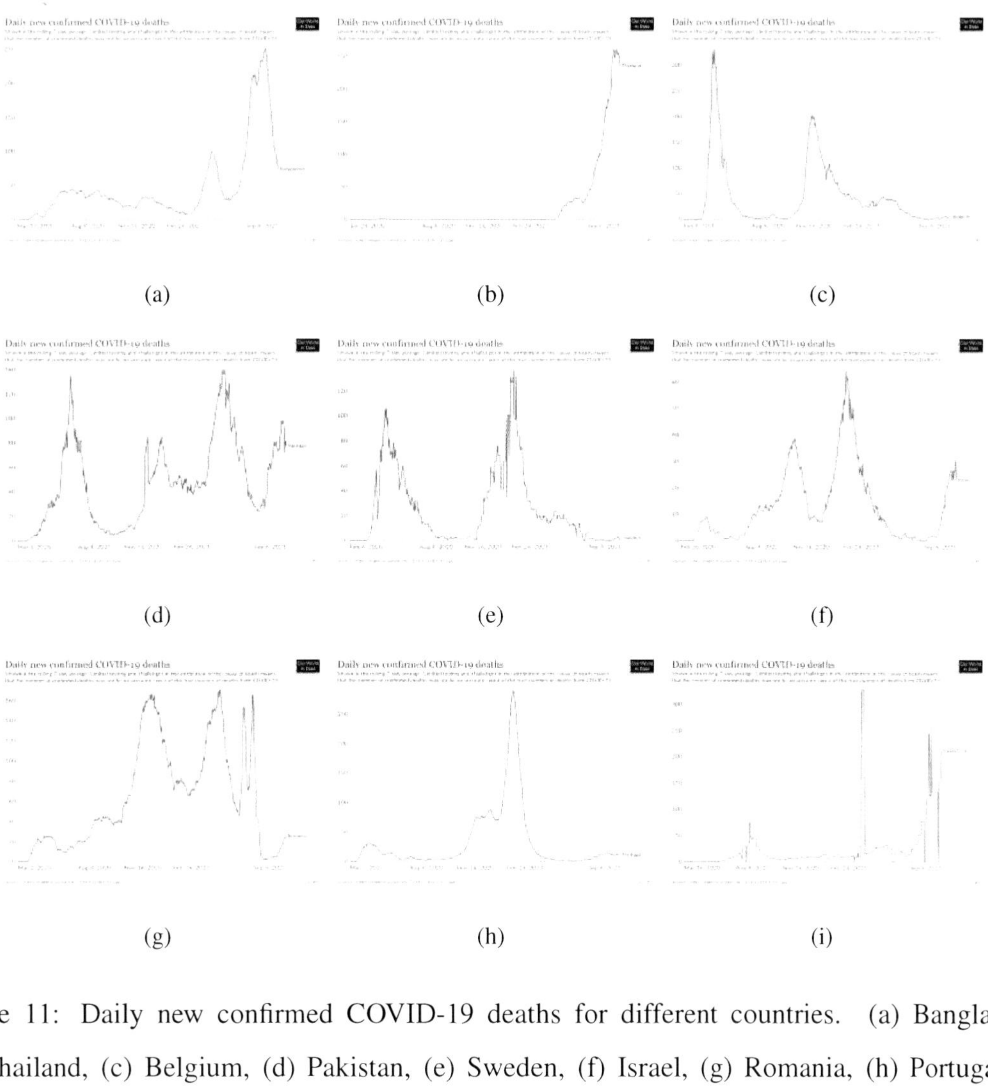

Figure 11: Daily new confirmed COVID-19 deaths for different countries. (a) Bangladesh, (b) Thailand, (c) Belgium, (d) Pakistan, (e) Sweden, (f) Israel, (g) Romania, (h) Portugal, (i) Kazakhstan

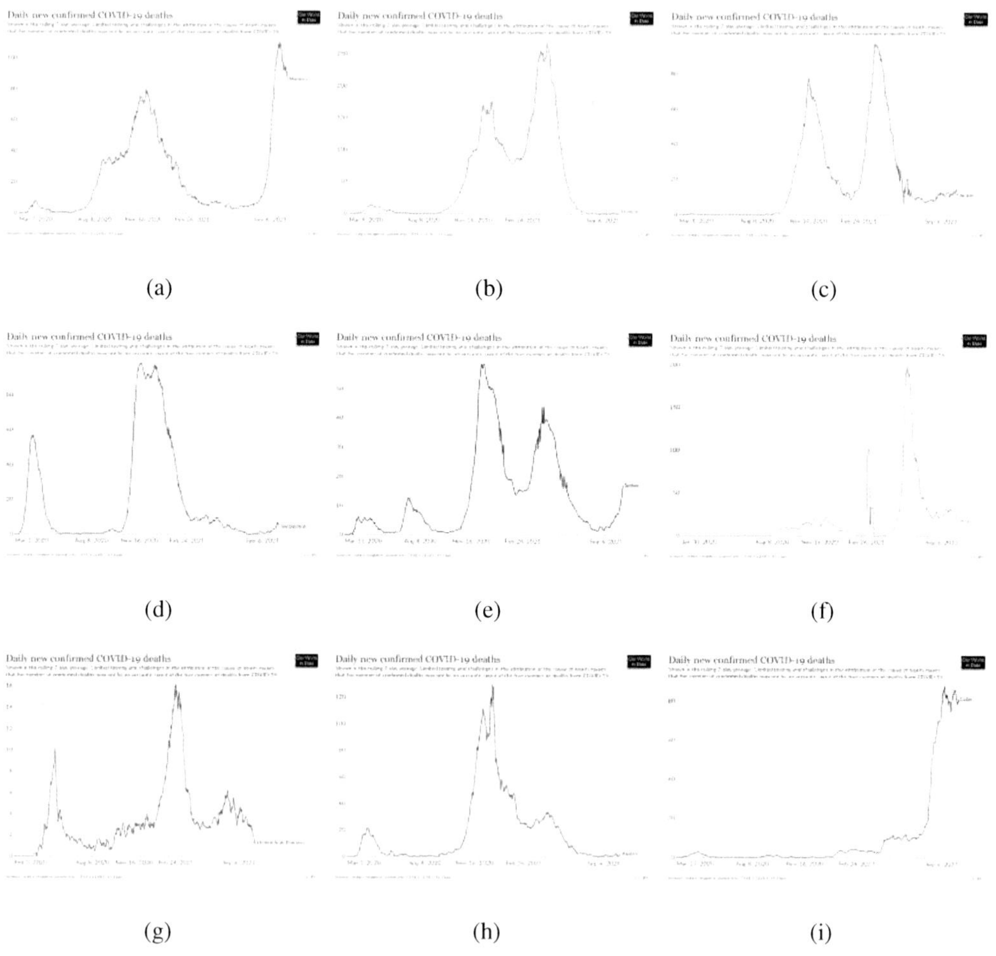

Figure 12: Daily new confirmed COVID-19 deaths for different countries. (a) Morocco, (b) Hungary, (c) Jordan, (d) Switzerland, (e) Serbia, (f) Nepal, (g) United Arab Emirates, (h) Austria, (i) Cuba

SUBJECT INDEX

A

B

D

E

F

G

H

L

M

N

O

P

R

S

Z

Made in United States
North Haven, CT
04 November 2026

21730357R00323